Current Developments in Anthropological Genetics

Volume 1

THEORY AND METHODS

Current Developments in Anthropological Genetics

Volume 1
THEORY AND METHODS

EDITED BY

James H. Mielke AND
Michael H. Crawford
University of Kansas
Lawrence, Kansas

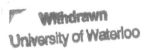
PLENUM PRESS • NEW YORK AND LONDON

Library of Congress Cataloging in Publication Data

Main entry under title:

Current developments in anthropological genetics.

Includes index.
CONTENTS: v. 1. Theory and methods.
1. Human population genetics—Addresses, essays, lectures. 2. Human evolution—
Addresses, essays, lectures. 3. Human genetics—Addresses, essays, lectures. I. Mielke,
James H. II. Crawford, Michael H., 1939-
GN289.C87   573.2   79-24900
ISBN 0-306-40390-0 (v. 1)

© 1980 Plenum Press, New York
A Division of Plenum Publishing Corporation
227 West 17th Street, New York, N.Y. 10011

Printed in the United States of America

Contributors

C. Cannings, Department of Probability and Statistics, University of Sheffield, Sheffield, England, and Department of Medical Biophysics and Computing, University of Utah, Salt Lake City, Utah

C. R. Cloninger, Department of Psychiatry, Washington University, School of Medicine, and the Jewish Hospital of St. Louis, St. Louis, Missouri 63110

J. C. DeFries, Institute for Behavioral Genetics, University of Colorado, Boulder, Colorado 80309

R. C. Elston, Department of Biometry, Louisiana State University, Medical Center, New Orleans, Louisiana 70112

H. Harpending, Department of Anthropology, University of New Mexico, Albuquerque, New Mexico 87131

L. B. Jorde, Division of Medical Genetics, Department of Pediatrics, University of Utah Medical Center, Salt Lake City, Utah 84132

J. M. Lalouel, Population Genetics Laboratory, University of Hawaii, Honolulu, Hawaii

C. C. Li, Graduate School of Public Health, University of Pittsburgh, Pittsburgh, Pennsylvania

F. B. Livingstone, Department of Anthropology, University of Michigan, Ann Arbor, Michigan 48104

J. W. MacCluer, Department of Biology, The Pennsylvania State University, University Park, Pennsylvania 16802

N. E. Morton, Population Genetics Laboratory, University of Hawaii, Honolulu, Hawaii 96822

D. C. Rao, Population Genetics Laboratory, University of Hawaii, Honolulu, Hawaii 96822

T. Reich, Department of Psychiatry, Washington University, School of Medicine, and the Jewish Hospital of St. Louis, St. Louis, Missouri 63110

J. Rice, Department of Psychiatry, Washington University, School of Medicine, and the Jewish Hospital of St. Louis, St. Louis, Missouri 63110

D. F. Roberts, Department of Human Genetics, University of Newcastle-upon-Tyne, England

M. S. Schanfield, American Red Cross, Blood Services, Washington, D.C. 20006

M. Skolnick, Department of Medical Biophysics and Computing, University of Utah, Salt Lake City, Utah

B. Suarez, Department of Psychiatry, Washington University, School of Medicine, and the Jewish Hospital of St. Louis, St. Louis, Missouri 63310

A. C. Swedlund, Department of Anthropology, University of Massachusetts, Amherst, Massachusetts 01003

E. A. Thompson, Department of Medical Biophysics and Computing, University of Utah, Salt Lake City, Utah and King's College, Cambridge, England

K. M. Weiss, Center for Demographic and Population Genetics, University of Texas Graduate School of Biomedical Sciences, Houston, Texas 77025

Preface

The papers in this volume were presented as part of the University of Kansas Department of Anthropology Distinguished Lecture Program on Anthropological Genetics. Consecutively, each contributor spent approximately a week on the campus at Lawrence participating in a seminar. The contributors to this volume were not on campus at one time, but visited us on alternating weeks; hence, a symposium-type interchange was not possible between all participants. However, the students and faculty of Kansas University acted as a sounding board.

This volume can be considered a companion and continuation of *Methods and Theories of Anthropological Genetics*, which was based upon a symposium on the state of the art in 1971. This present volume reflects what we consider to be some of the advances and current developments in anthropological genetics since 1973. Emphasis has shifted, to some degree, away from population structure analysis (as depicted in Crawford and Workman) to genetic epidemiology. However, population structure still remains a fertile and ongoing area of research with many theoretical questions still remaining unanswered.

The title, *Current Developments in Anthropological Genetics*, deserves some comment because a number of the contributors to this volume are not anthropologists. We have chosen the title to reflect the broader, integrating approach to the study of human genetics. The contributions to this volume all include some aspect of culture interacting with human genetics either on the population, familial, or individual levels. Obviously, we have not exhausted the full range of anthropological genetics, but have included a number of research areas that are presently undergoing both theoretical and methodological metamorphosis. In addition, the choice of topics is mediated by the availability of some contributors.

This volume begins with two contributions which set the frame for the remainder of the chapters -- the demographic and cultural framework in which human populations exist, or what we have called "Historical Approaches to Anthropological Genetics." Section II considers "Evolutionary Perspectives" ranging from natural selection and random variation to computer simulation.

vii

Sections III and IV are entitled "Analytical Theory," either with or without examples for illustration. In these sections topics such as segregation, path, and genetic distance analyses are considered. It may be of some help for the reader to peruse the final chapter by D. F. Roberts to gain a perspective prior to examining each of the selections.

Many colleagues and associates have contributed to the organization of the seminar series and to the publication of this volume. We thank Peter L. Workman for suggesting this type of seminar series during a visit to Lawrence in November, 1976. The administration of the University of Kansas (specifically Deans Robert Cobb and Robert Hoffman) has shared our vision of this unique educational and training experience for the faculty and graduate students of Anthropology. Anta Montet-White, Chair of Anthropology, has supported and encouraged this program. Mrs. Barbara Pirtle and Ms. Carol Dudgeon freed us from a multitude of administrative chores associated with the visit of 14 scholars from all over the United States and Europe. We acknowledge the participation of the graduate students in Biological Anthropology who attended all of the seminars, lectures, and informal discussions. In these interactions, our students asked probing questions and provided the important feedback necessary for a successful exchange of ideas. We thank the contributors for their time, expertise, and the prompt submission of their manuscripts for publication. Kirk Jensen, Michael Dardia, and Peter Strupp of Plenum Press made this volume possible.

One of the editors, Michael H. Crawford, was on a P.H.S. Research Career Development Award, 1K04DE0028-03.

Contents

PART III: ANALYTICAL THEORY

Chapter 7. The Genetic Structure of Subdivided Human Populations: A Review

Lynn B. Jorde

Chapter 8. Distance Analysis and Multidimensional Scaling

J.-M. Lalouel

Chapter 9. Pedigree Analysis of Complex Models

C. Cannings, E. A. Thompson, and M. Skolnick

Chapter 10. Current Directions in Genetic Epidemiology

T. Reich, B. Suarez, J. Rice, and C. R. Cloninger

PART IV: ANALYTICAL THEORY: ILLUSTRATED BY EXAMPLE

Chapter 11.   Segregation Analysis
             R. C. Elston

Chapter 12.   Path Analysis of Quantitative Inheritance
             D. C. Rao and N. E. Morton

Chapter 13.   Half-Sib Analysis of Quantitative Data
             Ching Chun Li

Chapter 14.   Mental Abilities: A Family Study
              John C. DeFries

Chapter 15.   Current Developments in Anthropological Genetics:
              Achievements and Gaps
              Derek F. Roberts

PART I

HISTORICAL APPROACHES TO ANTHROPOLOGICAL GENETICS

1

Voices of Our Ancestors

Kenneth M. Weiss

1. Introduction

It may seem unusual to deal with paleodemography in a series of presentations on anthropological genetics, since skeletons bear no genes for us to examine, and skeletal measurements, only weakly genetic to begin with, are only slightly related to demographic studies. On the other hand, there are only two basic questions asked by geneticists: How was present genetic diversity produced? and What are the genetic mechanisms behind present human biological characteristics? Both of these questions can be answered at least superficially through the use of paleodemographic data.

It should be kept in mind that of all anthropology, archeology, and genetics, only paleodemography deals with the actual ancestors of present human beings; the degree of inference made by all other sources of data is one step (or more) removed as compared with the use of the actual skeletons of past individuals. While skeletons may not reveal any genes, they at least reveal some aspects of what happened to genes in ancestral times.

There has been a flurry of activity in paleodemography over the past decade or so. This activity has centered on certain basic questions about the history of demographic parameters during the course of human biological and cultural evolution, both in relation to human biology directly and in relation to general theories of human social behaviour. Many questions have been answered,

KENNETH M. WEISS ● Associate Professor of Genetics, Center for Demographic and Population Genetics, University of Texas Graduate School of Biomedical Sciences, Houston, Texas 77025.
This work was accomplished with financial support from the following sources: National Institute General Medical Sciences, Grant number K04 6M00230, National Institute General Medical Sciences, Grant number GM19513, and National Cancer Institute, Grant number CA19311, which are gratefully acknowledged.

probably as well as they can be, while others have been opened in a quantitative way such that future data can be used to illuminate them further.

In addition to this description of our past, paleodemographic data and methods have been used by a few of us to provide base-line data on the nature of human biology as it relates to vital events (birth and death) by age. Many of us are now working on studies of human variation in such events at the present time in history, but need the results from paleodemography to provide the logical foundation for our work.

In this presentation, I will review some of the specific questions which have been asked, discuss the answers which have resulted, and evaluate the state of affairs in that area of study. I will try to point out areas in which we know as much as we are likely to know and those in which hope for future advances seems greatest.

Then I will turn to a discussion of ways in which paleodemographic data may be applied to certain questions of biomedical and genetic importance (naturally, to those issues in which I am presently engaged in active research). As it turns out, this will lead me to refer neatly to some topics which are to follow in this volume: the use of pedigrees in assessing the genetic control or causation of human disease. In doing this, I hope to show how we have come to an understanding of the general demographic conditions of our past history, and to show that this can be used directly in studies of very important areas of contemporary biomedical research: the study of the aging process and the understanding of the degenerative diseases of older life which are responsible for most deaths today. These issues are, to a rather great extent, issues of a genetic nature.

2. Basic Questions

Throughout its history as an area of investigation, paleodemography has sought to answer several basic questions:

1. What has population size and growth rate been like for various times, and areas of different sizes, in the past?

2. What have (average) age-specific birth and death rates been for various cultural stages or population units in our past?

3. What has been the life expectancy at birth during the course of human cultural evolutionary history?

4. What have been the areal distribution and migrational interconnections among population subunits?

5. Can pathology in skeletal material, along with ages and sexes of the dead, be used to make inferences about general health and longevity conditions in the past in ways useful for comparison with the present?

3. Methodological Approaches

Various methodological approaches have been used to attack these problems, based primarily on the analysis of skeletal materials, but also including analysis of archeological data relating to site number, size, and duration of occupation. These techniques primarily are as follows:

1. Ways of aging and sexing skeletal remains,

2. Application of mathematical techniques developed by demographers in order to derive parameter estimates indirectly when data were insufficient to evaluate them directly (e.g., age-specific mortality rates),

3. Use of contemporary bone pathological knowledge to study past populations along with the assumption that the basic biology of both times is unchanged,

4. Use of data from tribal populations in the ethnographic present, along with the assumption that past populations progressed through similar cultural forms when the material aspects of culture appear similar,

5. Models from geographic and ecological theory to analyze the processes by which hierarchical patterns of site size and areal distribution would be generated and maintained.

These methods have been applied to a set of specific questions, and these can be briefly summarized, along with my estimation of the state of affairs at present in the following areas.

3.1. Aging and Sexing of Skeletal Material

A chaotic and rather *ad hoc* set of age and sex criteria for assessing skeletal remains has dominated physical anthropology for decades, if not centuries (Hrdlicka, 1952; Bass, 1971), and it has become clear that better means need to be devised. No longer can it be said that subjective judgment is the best method (e.g., as Hrdlicka and Stewart, 1952, once claimed); now, multiple variable methods are available along with statistical tests. The composite methods presented by Acsadi and Nemeskeri (1970) are probably the best, but it still is true that without a known population or other comparative material, there is a lot of guesswork about the individuals near the cutoff points. Recently, age refinements based on osteological remodeling and properties of the Haversian system, etc. (e.g., see Ubelaker, 1974; Kerley and Ubelaker, 1978; Bocquet, 1977; S. Pfeiffer, 1980), have improved aging.

Nonetheless, some problems remain. First, many of the refinements, such as the histological ones, are effective mainly in specimens of older age — in paleodemographic materials these are both rare and relatively unimportant to the reconstruction of the life table. Second, in the absence of a reference population of the same biological/cultural type as that under study, there is no way to be sure of the aging/sexing done. Without an ability to check age criteria against bones of known age at death, systematic mis-sexing and mis-aging can occur, and this can obscure the fine differences between populations or between ancient and modern populations which we seek. For example, it can easily obscure our knowledge of whether male or fermale mortality rates were higher in the past. Masset (1971, 1973) has discussed this at length (and his work has been followed up by Bocquet, 1977); he suggests a fallback position of using a known population as a reference, and it is important that the age distribution of the reference population be known, so Masset suggests a standard population in which all age classes are of equal size. Since we can rarely have proper reference populations, we may forever be stymied in our desire to improve this area very much.

3.2. Improved Life Tables

Better aging and sexing of materials, and the use of more complete and larger sets of remains have greatly improved our understanding of life tables for early populations — mortality rates, fertility rates, and life expectancy. Good life tables, or at least serious attempts at them given very limited data, have been computed for Australopithecines (Mann, 1975), for many eastern and western European populations (Acsadi and Nemeskeri, 1970; Henneberg, 1976; Masset, 1971, 1973; Bocquet, 1977; Drenhaus, 1976), for Amerindian sites (Ubelaker, 1974; Buikstra, 1976; Asch, 1976; Weiss, 1973; Bennett, 1973), and for sites in Nubia by Swedlund and Armelagos (1975). There are, of course, others.

If there is a persistent failure it is the stubborn refusal to smooth data properly to account for stochastic elements in data and in the mortality rates actually operating (Weiss, 1973). Moore, Swedlund, and Armelagos (1975) showed that considerable variability in life tables could, in small populations, be produced simply by stochastic operation of mortality rates, while Smouse and ·Weiss (1975; Weiss and Smouse, 1976; Weiss, 1975) showed that when there is demographic feedback between population size and demographic rates (and there is), remains in cemeteries ought to be fairly reliable. Yet, sampling elements must be removed if really good life tables are to be derived from skeletal series.

The application of demographic theory to make accurate inferences about things we cannot observe in skeletal data — such as age-specific mortality rates — has been successfully done in recent years (Weiss, 1973; Asch, 1976; Drenhaus, 1976). In a work of mine (1973), I attempted to characterize tribal populations with a flexible series of model life tables which could be fitted to actual, incomplete, anthropological data. There has been some confusion about what was done there so that a brief word of explanation may be worthwhile. Those models provided for a set of juvenile mortality rates and a set of adult mortality rates and combined these in all possible ways. This was not meant to imply that any (high or low) juvenile mortality rate could be found with any (high or low) adult schedule: we know from ample experience that there is a connection and that mortality in general has connectedness. However, (1) this knowledge comes along almost exclusively from current populations of nation-states, and (2) we do not know the details of this connectedness from tribal populations, so that my purpose was to provide a labile set of life tables for data. Clearly if one fits one's data to a life table with very low juvenile mortality and very high adult rates, for example, one must be highly suspect of the data and not take the life table "fit" as evidence for the true mortality rates. There is still a major role to be played by judgment and an understanding both of one's data and of demographic facts. (I am grateful to that ever-alert critic, Dr. Nancy Howell, for pointing out this problem to me.)

These data-assessment problems notwithstanding, this work has been applied successfully to many populations, and from these applications there is a consistency of results in terms of typical life table values. While these vary considerably, they are all quite distinct from modern life tables, and I believe that we know now to a very good extent the general regimes of mortality which faced our ancestors. We may not ever know this in any significantly better detail, since a new population largely different from what has already been found (and confirmed often in the ethnographic present) would be so suspect as to be rejected as spurious or based on bad data. What we also do not know, and I do not have any idea how we will ever find this out, is what causes of death were responsible for mortality in tribal times. Paleopathological work will remain important in finding out about bone-manifest diseases, but other than that I do not see much room for useful work.

We do know things from present epidemiological studies which can relate to this issue, however:

(a) Some pathogens can exist in small, isolated tribal populations and these include *chronic* disease pathogens.

(b) Some pathogens can exist in nonhuman hosts and infect humans when they are available (malaria may be an example of this, as may have been the antecedents of some slow viruses now affecting humans, as well as measles, influenzas, or other diseases).

(c) Acute infectious diseases specific to humans, especially lethal or often-lethal ones, probably are a result of the later evolution of large, sedentary human populations and improved long-range transportation.

(d) Accidents, violence, and especially predation by other animals (including spiders and snakes) have taken a toll where they existed.

(e) The aging process, in terms of diseases we now identify, was probably little different in former times than it is now; however, physical (e.g., musculo-skeletal, dental, joint) wear and degeneration were heavier and may have been a major factor in mortality.

(f) The aging diseases, such as cancer, diabetes, heart disease, and so on, were probably relatively rare because they were preempted by earlier, more acute causes such as infection or injury.

(g) A sizeable fraction, certainly over 5%, of all infants were probably born with congenital defects, making death quick and inevitable, and doubtlessly these and many other newborns (e.g., twins, breech births) were killed by their mothers just after birth.

3.3. Locational and Distributional Aspects of Prehistoric Populations

Much work has been done to study the distribution of sites and of site sizes over culture areas in recent times, including attempts to determine the migrational patterns involved. This has generally been the realm of archeologists, and most stress has been placed on the study of neolithic patterns or those associated with early (or later) agricultural systems (e.g., Zubrow, 1976; Dumond, 1975; Sanders and Price, 1968; Bodmer and Cavalli-Sforza, 1976; Cohen, 1977; papers in Spooner, 1972). However, several investigators have attempted simulations of tribal or hunter—gatherer populations or empirical tests of the demographic dispersion of such peoples (e.g., Wobst, 1976; Birdsell, 1958; Williams, 1974). What has been found has been a hexagonal-territory matrix in which the villages composing a tribe are distributed. Such models have been questioned, and it is for future archeologists to determine their accuracy; they have at least some general resemblance to the ethnographic present, but this may not be valid as an analogy (e.g., Wobst, 1976).

Extensive study has been made of the demographic ramifications of the invention of agriculture. Whether population growth and its consequent pressure preceded and caused or followed and were caused by cultural improvements has been hotly debated (e.g., Boserup, 1965; and the works of Cohen, Spooner, Ammerman, Bodmer and Cavalli-Sforza, cited in references). This is a very important issue yet to be solved, although many problems lie ahead, in particular distinguishing between sporadic population growth and slower, steady growth (e.g., review by Weiss, 1976). The issues are important for they impinge on our understanding of present racial diversity and processes of population relationship which may apply to much earlier times as well. The geneticist is concerned with distinguishing between population expansion by the displacement or absorption of resident groups and gene flow with cultural diffusion (see Bodmer and Cavalli-Sforza, 1976, for discussion), and this will affect how we interpret trees of genetic differences among different human populations. Although it will probably remain in the realm of vague inference, much work can be done to help in this pursuit.

3.4. Social Stratification

Several workers have attempted in a crude and early way to use differences in age—sex composition of skeletal materials to make inferences about cultural/

status differences within or between populations. Buikstra (1976) has done this for Midwest Amerindian groups. Harper has done it to compare "biobehavioral adaptation" differences between Eskimo and Aleut populations. This work is tentative because sample sizes and age–sex accuracy limitations produce greater variance than the observed mean differences, and there have been uncorrected computational errors exaggerating the differences that do exist; however, it would be important if (or when) we could infer things about health or culture from differences in the ages at death of burial groups.

The temptation to overinterpret the social evidence from a fragmentary skeletal population should not be yielded to, however, and this seems to have happened with increasing frequency as our own society has gone more and more "public." Some of the abuses occur in introductory textbooks, where groundless flights of fancy are presented to bring the past to "life." A perhaps even more dangerous problem are blatant overclaims made to the press, or at least the way the press exploits anthropological findings. Recent silliness such as the claim in the popular press that because certain very old fossils were found in a group containing multiple adults and children that this demonstrates the first evidence of "family life" — and proof that it occurred early in human evolution and hence was a material factor in that evolution — is an example. This is too incredible to be blamed on the scientists themselves, who would know that many mammals, incidently including most primates, have had "family" life of this type for millions of years. We must beware of allowing ourselves or the popular media to make such nonsense of our work that we lose credibility when real evidence turns up.

3.5. Signal vs. Noise

I have argued in many places (e.g., 1976) that we must develop a much more sophisticated understanding of the way we interpret our data. In particular, we compute things such as population sizes, death rates, and so on from very small and fragmentary data, and we also use this demographic data for making statements about genetics and evolution. We must come to realize that we are in fact computing only *estimates* of *average* rates, under some specific assumptions, and that the variance about these estimates is very large. In fact, in many ways demographic processes are *essentially* stochastic, or probabilistic, in their nature. We must be fully aware that averages may tell us only a small part of the real story (for example, evolution may operate by sporadic, intense mortality selection rather than by gradual selection reflected in average mortality rates), and not only that, but contrasts we observe between populations are most often far from being statistically significant — and for this and other reasons far from statistically meaningful. Ten skulls do not a population make.

3.6. On the Possible Action of Natural Selection, and Population Control Mechanisms

The comparison of mortality curves derived from skeletal populations either with each other or with some standard curves has led several investigators to speculate on the possible genetic import of mortality in past times. From skeletal as well as tribal data, indices of natural selection's potential action have been derived (Weiss, 1973; Howell, 1979; Henneberg, 1976; Henneberg *et. al.*, 1978; Neel and Weiss, 1975; Spuhler, 1976). We now know in fairly concrete terms the degree to which mortality produced variation, amongst individuals in a given culture, in the number of offspring they produced. We know that mortality was more important than fertility in determining this difference − that is, that although fertility may have been regulated, more children were not produced because potential parents died than because of birth control.

We know that at about the time of the rise of agricultural states − say, classical and medieval times in regard to European history − that mortality became less effective and fertility more effective a force in determining the variance in reproduction. Both factors remained important, however, until the last few decades and the rise of medical science. Now, it seems that early mortality can select out but the few most defective individuals. Natural selection must now act mainly through fertility. Although paleodemographic work cannot show how much of the potential natural selection actually occurred, and how much variation in reproduction was not related to genes, it is clear that patterns of selection in the past probably worked more through mortality than they do now.

Some effort has been made to relate these facts between populations (e.g., Weiss, 1973; Henneberg, Piontek, and Strzalko, 1978), in the latter case to examine paleodemographic patterns with osteometric variation to test for genetic vs. cultural sources of variation. These efforts lead only to the most general, and suspect, conclusions. It does not seem likely that we can come to any useful understanding of the amount, or the mechanisms, of natural selection through paleodemographic data except insofar as that data can be related to contemporary epidemiological studies (see below).

3.7. General Results

The general result of all of this work is, in my opinion, a rather well-known answer to the basic questions about the *average* demographic rates which applied to our ancestral populations, their fertility patterns, their life expectancy, and the general nature of their spatial distributions. I believe it virtually impossible, with current data (or any I can conceive that we might acquire) to examine the nature of fluctuations in demographic rates or the way in which culturally induced growth actually occurred. I think also that our knowledge of spatial patterns, for example of hunting−gathering peoples, is rather shaky but that future investigations *can* illuminate this question. Certainly we can look forward to learning more about the spatial patterns of early versions of more complex cultural stages, such as states.

4. Implications for Modern Genetic Studies

A more interesting question, to me, now becomes: In what ways can we use data, methods, or results from traditional paleodemography in present studies of human biology and genetics?

One obvious answer, for those interested in mating patterns, is that further and vigorous pursuit of the spatial distribution question can lead to increased usefulness of migration–gene-flow–kinship analysis models of human genetic variation and its generation. This question makes use of archeological data as well as present patterns of gene frequency variation. Two examples of the use of demographic data for such problems can be cited (these are ones of particular interest to me and by no means exhaustive). Weiss and Maruyama (1976) have used settlement pattern data to examine questions related to the evolution and differentiation of human races over long time periods. Ammeman and Cavalli-Sforza (1971, 1973) have attempted to simulate the population effects of the neolithic "revolution" by looking at the way changed settlements and migration patterns would affect gene flow among groups, and relating this to present genetic diversity in Europe and the Middle East. For a general discussion see Weiss (1976) and Ward and Weiss (1976).

A second area is that of determining the general genetic nature of the basic mortality patterns found in human populations. Several questions along these lines arise as a natural consequence of studying the age patterns of diseases in contemporary populations:

1. Is the age of onset of a disease genetically determined?

2. Is the age pattern of mortality based on an active genetic program leading to death of an older generation in a population, or a passive process resulting from some other aspect of our evolution?

3. How much has our genetically based component of longevity changed in the course of our evolution?

4. What is the nature of human biological aging and its relation to diseases and causes of death, both in the present and in earlier days?

5. To what degree are specific disease susceptibilities based on genetic variation in human populations?

These are all biomedical questions about the genetic nature of human biology. To answer them, as with all genetic questions, one must have some means of comparing groups whose genetic makeup differs (if the item in question in fact has a genetic basis). Since we are asking questions about age patterns of diseases, we might think of comparing these between populations; however, in the absence of specific genes known to be related to disorders, it is impossible in between-population comparisons to isolate genetic as opposed to environmental or cultural factors related to mortality differences. Further, all populations experience a great variation in age patterns of mortality or morbidity — how much of this *within* population variation is itself genetically based? That is, without looking at individual variation in genes of the kind I am referring to, it seems difficult to make much sense out of average demographic rate differences between populations.

What can be done, then?

For several investigators, of which I am one, a beginning answer to these issues seems best found by understanding first that the evolutionary processes leading to longevity, disease susceptibility, and hence to the life table are ones involving stochastic risks whether or not heritable genetic variation is the basis for the results — that is, genes related to longevity and mortality patterns generally will not be deterministic genes such as those for eye color, but will merely lead to higher or lower, earlier or later, risks. This means that our problems can be examined only by studying large numbers of individuals — genes for risk differences of this type cannot be found by looking at a few families and testing for segregation of alleles (as one can do, for example, to find the cause for, say, PKU or sickle cell disease). We need large — very large — samples.

Yet in asking basically genetic questions, one's large samples must still be closely controlled for their genetic nature. This cannot be done, for example, by using various sets of national or regional demographic statistics; there, although the samples are very large, the genetic relationships and differences amongst the constituent individuals are completely unknown.

One answer to much of this seems to be in the use of extensive, numerous, very large pedigrees in populations that are virtually fully examined. This is something which could not be done until feasibly inexpensive computing facilities were available, and that has only been very recently. Examining many large pedigrees for genetic patterns simply cannot be done by hand — there are too many alternatives to consider at once.

This kind of application of paleodemographic methods and findings to contemporary biomedical questions is, perhaps, off the track that is being followed by many archeologically oriented paleodemographers. Yet it is a track being followed by many, if not most, of those of us who have spent the first part of this decade in developing paleodemographic data and methods (and by many others who spent that time doing demography among living tribal populations). This is so because we are now interested in questions which cannot be solved by paleodemographic data and because we feel that to a great extent the problems which such data can address have been solved.

Historical demography and a specialized branch, pedigree analysis, are a means of examining the vital processes of populations units which in many ways are quite similar to the burial populations of the paleodemographer except that they are better documented. First, the use of large historical demographic data bases, often using cemetery data and relating this to present populations, especially in tribal situations, and in particular pedigrees, involve populations of small size relative to what most demographers consider. Such size is, however, typical of the tribal populations of which paleodemographic data are representations.

Secondly, we are now dealing with populations of individuals related to each other in specific, close, and specifiable degrees. This is well controlled, but upon reflection any anthropologist might be expected to recognize that the tribal populations (e.g., villages) we have studied are also closely related, probably about in the same manner as a pedigreed population except that the paleodemographer does not know who is related to whom.

Paleodemographic studies have been inexorably leading to increased consideration of sampling variability in assessing life table variations such as death rates. Computer simulation and other approaches have been more often applied to understanding differences between or variability among village populations in their demography. Such methods are still crude, but their continued development is vital for application to the study of historical demographic or pedigree populations, for, to distinguish between vital events in different families (who, we hope, have different genes for important biological traits of interest to us) one must account for sampling variation. Thus, one direct feedback from paleodemographic work will be the use of sampling variation studies (of course, variation observed in the living tribal populations of the world is even more directly relevant).

A second direct usage which can be made of paleodemographic data is in our understanding of human aging as it is manifest in the age patterns of disease in our society. If we are to know the degree to which present disease patterns, now freed from being obscured by a heavy overload of early-onset infectious diseases, represent the biology of human aging, we must know the extent to which the patterns of the same diseases struck in the past millenia. Further, a knowledge of developmental rates, fertility, and so on will help us to understand how much of the timing of vital events which we see today may be culturally based.

It is fortunate that the evidence from paleodemography seems clear. Even without as yet having done much experimentation to decompose tribal age patterns of mortality, it is clear that the general age pattern of growth and development and that of aging and death have been the same for our ancestors for a very long time. If Mann (1975) is correct, in fact, development up through puberty has not changed in timing since Australopithecine times, one or more million years ago. In any case, it seems clear that the lifespan to which a person could live if he were not killed by an overload of infectious disease or by poisonous vermin or violence was basically the same as observed today.

This means that we can assume that age patterns of contemporary degenerative diseases, such as cancer and others, represent the inherent aging biology of man. Interindividual variability in risk of death to such disorders, by age, can then be put to environmental or genetic modifications of the same well-established risk pattern which has existed for a long time. We are thus freed from the hopeless situation we would be in if a majority of variability had to be attributed to local factors.

An example of the import of this conclusion based on paleodemographic research (which is still unknown to epidemiological workers) is the following: There is a great fear among most people that the conditions of industrial life — those things which we enjoy or which are byproducts of things we enjoy — are creating massive epidemics of terrible diseases such as cancer. Are food additives, for example, causing cancer in great numbers? Since we know that the age pattern of present degenerative diseases follows closely an old established pattern, we can rest assured that (with some very specific and notable exceptions) the deaths we experience are normal reflections of our basic biological aging and *not* due to the conditions of life. Were the latter responsible, the age pattern of mortality from cancers, etc., would be materially earlier than it would be in the absence of industrialization — this is not the case.

Thus, in understanding diseases we may look at basic human biology, and its variation and evolution, rather than trying to pin the burden on specific pollutants which, though they may be contributory, do not fully illuminate the disease process. This gives us hope that studying variation among people in aging processes we can study the general aging process first, and its manifestation as specific diseases second, and may actually come to understand the underlying causative nature of the diseases. This will, I believe, come to be a fundamental fact in the pursuit of the epidemiological understanding and the treatment of the diseases of old age.

5. Summary and Concluding Remarks

In summary, paleodemography has in the past decade become a quantitative field of endeavor with relatively rigorous quantitative methods. It has answered the basic questions of the average mortality and fertility regimes that existed during our evolutionary past. It has begun to open the doors to a better understanding of population distribution during cultural changes, and to demographic reflections of social structure and status; it has begun to examine the processes which may have accounted for the genetic variability observed today in our species, although many intractible questions in this area may remain forever unsolved. And paleodemography has revealed the degree to which we may use present day demographic facts in studies of human biology, evolution, and biomedicine, helping us to separate factors due to our present culture and those which are due to long-term evolution.

If future demographic studies of skeletal populations are largely relegated to describing small local differences in mortality, this is a sign of health and not of illness. Having now understood the levels of mortality, paleopathologists and cultural anthropologists/archeologists may now concentrate their efforts on other issues: the causes of death and the factors controlling population distribution and interaction.

It is a cliche that dead men tell no tales. Certainly, we cannot expect a few dead men to tell us everything we might wish to know from them. But, through a lot of work in recent years, voices have been heard. Our ancestors have spoken to us, if softly.

References

Acsadi, G., and Nemeskeri, J. (1970), *History of Human Life Span and Mortality*, Akademei Kiado, Budapest.

Ammerman, A. J., and Cavalli-Sforza, L. L. (1971), Measuring the rate of spread of early farming in Europe, *Man* 6:674–688.

Ammerman, A. J., and Cavalli-Sforza, L. L. (1973), A population model for the diffusion of early farming in Europe, in *The Explanation of Culture Change* (C. Renfrew, ed.), pp. 343–357, Duckworth, London.

Asch, D. (1976), The middle woodland population of the Lower Illinois Valley, monograph 1: Northwestern Archeological Program Scientific Papers.

Bass, W. M. (1971), *Human Osteology: A Laboratory and Field Manual of the Human Skeleton*, Missouri Archaeological Society, Columbia, Missouri.

Bennett, K. A. (1973), On the estimation of some demographic characteristics on a prehistoric population from the American Southwest, *Am. J. Phys. Anthrop.* 39:223–231.

Birdsell, J. B. (1958), On population structure in generalized hunting and collecting populations, *Evolution* 12 (2):189–205.

Bocquet, J. P., and Masset, C. (1977), Estimateurs en paléodémographie, *L'Homme* 17 (4):65–90.

Bodmer, W., and Cavalli-Sforza, L. L. (1976), *Genetics, Evolution, and Man*, W. H. Freeman, San Francisco.

Boserup, E. (1965), *The Conditions of Agricultural Growth: The economics of agrarian change under population pressure*, Aldine, Chicago.

Buikstra, J. (1976), Hopewell in the Lower Illinois Valley, Monograph 2, Northwestern Archeological Program Scientific Papers.

Cohen, M. N. (1977), *The Food Crisis in Prehistory*, Yale University Press, New Haven, Connecticut.

Drenhaus, U. (1976), Eine methode zur rekonstruktion und beschreibung von nicht-rezenten populationen in demographischer sicht, *Z. Morphol. Arthropol.* 67:215–230.

Dumond, D. E. (1975), The limitation of human population: a natural history, *Science* 187:713–721.

Henneberg, M. (1976), On the estimation of demographic variables from prehistoric populations, in *The Demographic Evolution of Human Populations* (R. H. Ward and K. M. Weiss, eds.), Academic Press, London.

Henneberg, M., Pointek, J., and Strzalko, J. (1978), Natural selection and morphological variability: the case of Europe from neolithic to modern times, *Curr. Anthrolol.* **19**: 67–82.

Howell, N. (1979), *Demography of the Dobe !Kung*, Academic Press, New York.

Hrdlicka, A. (1952) *Hrdlicka's Practical Anthropology* (T. D. Stewart, ed.), The Wistar Institute of Anatomy and Biology, Philadelphia.

Kerley, E., and Ubelaker, E. (1978), Revisions in the microscopic method of estimating age at death in human cortical bone, *Am. J. Phys. Anthropol.* **49**: 545–546.

Mann, A. E. (1975), Paleodemographic aspects of the South African Australopithecines, University of Pennsylvania Publications in Anthropology, No. 1.

Masset, C. (1971), Erreurs systematiques dans la determination de l'age par les sutures craniennes, *Bull. Mem. Soc. Anthropol.* **12**: 85–105.

Masset, C. (1973), La demographie des populations inhumees, *L'Homme* **13**: 95–131.

Moore, J. A., Swedlund, A. C., and Armelagos, G. J. (1975), The use of life tables in paleodemography, *Soc. Amer. Archaeol.* **30**: 57–70.

Neel, J. V., and Weiss, K. M. (1975), The genetic structure of a tribal population, the Yanomama Indians, *Am. J. Phys. Anthropol.* **42**: 25–51.

Pfeiffer, S. (1980), in preparation.

Sanders, W. T., and Price, B. J. (1968), *Mesoamerica: The Evolution of a Civilization*, Random House, New York.

Smouse, P. E., and Weiss, K. M. (1975), Discrete demographic models with density-dependent vital rates, *Oecologia* **21**: 205–218.

Spooner, B. (1972), *Population Growth: Anthropological Implications*, MIT Press, Cambridge.

Spuhler, J. N. (1976), Index of natural selection in human populations, in *Demographic Anthropology: Quantitative Approaches* (E. Zubrow, ed.), University of New Mexico Press, Albuquerque, New Mexico.

Swedlund, A., and Armelagos, G. J. (1975), *Demographic Anthropology*, Wm. C. Brown & Co., Dubuque, Iowa.

Ubelaker, D. H. (1974), Reconstruction of demographic profiles from ossuary skeletal samples: a case study from the tidewater Potomac, Smithsonian Contributions to Anthropology, No. 18, Sithsonian Institute Press, Washington, D.C.

Ward, R. H., and Weiss, K. M. (1976), *The Demographic Evolution of Human Populations*, Academic Press, London.

Weiss, K. M. (1973), Demographic models for anthropology, Memoirs, No. 27, Society for American Archaeology, Washington, D. C.

Weiss, K. M. (1975), Demographic disturbance and the use of life tables in anthropology, Memoirs, No. 30, Society for American Archaeology, Washington, D. C.

Weiss, K. M. (1976), Demographic theory and anthropological inference, *Ann. Rev. Anthropol.* **5**: 351–381.

Weiss, K. M., and Maruyama, T. (1976), Archeology, population genetics, and studies of human racial ancestry, *Am. J. Phys. Anthropol.* **44**: 31–49.

Weiss, K. M., and Smouse, P. E. (1976), The demographic stability of small human populations, in *The Demographic Evolution of Human Populations* (R. H. Ward and K. M. Weiss, eds.), Academic Press, London.

Williams, B. J. (1974), A model of band society, *Am. Antiq.* **39** (4), part 2.

Wobst, H. M. (1976), Locational relationships in paleolithic society, in *The Demographic Evolution of Human Populations* (R. H. Ward and K. M. Weiss, eds.), pp. 49–58, Academic Press, London.

Zubrow, E. B. W. (ed.) (1976), *Demographic Anthropology*, University of New Mexico Press, Albuquerque, New Mexico.

2

Historical Demography

Applications in Anthropological Genetics

ALAN C. SWEDLUND

1. Introduction

The incorporation of demographic data into genetic analysis is now an accepted tradition in research; but as recently as the late 1950s, and despite the early examples of Haldane (1927), Fisher (1930) and others, the merits of demographic data still required emphasis and only a few studies existed. Birdsell (1958), Bodmer (1965), Cavalli-Sforza (1962), Kirk (1966), Kiser (1965), Roberts (1956, 1965), Sutter (1963), Sutter and Tran-Ngoc-Toan (1957), Spuhler (1959), and others reminded us of the potential utility of demography by developing analytical models and in novel, empirical applications. Research in both applied (United Nations, 1962; Acheson, 1968) and basic (Crawford and Workman, 1973) genetics benefited from this rejuvenated interest in demography. More recently several investigators (e.g., Harpending, 1974; Harrison and Boyce, 1972; Roberts, 1973; Ward and Weiss, 1976; Workman, Mielke, and Nevanlinna, 1976) have reiterated the relevance of *historical* inference on populations, and despite several limitations and pitfalls, their utitlity has also been clearly demonstrated.

In this chapter I will consider some of those limitations which inhibit genetics research with historical data and discuss the role of historical demography in anthropological genetics. I will present a review of the types of data

ALAN C. SWEDLUND • Department of Anthropology, University of Massachusetts, Amherst, Massachusetts 01003.

derivable from historical sources and their traditional applications in population genetics. In conclusion, I will discuss some alternative applications which derive from my own research experiences and those of other current investigators. It is my contention that historical demographic data are simply that, *data*, and they do not offer solutions to major theoretical problems in anthropological genetics. However, they are a very underexploited source of inference on a host of important questions, and can be used to test assumptions that might otherwise go unchallenged for lack of suitable cases. Anthropology's tendency to focus on nonliterate societies and short-term observation periods leaves a gap which historical studies can help to fill.

Certainly one of the most evident limitations in studying the genetics of historical populations is that there are no genes — a fact that must be disconcerting to the most optimistic researcher. There is little one can do about this problem except in cases where contemporary representatives of a population can be bioassayed and the population history then be used to account for the variation observed. This is a goal common to many studies and one of the more productive applications of historical data. Nevertheless, this approach itself is restrictive since it eliminates many potential data bases from consideration and also other kinds of applications. Therefore, in lieu of concrete genetic inference, it is often desirable to consider historical population data as a reflection of a wide variety of evolutionary processes to which specific genetic variants can only be nominally and somewhat artificially bestowed.

A second limitation has to do with the fact that the demographic records themselves have usually been gathered for entirely different, and essentially nonbiological reasons. The purpose may be political, ecclesiastical, or economic, but it is seldom medical or biological. However, this does not preclude our consideration of their genetic significance. In fact, some demographers (Van de Walle, 1976) argue that using data for purposes other than for which they were collected may be very appropriate since the original collectors and respondents would not be systematically biased for such questions.

The third major limitation is also characteristic of other areas of human genetics, but is compounded in historical contexts; that is, the lack of experimental controls. Research designs require the development of controls on a *post hoc* basis and many factors do not provide for a method of control. At times it is necessary to postulate several explanations for the same outcome without being able to reject any.

In spite of these rather substantial limitations it is clear that historical demography has an important role to play in anthropological genetics research. Evolution is history and Harrison and Boyce (1972), Workman *et al.* (1976), and others note that understanding of the *processes* governing human evolution is considerably enhanced by observing past trends in human population change and structure. It is perhaps the best focal point from which to view the interaction between cultural and biological change.

Sivi, 1976). Reconstitution studies have grown largely out of historical research and involve linkage of vital events, census, and/or other sources into families, sibships, or most importantly, whole genealogies. This approach allows one to investigate the complete life history of specified individuals, but also to correlate a host of variables directly with their occurrence among affine, consanguineous, and nonkin pairs or clusters. From reconstituted data inbreeding, "heritability" patterns and a number of other problems of genetic interest can be studied. Computer linkage of records has made reconstitution feasible in many more instances than previously possible, but it is still a very costly procedure in time and money. Both aggregated and reconstituted data are amenable to cohort and time-specific treatments. In the former one usually sacrifices certain controls for larger sample size. In the latter sample, sizes often must be small, but much more is known about the status of each observation (subject).

The information available in historical materials can be utilized to consider a number of determining variables. Three general demographic categories can be established: (1) cause of death/morbidity, (2) fertility behavior, and (3) population structure. Each of these categories, in turn, has correlates that can be partitioned into (a) genetic, (b) environmental, or (c) social classes on the basis of our analytical purposes or *their* principal characteristics. Examples would be hereditary diseases, climate, and occupational status, respectively. These will not necessarily be mutually exclusive, but will allow one to test a series of relationships with observed demographic patterns.

A consistent question which arises in population research is, "should a given demographic event be considered as the independent or dependent variable?" It is silly to ask this question without a specific hypothesis in mind, of course, since population processes can act as cause or consequence, or both through systemic feedback. In general, however, population processes are treated as independent variables in the analysis of gene flow and genetic drift, and as dependent variables for the mutation rate and in the presence of selection.

3. Research Problems

Although there are a number of problems that can be identified as appropriate for historical consideration, the majority can be subsumed under headings which reflect deviations from Hardy–Weinberg assumptions. Two major topics typically emerge: (1) the study of deviations from panmixia brought about by finite population size and nonrandom mating — population structure and (2) selection. Population structure and selection are interactive, of course. An obvious example is when inbreeding load decreases the fitness of one subgroup by comparison to another. It is not uncommon to incorporate selection and mutation as systematic pressures in population structure models, or to consider population structure as a cause of isolation of subdivided populations into

I suppose that historical demography is a sufficiently broad top.
it might include cases like the classic study of Livingstone (1958) s
culture history and population distributions of the west African gr
question were instrumental in understanding the frequency of sickle cell
wise, historical demography might include works of the nature that are re
exemplified by Cavalli-Sforza and associates (e.g., Menozzi, Piazza, and Ca
Sforza, 1978) on the spread of populations and agriculture in neolithic Eur
However, I would like to confine the discussion in this essay to those case
which specific, written demographic records of pre-20th century groups ha
been consulted. This can include cases where genetic inference on the d
scendant populations may or may not exist. In this way my area of concer
more closely conforms to the notion of historical demography that other socia
and biological scientists hold than would be true otherwise.

2. Data Sets

Historical data can come from a multitude of sources. Probably the most
common sources are vital registrations and censuses. Vital registrations usually
contain births or baptisms (date, place), deaths (date, place, and sometimes
cause), and marriages (date, place). Occasionally there will be additional information on occupation, residence, etc., and in some countries (e.g., Sweden)
migration, other than at marriage, is recorded. Census lists usually summarize
total population, household size and structure, and a variety of socioeconomic
variables for a single point in time.

Many of these records are available in their original format for historical
populations, whereas access to the original data (with named individuals) is pro-
hibited by law for the recent and contemporary citizens. Opportunities for
analysis of these data are considerably augmented by the presence of a wide
range of other sources including tax lists, wills and probates, deeds, maps, medical records, genealogies, diaries, etc. It is thus possible to reconstruct a number
of important aspects of the population in question.

For purposes of analysis the primary data are normally subjected to one of
two kinds of reduction. The easiest and most common is simple aggregation of
data covering a specified point or series of points in time. Aggregated data are
generally used to estimate the incidence of an event as a function of those
"exposed to risk." A time series of such estimates will describe change in the
population. Common outcomes of aggregate techniques include such tools as
migration matrices, cohort and time-specific fertility schedules and cohort and
time-specific life tables (see Shryock and Siegel, 1973, for a description of the
major demographic techniques).

A second method which is of considerable importance in genetics is
reconstitution (e.g., see Wrigley, 1969; Skolnick, Cavalli-Sforza, Moroni, and

ecologically diverse territories where selection acts differentially, but in most cases the two are treated essentially independent of one another.

3.1. Population Structure

Population structure (Cannings and Cavalli-Sforza, 1973; Carmelli and Cavalli-Sforza, 1976; Harrison and Boyce, 1972; Morton, 1969; Yasuda and Morton, 1967) includes the effects of inbreeding (consanguinity), assortative mating, random genetic drift, and migration, and takes account of such factors as the size and distribution of subdivided populations. The more sophisticated models consider some or all of these deviations occurring simultaneously. It is not my responsibility to describe or criticize the available models here (see Harpending, 1974; Harrison and Boyce, 1972; Jorde, this volume), but to indicate their application in historical populations.

Consistent with the discussion above, it is logical to utilize historical data in those cases where change over time is a primary consideration. Several models assume constant rates of migration, population size, inbreeding, etc. However, historical populations provide the opportunity to investigate changing rates, to estimate their effects, and to test the robustness of models employing assumptions of constant conditions. Spuhler (1973) describes three types of changes in gene frequency: (a) systematic, (b) random, and (c) nonrecurrent. Nonrecurrent change is interesting empirically as an incident explaining a particular case. For example, population bottlenecks (which may be random but sufficiently rare so as to be treated as nonrecurrent) have been shown to account for significant changes in gene frequencies (Roberts, 1973). For general theoretical purposes, however, it is the systematic and random modes of change which are most important in past populations.

Although there are a few early studies of population structure which employ historical data (e.g., Sutter and Tabah, 1955) the major impetuses have been computer technology and reconstitution methodology of the past 15 or so years. Major contributions appeared in the mid-1960's with the work or Alström and Lindelius (1966), Küchemann, Boyce, and Harrison (1967), Cavalli-Sforza (1962), Cavalli-Sforza and Zei (1967), and Roberts (1968). Since that time numerous studies have been done in western Europe (e.g., Hiorns, Harrison, Boyce, and Küchemann, 1969; Dobson and Roberts, 1971; Roberts and Sunderland, 1973; Roberts and Rawling, 1974; Cavalli-Sforza, 1969; Hussells, 1969; Morton and Hussells, 1970; Ellis and Starmer, 1978), Scandinavia (Mielke, Workman, Fellman, and Eriksson, 1976; Workman et al., 1976); Japan (Yasuda, 1975; Yasuda and Kimura, 1973), North America (Crawford, 1976; Halberstein and Crawford, 1972; Morgan, 1973; Swedlund, 1972; Workman, Harpending, Lalouel, Lynch, Niswander, and Singleton, 1973; Steinberg, Bleibtrau, Kurczynski, Martin and Kurczynski, 1967), and elsewhere.

To summarize the findings in these various studies is difficult indeed.

Different approaches are performed on populations which vary greatly in time, space, and cultural ecology. Perhaps the most meaningful evaluation of the work done to date can be focused on methodological assumptions and on the magnitude of the estimates themselves. Virtually all methods and their empirical cases have in common the estimation of a coefficient of relationship. This coefficient may refer to the degree of genetic similarity (identity) between individuals of the same population or between (among) population subdivisions.

According to Yasuda and Morton (1967), the degree of relationship can be estimated by a number of models ranging from pedigree analysis in a simple breeding isolate (genealogical model) through various interactive models of two or more breeding populations (hierarchical, partitioned, and spatial). Each model, of course, has a set of assumptions. The spatial model is generally thought to most closely approximate the behavior of real human populations, and to reflect their genetic history.

It is important to emphasize that processes of population structure largely depend on population characteristics, not genetic characteristics. Polymorphic systems in which the alleles (or phenotypes) are of approximately equal fitness are generally assumed, and presumably frequencies reflect the results of varying population size, intensity of interactions, and nonrandom mating. Estimates of the effects can thus be made independently of genetic data. Comparisons with genetic data will provide inference on the importance of structure in explaining contemporary gene frequencies, and the source of that variation (e.g., genetic drift and gene flow, etc.).

The contemporary members of a population can be bioassayed with regard to serological loci or by anthropometric series, data which are clearly absent for historical populations (although some early military documents do contain some anthropometrics). However, matrimonial distances, parent—offspring distances, isonymy, geographical distances between communities, and a host of other variables can be very well represented in historical sources. Moreover, the longitudinal study of these variables opens the possiblity for witnessing changing trends of genetic significance.

From the earlier works of Sewall Wright and consistently reiterated since, a significant cause of deviation from random mating appears to be differing mating opportunities as a result of isolation by distance. The distances between individuals within a population and the distances between subpopulations have a strong effect on potential mate selection. Isolation by distance thus estimates the potential for drift and flow and their combined effects, when breeding size is accounted for. Malécot (1969; also in Morton, 1969, and Workman et al., 1976) has derived the relationship between distance and the coefficient of kinship for a number of theoretical distributions of mating distance:

$$\phi_{(d)} = ae^{-bd}$$

where a is the estimate of local kinship and b is the systematic pressure from long-range migration. Numerous related models and methods for estimation have subsequently been developed, some of which assume no specific form of migration (see Morton, 1969; Morton, 1973; Cannings and Cavalli-Sforza, 1973; Harpending, 1974; Jorde, this volume for reviews) and behavioral models have been proposed (e.g., Boyce, Küchemann, and Harrison, 1967). Isolation by distance is the most useful construct for consideration of historical population structure studies.

If migration rates between subdivisions of a population have remained essentially constant, and certain other assumptions are met, the variation and covariation of gene frequencies among these populations are a reflection of population history. Several studies have thus been undertaken to either confirm or reject this observation. After bioassaying the contemporary population and determining the degree of relatedness by one of the distance models, the results are compared with inferences from historical demographic or other data.

3.1.1. Data

Several kinds of data can be used to compare with expectations: (1) parent—offspring migration, (2) matrimonial migration, (3) isonymy, and of course (4) genealogical pedigrees. Correlation can then be used to evaluate congruence between any two sets of results. Parent—offspring distances provide one of the best estimates, since differential fertility can also be incorporated in the matrix. Matrimonial distances between subpopulations can be utilized if fertility is assumed to equal two children for each marriage. Matrimonial distances are easier to collect and apparently provide comparable results in a variety of cases (Cavalli-Sforza, 1962; Mielke *et al.*, 1976; Hiorns, Harrison, Boyce, and Küchemann, 1973); in some cases the two may differ significantly, however (Yasuda and Kimura, 1973).

Isonymy estimates have been performed on a number of historical populations (e.g., Morton and Hussells, 1970; Ellis and Friedl, 1976; Lasker, 1969; Roberts and Rawling, 1974; Swedlund, 1971; Yasuda and Furusho, 1971). In addition, the recognition that surnames can be used for genetic inference has led to other useful applications (e.g., Dobson and Roberts, 1971; Lasker, 1977; Yasuda, Cavalli-Sforza, Skolnik, and Moroni, 1974). Crow and Mange (1965) presented the formal method of isonymic analysis and applied it to a case study of Hutterite data. The inbreeding coefficient (F) is estimated by

$$F = P/4$$

where P is the probability of isonymous marriages (based on their frequency distribution) in a population. From observed isonymy it is possible to estimate a nonrandom component of inbreeding (Crow and Mange, 1965) that reflects consanguineous matings in excess of or below the rate predicted by random combinations. There are several assumptions necessary in applying isonymy to historical populations (Swedlund, 1975; Ellis and Starmer, 1978), probably the most restricting of which is that the surnames must be monophyletic in origin.

Several studies (e.g., Morton and Hussells, 1970; Roberts and Rawling, 1974) have shown isonymy estimates to be somewhat higher than those from other methods, very possibly as a result of the monophyletism assumption. However, the overestimate from isonymy may be no worse than the underestimate of other methods, which can result from remote consanguinity and other unknowns about the founder population. In general, the estimates from isonymy are roughly comparable to other methods, are very useful in historical populations, and when available for several communities, can be treated in matrix forms analogous to other inferences on kinship.

The traditional method of pedigree analysis can also be utilized. Random pairs of sibships within generations can be sampled and a mean coefficient of kinship estimated.

3.1.2. Assumptions

The spatial models incorporating isolation by distance require the least rigid assumptions and therefore probably have the greatest generality in explaining a variety of cases. Assumptions that are usually necessary include the following: (1) the subdivisions ultimately have the same founder population and there is thus some phylogenetic relationship between all subdivisions; (2) the population is distributed more or less uniformly in space; (3) growth rates are equal; (4) migration rates are constant for the period being considered; (5) "outside" migration, selection, and mutation are either absent or can be treated as linear systematic pressures; and (6) geographic distance can be expressed in two dimensions.

Historical evidence and intuition alone would suggest that these assumptions are often violated. Thus, Workman *et al.* (1976) and others have pointed out that bias is introduced by the fact that many populations do not fit the phylogenetic model. Knowledge of the origins of founder populations and of the effects of regional fission—fusion processes can lead to quite different conclusions than those based on structural models alone. The various assumptions can be treated under the traditional demographic topics of population *size, distribution,* and *composition.*

Population size, or more appropriately, effective population size (N_e) is normally assumed to be constant in time in the estimation of coefficients of relationship. In historical studies a common convention is to divide the data into separate time periods and compute effective size for each of the subdivided populations and for each of the periods. Based on a number of empirical studies, the estimate often used is 1/3 the census size. If growth is stationary and net migration is effectively zero, this estimate is probably valid. However, historical studies of human populations (e.g., Eaton and Mayer, 1953; Küchemann *et al.*, 1967; Swedlund, 1971; Swedlund, Temkin, and Meindl., 1976) have shown clearly that neither stationary nor stable rates can be assumed. Moreover, deviations from stability are not necessarily the result of purely stochastic processes, but in fact often result from systematic changes in ecological and demographic potentials. While growth cannot proceed indefinitely, it appears that size equilibrium is seldom a long-term state in regional human populations.

The determination of effective population size (Crow and Morton, 1955; Kimura and Crow, 1963) is usually based on equations that parameterize the population at replacement levels. Few empirical applications exist in which this stationary assumption is challenged, but in at least one case (Swedlund, 1971: 18, 19) the resulting estimate was only 13.6% of total population size instead of the predicted 35.8%; a result of high fertility rates.[†] Even this deviation does not necessarily present a problem in estimating coefficients of relationship, since effective size is usually only used to weight the relative contributions of each subdivided population. So long as there are not drastic differences in the growth characteristics of the respective subpopulations, any reasonable percentage would do if applied systematically. However, *over time* high fertility (Swedlund, 1971) or high migration (Morton and Hussells, 1970) can cause the effective size to change. The effect would be to alter the kinship estimates; the magnitude and full nature of the effects will probably best be understood when several historical studies (or simulations based on known rates) have tackled this problem.

Population distribution has received more attention than size in the genetics literature. The spatial model treats population subdivisions as though migration was essentially isotropic, with population clusters located uniformly in space. The two mitigating factors of obvious interest are variations in population density and the irregular spacing of communities (Cavalli-Sforza, 1962). As noted, some aspects of population density can be controlled for by weighting estimates with census, breeding, or effective size. However, a more subtle problem may exist when communities of greatly differing scale and function are simultaneously considered, or when the "communities" sampled do not conform to the "subdivided," local populations of Malécot's model. Thus, Yasuda and Morton (1967) point out that the use of prefectures in Japanese studies yielded poor fits because of imprecise sampling at small distances. It has also been noted that the pooling of within-community matings as marriages that occur at essentially 0 distance exaggerates the leptokurtic nature of mating distributions.

The spacing of communities can result from a combination of historical and environmental factors, and a few anthropological studies (e.g., Cavalli-Sforza, 1962; Mielke *et al.*, 1976; Swedlund, 1975) have attempted to describe community formation and settlement distribution. Normally the effects of isolation by distance are given by the mean of the covariances in gene frequencies or migration frequencies. The potential atypical patterns which do exist are masked by the overall trend. Mielke *et al.* (1976) and Workman *et al.* (1976) have shown how disaggregation into smaller series can reveal significant deviations from this overall trend.

[†] This value corrects a simple arithmetic error in the original.

Directionality and distance in migration patterns is in part affected by the topography and transportation networks present, as well as by the density and hierarchical diversity in functions of various communities. Roads, rivers, and other corridors and barriers tend to orient migration along specific axes. Biases in orientation have been observed in England (Boyce, Küchemann, and Harrison, 1968), the United States (Swedlund, 1972), Japan (Yasuda and Kimura, 1973), and elsewhere. Mielke *et al.* (1976) were able to document the effects of modernization in transportation networks as a contributing factor in the breakdown of isolation by distance in the Åland Islands. The migration matrix methods and Malécot model obviously work best where the assumptions are most closely approximated – this is apparently the case for village agricultural populations (Cavalli-Sforza and Bodmer, 1971: Chapter 8; Harrison and Boyce, 1972). In cases where communities are highly disparate in size and socioeconomic functions (i.e., central place hierarchies), the model will be less appropriate.

Population composition incorporates a very large number of variables including age, sex, marital status, social class, income, etc. Composition is important to population effective size estimates since N_e is in part determined by the age structure, proportion marrying, and marital age, but perhaps the utility of historical studies has been most clearly evidenced in analysis of differential migration by compositional factors. Age at marriage (e.g., Yasuda, 1975; Jeffries, Harrison, Hiorns, and Gibson, 1976), social class (e.g., Harrison, Hiorns, and Kücheman, 1970; 1971; Harrison, Küchemann, Hiorns, and Carrivick, 1974; Küchemann, Harrison, Hiorns, and Carrivick, 1974; Abelson, 1977; Mielke *et al.*, 1976: 286), and sex (e.g., Cavalli-Sforza, 1969; Coleman, 1977; Yasuda, 1975; Harrison *et al.*, 1971) of migrants have been considered. As noted, it is difficult to generalize from these findings, and different cultures from varying time periods are involved, but patterns do emerge. For example, Yasuda (1975) notes that females migrate at higher rates than males, and this is also observed by Cavalli-Sforza and others. It can probably be generalized that in sedentary agricultural populations, the tendency for males to inherit land will precipitate a somewhat higher mobility rate for females. Yasuda (1975) also notes that age at marriage is not highly correlated with mobility, but since different social classes tend to have differing mean ages at marriage and differing mobility rates (Jeffries *et al.*, 1976) some age-dependent effects can be assumed, especially where class and occupation are not strongly associated with agriculture.

3.1.3. Coefficients of Relationship

Notwithstanding the acknowledged ambiguities and common confusion about the precise meaning of various estimates of inbreeding or consanguinity (Reid, 1973, and Weiss, 1976, discuss this), a characteristic feature of such estimates is that they seldom indicate high levels in human populations. Mating in most populations is essentially random. Local variation resulting from drift is commonly observed, but migration, and presumably some selection, tends to maintain heterozygosity and prevail against trends toward fixation. In light of this observation it is clear that methods which permit investigation of the cultural and ecological factors that affect population structure are most important. By these methods the processes that maintain variability and random mating can be detected and understood, thus offsetting the lack of inference that is sometimes carried in the estimates themselves.

While population structure can have important effects on gene and genotype frequency distributions, its overall evolutionary significance is still debated. From a macroevolutionary point of view, deviations from panmixia would not be expected to have much long-term significance except for neutral alleles or unless these deviations interacted with selection. In microevolutionary contexts, however, we frequently can account for virtually all of the genetic variation on the basis of population structure alone. Most historical studies document the eventual breakdown of isolation by distance and the gradual homogenization of subdivided populations as mobility increases.

These observations have promoted Harpending (1974) and others to comment that the study of the genetic structure of small populations has contributed to our understanding of regional history, but very little has been contributed toward our understanding of the evolution of the whole species. Studies such as those conducted by Cavalli-Sforza and associates in the Parma Valley or by Workman and associates in Finland have convincingly demonstrated the effects of population structure on local and regional genetic variability. Perhaps this should be sufficient, but there is an aggravating truth to what Harpending says, and most structure studies contribute little to this larger problem.

3.2. Selection

Far less attention has been placed on the study of selection in historical, or for that matter, contemporary human populations. Natural selection is the result of differential fertility and mortality and is thus of obvious demographic interest. Differential fertility and mortality can be measured on a number of different levels (Spuhler, 1976:185): (1) individual, (2) phenotype, (3) genotype, (4) gene. Clearly the more specific the level is that we can analyze, the more likely it is that we are actually measuring genetic *fitness*. It is also true, however, that with the exception of a host of rare inherited diseases, most gene markers known today have relatively high and similar fitnesses. Moreover, selection occurs on the genome and is seldom strong for any one specific allele or genotype, so that selection against any one genotype at a particular locus may be mediated somewhat by the overall genotype of the individual. Thus, the study of selection must often be undertaken at the least precise levels of inference. For historical populations, of course, even phenotypic levels can rarely be investigated and selection must be almost solely viewed from the individual level.

With very few exceptions the study of selection in historical populations has been done without regard to tracing the fertility and mortality profiles of specific individuals, but rather, the analysis of aggregate profiles of mean and variance in fertility and survivorship. The conventional method of analysis has been *Crow's index of total selection* (1958). Genetic fitness is usually defined as the contribution of one genotype in a population relative to the contributions of other genotypes present in the same population. According to Fisher's fundamental theorem of natural selection (1958), intensity of selection will therefore be proportional to the variability in fitness. Crow's index employs the means and variances of fertility and mortality for the whole population, and would measure actual genetic selection only when the mean–variance ratios are completely due to heredity, so that the Index I_t has been called the "opportunity for selection" or the "maximum opportunity for selection" (Swedlund, 1978; Spuhler, 1976). The index is given by

$$I_t = I_m + \frac{I_f}{ps}$$

where I_m is the index of mortality, given by

$$I_m = \frac{pd}{ps}$$

where pd is the proportion dying before age 15, ps the proportion surviving to age 15, and the index of fertility I_f is given as

$$I_f = \frac{V_f}{\bar{x}^2}$$

where $\bar{x}$ and V_f are the mean and variance in offspring to women reaching reproductive age.

According to Spuhler (1976), Crow's index has been modified and extended to consider prenatal mortality separately (Crow, 1973) and for women dying before the age of menopause but after reproductive maturity (Kobayashi, 1969). Use of the index has recently been reviewed by Spuhler (1976) and Ward and Weiss (1976). Spuhler has provided an exhaustive list of values for the index computed for various populations.

While this method affords the investigator with a means of estimating selection potential, the inherent weaknesses in the estimate should be obvious. Much of the variance in fertility and mortality can and probably does result from cultural and nongenetic environmental factors. Nevertheless, it does provide some inference on selection where genotypic data are lacking. A single estimate from one population is a somewhat meaningless value. However, when cross cultural comparisons are made, or temporal trends observed, the parameters are useful.

Spuhler (1976) and Jacquard and Ward (1976) observe that modernization tends to lower the index, both through lower mortality rates and also the

Table 1. Secular Trends in Crow's Index for Three
Historical Populations

	I_m	I_f	I_t
A. Deerfield[a]			
1721–1740	0.302	0.165	0.517
1741–1760	0.193	0.224	0.460
1761–1780	0.346	0.287	0.732
1781–1800	0.435	0.292	0.854
B. Ramah Navajo[b]			
1844–1889	0.125	0.239	0.450
1890–1909	0.203	0.643	0.977
1910–1924	0.366	0.518	1.073
C. Polish Hill[c]			
Before 1905	2.98	0.99	4.31
1906–1925	1.33	0.89	3.39
1926–	0.14	0.78	1.03

[a] Meindl Swedlund and Temkin-Greener (1976).
[b] Morgan (1973).
[c] Crawford and Goldstein (1975).

reduction of fertility size and variances through family planning. It is also noted that fertility has become increasingly important in the opportunity for selection as modern medicine and public health have so successfully reduced infant mortality. A comparison of three historical populations over time reveals a range of possible trends (Table 1).

Deerfield represents a recently colonized and rapidly growing population of 18th century New England; the Ramah Navajo a rapidly growing native American population of the Southwest; and the Polish Hill a declining, migrant population of the industrial Northeast. The most striking comparison is the generally similar trend and magnitudes for the total index for the Deerfield and Ramah samples, as opposed to the large, but declining values for Polish Hill. The first two might be expected to be typical of growing populations; however, the Deerfield estimate of I_f includes only women with at least one child. Thus, the variances may be somewhat low. In both samples the increase in the mortality component is noteworthy and probably reflects the effects of increasing population density and exposure to infectious disease (Meindl and Swedlund, 1977; Morgan, 1973:289–290). The Polish Hill population reflects a case where intense crowding and high rates of infectious disease were gradually alleviated by population emigration, sanitation measures, and improved access to medical care. The decrease in variation of fertility is characteristic of other modern populations.

In summary, Crow's index and other general methods such as the use of r (intrinsic growth rates; e.g., see Roberts, 1968) provide some inference on the potential for selection in historical populations. Their utility is probably maximized when trends over time are considered rather than a single estimate, but there is still very little one can say about fitness differences among individuals in the populations being studied. At best, an overall picture of the contributions by mortality and fertility is achieved.

4. Alternative Approaches for Historical Populations

If analyses of historical populations were confined to the population structure and selection methods discussed above, then I would argue that we have little further to gain from the study of historical demography. The major lessons would already have been learned. However, a reevaluation of the concept of fitness and a more creative treatment of historical data afford additional opportunities in anthropological genetics.

As indicated at the beginning of this chapter, the student of historical demography has to accept certain inadequacies of the data that are by no means minor. We can make this bitter medicine go down a little easier if we keep in mind a few points about the nature of human variation and of our roles as anthropologists.

Selection is on the Phenotype. Selection occurs at the level of the phenotype and on individuals. Thus, the entire genome is important and there are ways that historical records can be used to make reasonable distinctions between individual "types." Furthermore, as Weiss (1980) has pointed out, for any age an individual attains there are probably several competing causes of death or infertility, each with its own coefficient of selection. The one that any individual succumbs to results from a combination of genotypic and environmental factors, and will not necessarily be the one that the individual is most susceptible to genetically.

Complex Traits vs. Complex Etiologies. Realistically, we are aware that many of the most interesting genetic responses in human populations result from complex, polygenic traits which also may show considerable phenotypic plasticity. In addition, a specific morbid or mortal event can very often involve a very complex etiology of both environmental and genetic factors. It is my impression that we often confuse complex traits with complex etiologies. While there may be little we can do with historical data to tell us the specifics of the components of complex traits, we can measure and partition components of individual variation and environmental variability.

Social Biology. In almost ritualistic fashion anthropologists continually mention the importance of culture in determining biology and vice versa. But it cannot be repeated too often and we should not underestimate the importance of a successful behavioral adaptation in conferring a long-term advantage that ultimately affects the distribution of genes. In turn, we must be careful not to invoke some grandiose sociobiological scheme to explain a natural demographic phenomenon that has little or nothing to do with the actual fitnesses of the genotypes in question. Historical demography affords many opportunities to view the interaction between biology and culture, and begs for careful research designs rather than untested generalizations.

Fitness and Heritability in the Larger Sense. The difficulties attending the measurement of fitness and heritability in historical populations have prompted the need for those who do historical research to be somewhat circumspect. My associates and I find ourselves using such terms as "constitution" of the individual to avoid too much in the way of genetic implication. But there is no danger in this so long as we are not deluded into believing we are measuring something that we are actually not. If, after all, we are interested in the general area of human ecology and adaptation, then our role as historical, biological anthropologists is to measure the things we can, provide as much in the way of genetic inference as possible, and accept the limitations. To demand greater precision in the genetic analysis of these data is "to throw out the baby with the bathwater." Moreover, we can take comfort in the difficulties of estimating heritability for almost any data involving human populations and complex traits (see Lewontin, 1974; Kempthorne, 1978).

Games We Can Play

In this final section, I will very briefly outline a couple of the approaches currently being tested by my associates and me on data from the Connecticut River Valley in western Massachusetts. These analyses are not necessarily unique (most are not) but they exemplify the more detailed treatment of historical data that is currently underway by a number of investigators. For illustrative purposes, I will consider mortality events as opposed to fertility or interactive patterns.

For a given vital event we can arrange the data in a variety of ways, but the two utilized here are to establish cohorts (individuals experiencing an event at roughly the same time) and families/genealogies (individuals related but not necessarily contemporary). In the examples below the use of grouped, family data is illustrated but no genealogical models are utilized. We currently have over 800 family histories linked for the community of Deerfield, Massachusetts, between the years 1720 and 1910, and several of these are in genealogical form. However, analysis of these files is only just now underway.

Mortality. In the study of mortality it is well to keep in mind a general, and usually unsolvable equation of life expectancy:

$$e_x = f$$

where f stands for genome, social heredity, environment, and social factors acquired independently of "family." In any particular case of life expectancy, or survivorship, a given value should be determined by these four factors. We are usually restricted from having inference on all four simultaneously in historical populations, but should design experiments with these in mind.

One cohort study we have recently completed is based on estimating the effects of childhood mortality on subsequent survivorship in cohorts undergoing "severe" and "normal" regimes of mortality before the age of 10 (Meindl and Swedlund, 1977). The samples come from Deerfield and Greenfield, Massachusetts, and our concern centers on whether or not survivors of cohorts "screened" (stressed) at an early age by heavy mortality will show higher life expectancies on the average than unscreened (unstressed) groups. The Deerfield and Greenfield populations have recorded their vital statistics beginning in 1670 and 1750, respectively, and therefore even the longest of life spans are observable. In addition, the historical periods are marked with several epidemics of virulent childhood dysentery. Two of these (Deerfield 1803 and Greenfield 1802) have formed the basis of a test of the hypothesis just stated, i.e., populations subjected to high childhood mortality will display greater longevity after childhood if all other factors are constant.

All individuals who were born in Deerfield during the decade prior to the 1803 epidemic (and who lived out their lives in that town) may be considered members of a "stressed" cohort. Membership in this group simply assumes that the individual was exposed early in life to the epidemic at the time of his greatest risk. Another birth cohort, hopefully similar in every respect to the first, was selected from the same location directly *after* the occurrence of the epidemic. These form the "unstressed" or control cohort. A pair of life tables was then constructed in which expectation of life was compared at every age after ten. The entire procedure was repeated for Greenfield.

The group in Deerfield exposed to an epidemic lost 37% of their number by age 10; the figure for their unstressed counterparts was 28%. The Greenfield epidemic, which was by far the more severe of the two, contributed to a 41% mortality rate in the selected cohort; the postepidemic group lost only 18%. All four figures are probabilities of dying in ten-year intervals.

The four groups were then redefined on the basis of attaining the age of ten. In other words, the events of childhood mortality were removed, with reduction in survivorship commencing only after this age (Fig. 1). The normalized survivorships are shown for the paired cohorts in this figure. The upper graphs show the comparisons in each of the towns. The lower figures represent the same data recombined to compare response within the sexes.

The entire design can best be explained using these figures: (1) If the epidemics neither "screened" nor "strengthened" the stressed cohorts, the two normalized survivorships for each of the graphs would be the same (or at least very close). (2) If, on the other hand, they *did* have one of those effects, the stressed group would display higher survivorship. This is essentially what was found. In the figures, the higher of the two curves represents the survivorship of a group exposed to the epidemic (in all four cases). Comparisons of expectation of life at the end of risk to dysentery were also very informative. In Greenfield a ten-year-old survivor of the epidemic had a six-year advantage over his

Survivorship from Age Ten

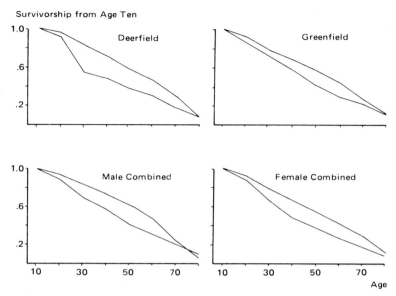

FIGURE 1. Survivorship from age ten in the Deerfield and Greenfield cohorts. Bottom survivorships are of combined males and females from both towns. In each case the upper curve is the "screened" cohort. From Meindl and Swedlund (1977). Reprinted with permission of Wayne State University Press.

counterpart in expectation of life. The Deerfield survivor enjoyed a ten-year difference. In *that* community, the longevity of the adults who survived exposure was of such great magnitude that their expectation of life at *birth* was actually over a year higher than that of the control!

Another interesting point to come out of the Deerfield comparison concerns the later cohort's loss of individuals during reproductive years. You can see the sharp descent in the lower survivorship curve in the upper left figure (Fig. 1). This has some implications concerning the *cost* of mortality to a society. Populations experiencing an early loss of individuals might be later spared more expensive disruptions. The loss of young adults (who in agricultural societies represent valuable producers) has additional effects on the stability of the family and household. These effects are not well buffered by other mechanisms, such as fertility, because young adults are not as easily or immediately replaced as children.

Of course, other factors may have contributed to the magnitude of the differences in these paired survivorships. Demographic events have many determinants and the selection of a "perfect" control is very difficult if not impossible to obtain from small populations. The differences between the paired age-at-death distributions appear to be the result of either differential composition and/or *average individual constitution*, i.e., selective or developmental effects of an epidemic. But these internal differences are only part of the picture. We

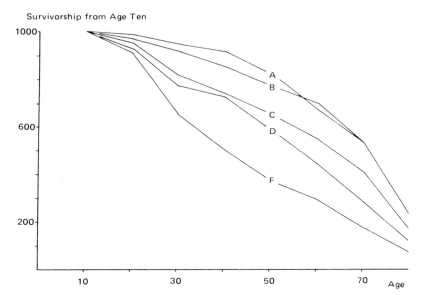

FIGURE 2. Cohort survivorship of four cohorts (*A—D*) prior to the epidemic and one
following (*F*), each representing a decade's mortality. The epidemic cohort, *E*, would
fall near *C* in rates. From Meindl and Swedlund (1977). Reprinted with permission of
Wayne State University Press.

might refer to the general increase over time in Deerfield and Greenfield mortality as the increase in the forces of mortality *external* to the cohort. Then any
group would be expected to display a given mortality schedule simply because of
its position in time.

To emphasize this point, four additional cohorts were selected for Deerfield
from the four decades previous to that of the epidemic group (Fig. 2). Survivorship was normalized as before and the schedules are depicted in this figure. *A*
through *D* represent the new data. *F* is Deerfield's original postepidemic birth
cohort; *not* shown is survivorship *E*, which is that of the Epidemic group. You
can see the regular increase in adult mortality by this ordered reduction in
survivorship schedules.

If the increase in adult mortality were as regular as suggested by all but the
epidemic cohort, we might say that the "expected" survivorship of cohort *E*
would lie between those of *D* and *F*. But *E* represents the adult survivorship of
the epidemic group and its actual position is near survivorship *C*. The reason for
this may be that external and internal forces of mortality (as defined above)
have acted in different directions in cohorts *E* and *C* to produce similar distributions.

In sum, the trends reveal distinctive patterns for the stressed and unstressed
cohorts, and they remain after controlling for overall trends in mortality over
time. Although we cannot specify the constitutional components that confer

greater longevity on the stressed survivors, it is logical to assume that it is, in part, the result of physiological and immunological factors of genetic origin. A further test of this model is being undertaken in which we are comparing the survivorships of known offspring of the stressed cohort with control samples of the same age from the general population.

Another approach we are experimenting with, which involves grouped family data, is to compare correlates of longevity for a large sample of Deerfield deaths. Several previous studies have demonstrated the relatively low heritability of fertility and longevity (see Cavalli-Sforza and Bodmer, 1971). Nevertheless, some vague but tantalizing observations can be made. In this analysis mortality events are grouped by surname, occupation, wealth status, and the number of children per sibship. In the first test an individual of surname x is drawn, a second individual of the same surname is randomly drawn, another pair is drawn, and the ages at death plotted. The expected distribution would be random, with no correlation between pairs. The results are summarized by values of Kendall's tau (correlation coefficient) for determination of significance.

Any correlation would presumably reflect the combined effects of social and biological inheritance of longevity. Further tests can then be performed to note associations within occupational and wealth status. The initial runs on Deerfield are shown in Table 2.

Table 2. Surname and Sib Pair Correlations for Longevity: Deerfield, Massachusetts, Using Kendall's Tau

Test	N^a	τ	$P<$
Deerfield before 1850	(612)	0.0533	0.049
Deerfield before 1850–1910	(603)	0.0573	0.036
Deerfield 0–21 yrs.	(603)	0.0632	0.021
Sib correlations			
number of children			
2, 3	(114)	0.1268	0.05
4, 5, 6	(340)	0.1126	0.002
7, 8, 9	(235)	0.1040	0.02
wealth			
poor	(292)	0.1396	0.02
rich	(288)	0.0676	n.s.[b]
father's occupation			
unskilled	(303)	0.1231	0.002
farmers	(457)	0.0671	0.033
professional	(272)	0.1211	0.003

[a] N is the number of pairs used in each comparison.
[b] n.s. = not significant.

That surnames alone would give weak, but positive correlations at significant levels was somewhat unexpected. Different samples were drawn so that deaths occurring before 1850 and after 1850 could be compared. In the third test, the 1850–1910 data were standardized in such a way so that all individuals who survived beyond age 21 were collapsed to age category 21. This was done since it was expected that the distribution of deaths beyond age 21 might unduly weight the positive associations. By collapsing in this way, all deaths at ages greater than 21 do not enter the correlation. It can be observed that the N's are hefty in virtually all of the tests.

The second set of tests involved pairing sibs by family size, wealth, and occupation. In each case (except for two-children families) the sibships were jumbled and random pairs drawn without replacement. It appears that there are significant correlations in longevity in all classes except among the rich, wealth class. Although the possibility of a type II error is great here, it is tempting to speculate that among the wealthy, the economic advantages (nutrition, uncrowded living conditions, etc.) mediate the environmental screening on what are already relatively high fitnesses, and thus correlations are weakest.

Thus, the hypothesis that there is a genetic component to longevity should not be rejected on the basis of these tests. The next step we are currently undertaking is to partition the variances associated with mean differences in longevity between groups, and to develop appropriate analysis of variance models. Low, positive correlations are just what one might expect if a genetic component were operating and further tests involving various socioeconomic categories and biological relationships seem warranted.

These brief examples are admittedly very tenuous in substance from a genetic perspective, but they indicate possibilities for analysis that can be significantly elaborated upon, and from which some hints at the nature of genetic adaptation in historical populations are possible. They are necessarily "rough" because that is the status of our available data in these early stages of the research. As our genealogical files are completed and additional variables can be linked to the fertility and mortality files, more powerful and meaningful tests will be feasible.

Possibly the best opportunities for the application of genetic models will be in the analysis of distributions of specific diseases along family lines. Coefficients of heritability may be estimated for several diseases where the genetic component is presently unclear. Many historical sources contain cause-of-death information of reasonable accuracy and interpretable in terms of modern diagnoses. Infectious diseases such as tuberculosis (Burnet and White, 1972), metabolic conditions such as diabetes, and degenerative diseases like various neoplasms can often be traced over several generations. The projects of K. Weiss and his associates using data from Laredo, Texas and of M. Skolnick and associates on the Mormon genealogies (Bean, May, and Skolnick, 1977; Cannings, Thompson, and Skolnick, this volume) should contribute significantly in this regard.

5. Summary and Conclusions

In this chapter I have reviewed past and current trends in the study of historical demography and outlined the kinds of data available. I have indicated some of the strengths and limitations of these data for research in anthropological genetics. By far the greatest attention has been paid to questions regarding the effects of population structure on nonrandom mating. Far less attention has been addressed to questions of selection and this is largely due to the difficulties encountered in attempting to measure selective processes. Nevertheless, differential fertility and mortality can be observed in many instances and greater attention should be focused on selection in the future. We are not necessarily going to find concrete cases of gene and genotypic change so much as we are going to be able to observe the modes in which demographic change occurs.

Past populations from a variety of geographic regions reveal similar trends in mating patterns and the eventual breakdown of isolation by distance. There is a remarkable amount of localized mating in populations of fairly recent times, and much regional variation in gene frequencies can be accounted for by this regional differentiation. On the other hand, coefficients of relationship from many samples suggest that, while variation in the gene frequencies of subdivided populations can largely be accounted for by the stochastic process of drift, migration is an extremely important factor. Frequency differences are seldom very large.

Mating, by genotype, would appear to be essentially random in the populations investigated. More interesting from the standpoint of applying historical data are studies on assortative mating by class and other social indicators. In England, at least (Harrison *et al.*, 1974), it would appear that there is little genetic isolation between classes; both class mobility and intermarriage serve to insure that the classes will share a high degree of relatedness in only a few generations. Further studies of this type for other regions would be desirable and some are currently underway.

About the only way that selection has been measured in historical populations is by Crow's index (Crow, 1958). These studies have recently been reviewed elsewhere (Spuhler, 1976). It is clear that the effects of "modernization," that is, increased life expectancy, decreased fertility, and decreasing variance in fertility have been to reduce the *maximum opportunity for selection*. But selection can still be significant, especially at the prenatal level. The best use of historical data for the study of Crow's index is when the index is calculated for various points in time and the results related to changing demographic and social patterns.

One of the most significant areas for future work in historical demography will be in the study of the distribution of fatal diseases along family and community lines. This could enhance our understanding of the heritability of certain diseases in the past, and be informative regarding the fitness of past populations.

Finally, it is important to emphasize a point made earlier in this chapter, which is that when we are dealing with models for genetic inference we are probably utilizing historical demographic data in one of its weakest contexts. It is difficult to draw the line on what constitutes anthropological genetics (as the topics in this volume attest), but obviously the central focus is the genetic basis for human variation. Population ecology is a larger arena for the study of human variation and biocultural interaction, of which genetics is one part. Population ecology also embraces many nongenetic biological processes as well as cultural and environmental factors. I am not a critic of reductionism in human biology, but the historical demographer's perspective must include the observations that many genetic problems require nongenetic sources of inference, and that many of the most interesting demographic problems regarding human variation and adaptation have very little to do with genetics. Historical demography is perhaps most effectively exploited in the analysis of demographic responses, at the family and community level, to general patterns of economic, social, and environmental change. The other side of the coin is that methodologies largely developed in genetics have much to offer in addressing such questions.

ACKNOWLEDGMENTS

I would like to thank Kenneth Morgan, University of Alberta, for criticism and suggestions on this paper. Conversations with him and Peter Workman, University of New Mexico, have made important contributions to my thinking about the role of historical demography in genetics. Any errors or misinterpretations are my own, however. Richard Meindl, Kent State University, has provided several ideas on methodology and made the statistical comparisons. This research has been supported by the National Institutes of Health (NICHD 08979) and the National Science Foundation (BNS 7907369).

References

Abelson, A. (1978), Population structure in the western Pyrennees: social class, migration and frequency of consanguineous marriage, 1850–1910, *Ann. Hum. Biol.* 5:165–178.

Acheson, E. D. (ed.)(1968), *Record Linkage in Medicine*, Livingstone, Edinburgh.

Alström, C. H., and Lindelius, R. (1966), *A study of the population movement in nine Swedish subpopulations in 1800–1849 from the genetic-statistical viewpoint*, S. Karger, Basel.

Bean, L. L., May, D., and Skolnick, M. (1977), The Mormon historical demography project: structure and data evolution, presented at Colloque International de Demographique Historique, Florence, Italy.

Birdsell, J. B. (1958), On population structure in generalized hunting and collecting populations, *Evolution* 12:189–205.

Bodmer, W. F. (1965), A program for genetic demography based on data from large-scale surveys, *Eugen. Q.* 12(2):85–89.

Boyce, A. J., Kücheman, C. F., and Harrison, G. A (1967), Neighbourhood knowledge and the distribution of marriage distances, *Ann. Hum. Gen.* **30**:335–338.

Boyce, A. J., Küchemann, C. F., and Harrison, G. A. (1968), The reconstruction of historical movement patterns, in *Record Linkage in Medicine* (E. Acheson, ed.), pp. 303–319, Livingstone, Edinburgh.

Burnet, M., and White, D. O. (1972), *Natural History of Infectious Disease*, Cambridge University Press, Cambridge.

Cannings, C., and Cavalli-Sforza, L. L. (1973), Human population structure, *Adv. Hum. Gen.* **4**:105–172.

Carmelli, D., and Cavalli-Sforza, L. L. (1976), Some models of population structure and evolution, *Theor. Popul. Biol.* **9**(3):329–359.

Cavalli-Sforza, L. L. (1962), The distribution of migration distances: models and applications to genetics, in *Les Desplacements Humain* (J. Sutter, ed.), pp. 139–158, Hatchette, Paris.

Cavalli-Sforza, L. L. (1969), "Genetic drift" in an Italian population, *Sci. Am.* **221**(2):30–37.

Cavalli-Sforza, L. L., and Zei, G. (1967), Experiments with an artifical population, in *Proceedings of the Third International Congress on Human Genetics* (J. F. Crow and J. V. Neel, eds.), pp. 473–478, Johns Hopkins Press, Baltimore.

Cavalli-Sforza, L. L. and Bodmer, W. F. (1971), *The Genetics of Human Populations*, W. H. Freeman, San Francisco.

Coleman, D. A. (1977), The geography of marriage in Britain, 1920–1960, *Ann. Hum. Biol.* **4**(2):101–132.

Crawford, Michael H. (ed.) (1976), *The Tlaxcaltecans: Prehistory Demography, Morphology, Genetics*, University of Kansas Publications in Anthropology, Vol. 7, University of Kansas Press, Lawrence, Kansas.

Crawford, M. H., and Goldstein, E. (1975), Demography and evolution of an urban ethnic community: Polish Hill, Pittsburgh, *Am. J. Phys. Anthropol.* **43**(1):133–140.

Crawford, M. H., and Workman, P. L. (eds.) (1973), *Methods and Theories in Anthropological Genetics*, University of New Mexico Press, Albuquerque.

Crow, J. F. (1958), Some possibilities for measuring selection intensities in man, *Hum. Biol.* **30**(1):1–13.

Crow, J. F. (1973), Some effects of relaxed selection, in *Proceedings of the Fourth International Congress on Human Genetics*, J. De Grouchy, F. J. G. Ebling, and I. W. Henderson (eds.), pp. 155–166, Excerpta Medica, Amsterdam.

Crow, J. F., and Mange, A. P. (1965), Measurement of inbreeding from the frequency of marriages between persons of the same surname, *Eugen. Q.* **24**(4):454–477.

Crow, J. F., and Morton, N. E. (1955), Measurement of gene frequency drift in small populations, *Evolution* **9**:202–214.

Dobson, T., and Roberts, D. F. (1971), Historical population movement and gene flow in Northumberland parishes, *J. Biosocial Sci.* **3**:193–208.

Eaton, J. W., and Mayer, A. J. (1953), The social biology of very high fertility among the Hutterites: the demography of a unique population, *Hum. Biol.* **25**(3):206–64.

Ellis, W. S., and Friedl, J. (1976), Inbreeding as measured by isonymy and by pedigrees in Kippel, Switzerland, *Soc. Biol.* **23**:158–167.

Ellis, W., and Starmer, W. T. (1978), Inbreeding as measured by isonymy, pedigrees and population size in Torbel, Switzerland, *Am. J. Hum. Gen.* **30**:366–376.

Fisher, R. A. (1930), *The Genetical Theory of Natural Selection*, Oxford University Press, Oxford.

Halberstein, R. A., and Crawford, M. H. (1972), Human biology in Tlaxcala, Mexico: demography, *Am. J. Phys. Anthropol.* **36**(2):199–212.

Haldane, J. B. S. (1927), A mathematical theory of natural and artifical selection, Part IV, *Proc. Cambridge Philos. Soc.* **23**:838–844.

Harpending, H. (1974), Genetic structure of small populations, *Ann. Rev. Anthropol.* **3**:229–243.

Harrison, G. A., and Boyce, A. J. (1972), Migration, exchange, and the genetic structure of populations, in *The Structure of Human Populations* (G. A. Harrison and A. J. Boyce, eds.), pp. 128–145, Clarendon Press, Oxford.

Harrison, G. A., Hiorns, R. W., and Küchemann, C. F. (1970), Social class relatedness in some Oxfordshire parishes, *J. Biosoc. Sci.* **2**:71–80.

Harrison, G. A., Hiorns, R. W., and Küchemann, C. F. (1971), Social class and marriage patterns in some Oxfordshire populations, *J. Biosocial Sci.* **3**:1–12.

Harrison, G. A., Küchemann, C. F., Hiorns, R. W., and Carrivick, P. J. (1974), Social mobility, assortative marriage and their interrelationships with marital distance and age in Oxford City, *Ann. Hum. Biol.* **1**(2):211–223.

Hiorns, R. W., Harrison, G. A., Boyce, A. J., and Küchemann, C. F. (1969), A mathematical analysis of the effects of movement on the relatedness between populations, *Ann. Hum. Gen.* **32**:237–250.

Hiorns, R. W., Harrison, G. A., Boyce, A. J., and Küchemann, C. F. (1973), Factors affecting the genetic structure of populations: an urban rural contrast in Britain, in *Genetic Variation in Britain* (D. F. Roberts and E. Sunderland, eds.), pp. 17–32, Taylor and Francis, London.

Hussells, I. (1969), Genetic structure of Saas, a Swiss isolate, *Hum. Biol.* **41**(4):469–479.

Jacquard, A., and Ward, R. H. (1976), The genetic consequences of changing reproductive behaviour, *J. Hum. Evol.* **5**(1):139–154.

Jeffries, D. J., Harrison, G. A., Hiorns, R. W., and Gibson, J. B. (1976), A note on marital distance and movement, and age at marriage, in a group of Oxfordshire villages, *J. Biosocial Sci.* **8**:155–160.

Kempthorne, O. (1978), Logical, epistemological and statistical aspects of nature-nurture data interpretation, *Biometrics* **34**:1–23.

Kimura, M., and Crow, J. F. (1963), The measurement of effective population number, *Evolution* **17**(3):279–288.

Kirk, D. (1966), Demographic factors affecting the opportunity for natural selection in the United States, *Eugen. Q.* **13**:270–273.

Kiser, C. V. (1965), Types of demographic data of possible relevance to population genetics, *Eugen. Q.* **12**(2):72–84.

Kobayashi, K. (1969), Changing patterns of differential fertility in the population of Japan, in Proceedings of the Eighth International Congress on Anthropological and Ethnographic Science, Vol. 1, pp. 345–57, Science Council of Japan, Yeno Park, Tokyo, Japan.

Küchemann, C. F., Boyce, A. J., and Harrison, G. A. (1967), A demographic and genetic study of a group of Oxfordshire villages, *Hum. Biol.* **41**:309–321.

Küchemann, C. G., Harrison, G. A., Hiorns, R. W., and Carrivick, P. J. (1974), Social class and marital distance in Oxford City, *Ann. Hum. Biol.* **1**(1):13–27.

Lasker, G. W. (1954), Human evolution in contemporary communities, *Southwest. J. Anthropol.* **10**(4):353–365.

Lasker, G. (1969), Isonymy: a comparison of rates calculated from pedigrees, grave markers, and death and birth registers, *Hum. Biol.* **41**:309–21.

Lasker, G. W. (1977), A coefficient of relationship by isonymy: a method for estimating the genetic relationship between populations, *Hum. Biol.* **49**(3):489–493.

Lewontin, R. C. (1974), The analysis of variance and the analysis of causes, *Am. J. Hum. Gen.* **26**:400–411.

Livingstone, F. B. (1958), Anthropological implications of sickle cell gene distribution in West Africa, *Am. Anthropol.* **60**:533–562.

Malécot, G. (1969), *The Mathematics of Heredity*, W. H. Freeman, San Francisco.

Meindl, R. S., Swedlund, A. C., and Temkin-Greener, H. (1976), Mortality and fertility trends in an historical population, paper presented at American Association of Physical Anthropologists, St. Louis, Missouri (April, 1976).

Meindl, R. S., and Swedlund, A. C. (1977), Secular trends in mortality in the Connecticut Valley, 1700–1850, *Hum. Biol.* **49**(3):389–414.

Menozzi, P., Piazza, A., and Cavalli-Sforza, L. (1978), Synthetic maps of human gene frequencies in Europeans, *Science* **201**:786–792.

Mielke, J. H., Workman, P. L., Fellman, J., and Eriksson, A. W. (1976), Population structure of the Åland Islands, Finland, in *Advances in Human Genetics*, Vol. 6 (H. Harris and K. Hirschhorn, eds.), pp. 241–321, Plenum Press, New York.

Morgan, K. (1973), Historical demography of a Navajo Community, in *Methods and Theories of Anthropological Genetics* (M. H. Crawford and P. L. Workman, eds.), pp. 263–314, University of New Mexico Press, Albuquerque.

Morton, N. E. (1969), Human population structure, *Ann. Rev. Gen.* **3**:53–74.

Morton, N. E. (ed.) (1973), *Genetics of Population Structure*, University of Hawaii Press, Honolulu.

Morton, N. E., and Hussels, I. (1970), Demography of inbreeding in Switzerland, *Hum. Biol.* **42**(1):65–78.

Reid, R. M. (1973), Inbreeding in human populations, in *Methods and Theories of Anthropological Genetics* (M. Crawford and P. Workman, eds.), pp. 83–116, University of New Mexico Press, Albuquerque.

Roberts, D. F. (1956), A demographic study of a Dinka village, *Hum. Biol.* **28**:323–49.

Roberts, D. F. (1965), Assumption and fact in anthropological genetics, *J. R. Anthropol. Inst.* **95**:87–103.

Roberts, D. F. (1968), Genetic fitness in a colonizing human population, *Hum. Biol.* **40**: 494–507.

Roberts, D. F. (1973), Anthropological genetics: problems and pitfalls, in *Methods and Theories of Anthropological Genetics*, (H. Crawford and P. Workman, eds.), pp. 1–17, University of New Mexico Press, Albuquerque.

Roberts, D. F., and Rawling, C. P. (1974), Secular trends in genetic structure: an isonymic analysis of Northumberland parish records, *Ann. Hum. Biol.* **1**(4):393–410.

Roberts, D. F., and Sunderland, E. (eds.) (1973), *Genetic Variation in Britain*, Taylor and Francis, London.

Shryock, H. S., and Siegel, J. S. (1973), The methods and materials of demography, U.S. Department of Commerce, Washington, D. C.

Skolnick, M., Cavalli-Sforza, L. L., Moroni, A., and Sivi, E. (1976), A preliminary analysis of the genealogy of Parma Valley, Italy, in *The Demographic Evolution of Human Populations* (R. H. Ward and K. M. Weiss, eds.), pp. 95–115, Academic Press, London.

Spuhler, J. N. (1959), Physical anthropology and demography, in *The Study of Population* (P. Hauser and O. Duncan, eds.), University of Chicago Press, Chicago.

Spuhler, J. N. (1973), Anthropological genetics: an overview, in *Methods and Theories of Anthropological Genetics*, (M. Crawford and P. Workman, eds.), pp. 423–451, University of New Mexico Press, Albuquerque.

Spuhler, J. N. (1976), The maximum opportunity for natural selection in some human populations, in *Demographic Anthropology* (E. Zubrow, ed.), pp. 185–226, University of New Mexico Press, Albuquerque.

Steinberg, A. G., Bleibtreu, H. K., Kurczynski, T. W., Martin, A. O., and Kurczynski, E. M. (1967), Genetic studies in an inbred human isolate, in *Proceedings of the Third*

International Congress on Human Genetics (J. F. Crow and J. V. Neel, eds.), pp. 267–290, Johns Hopkins Press, Baltimore.

Sutter, J. (1963), The relationship between human population genetics and demography in *Genetics of Migrant and Isolate Populations* (E. Goldschmidt, ed.), pp. 160–168, Williams and Wilkins, Baltimore.

Sutter, J. and Tran-Ngoc-Toan (1957), The problem of the structure of isolates and of their evolution among human populations, *Cold Spring Harbor Symp. Quant. Biol.* **22**: 379–383.

Sutter, J. and Tabah, L. (1955), L'evolution des Isolates de deux Departments Francais, *Population* **22**:709–34.

Swedlund, A. C. (1971), The genetic structure of an historical population: a study of marriage and fertility in Old Deerfield, Massachusetts, University of Massachusetts Research Report 7.

Swedlund, A. C. (1972), Observations on the concept of neighborhood knowledge and the distribution of marriage distances, *Ann. Hum. Gen.* **35**:327–330.

Swedlund, A. C. (1975), Isonomy: Estimating inbreeding from social data, *Eugen. Soc. Bull.* **7**:67–73.

Swedlund, A. C. (1978), Historical demography as population ecology, *Ann. Rev. Anthropol.* **7**:137–173.

Swedlund, A. C., Temkin, H., and Meindl, R. (1976), Population studies in the Connecticut Valley: Prospectus, in *The Demographic Evolution of Human Populations* (R. H. Ward and K. M. Weiss, eds.), pp. 75–93, Academic Press, London.

United Nations (1962), *The Use of Vital and Health Statistics for Genetic and Radiation Studies*, United Nations, New York.

Van de Walle, E. (1976), The current state of historical demography, *Public Data Use* **4**:8–11.

Ward, R. H., and Weiss, K. M. (1976), The demographic evolution of human populations, in *The Demographic Evolution of Human Populations* (R. H. Ward and K. M. Weiss, eds.), pp. 1–24, Academic Press, London.

Weiss, K. M. (1976), Demographic theory and anthropological inference, *Ann. Rev. Anthropol.* **5**:351–381.

Weiss, K. M. (1980), Evolutionary perspectives on human aging, in *Other Ways of Growing Old* (P. Amoss and S. Havre, eds.), Stanford University Press, Stanford, California.

Workman, P. L., Harpending, H., Lalouel, J. M., Lynch, C., Niswander, J. D., and Singleton, R. (1973), Population studies on southwestern Indian tribes VI. Papago population structure: a comparison of genetic and migration analyses, in *Genetic Structure of Populations* (N. E. Norton, ed.), pp. 166–194, University of Hawaii Press, Honolulu.

Workman, P. L., Mielke, J. H., and Nevanlinna, H. R. (1976), The genetic structure of Finland, *Am. J. Phys. Anthropol.* **44**:341–367.

Wrigley, E. A. (1969), *Population and History*, McGraw-Hill, New York.

Yasuda, N. (1975), The distribution of distance between birthplaces of mates, *Hum. Biol.* **47**:81–100.

Yasuda, N., and Morton, N. E. (1967), Studies on human population structure, in *Proceedings of the Third International Congress on Human Genetics* (J. F. Crow and J. V. Neel, eds.), pp. 249–266, Johns Hopkins Press, Baltimore.

Yasuda, N., and Furusho, T. (1971), Random and nonrandom inbreeding revealed from isonymy study. I. Small cities of Japan, *Am. J. Hum. Gen.* **23**(3):303–316.

Yasuda, N., and Kimura, M. (1973), A study of human migration in the Mishima district, *Ann. Hum. Gen.* **36**:313–322.

Yasuda, N., Cavalli-Sforza, L. L., Skolnick, M., and Moroni, A (1974), The evolution of surnames: an analysis of their distribution and extinction, *Theor. Popul. Biol.* **5**(1): 123–142.

PART II

EVOLUTIONARY PERSPECTIVES

3

Perspectives on the Theory of Social Evolution

HENRY HARPENDING

1. Introduction

In this chapter I wish to discuss the role of population genetics theory in sociobiology and anthropology and to describe some of the more interesting and useful areas where population genetics and anthropology should interact. As anthropologists we are in a position to make important contributions to sociobiology because of our intricate knowledge of the behavior, social patterns, and population biology of man. These contributions will be most coherent if they address pertinent problems and issues of current evolutionary theory.

In biology faults and gaps often separate an algebraic theory and a verbal understanding of the content of that theory. Misunderstandings also arise over the utility and applicability of theoretical assertions for data analysis and interpretation. Many of us regard one of these aspects of scientific procedure as central and the others as secondary, but sensible science requires concern both with theory and with interpretations and applications. It is widely appreciated that observations and induction lead to theory building; it is not so widely appreciated that mathematical understanding in its turn shapes and conditions common understanding and viewpoint.

For example, many biologists are convinced of the overwhelming predominance of selection at the level of the individual for determining the course of evolution (Williams 1966). Much of this conviction is due to the early theory

HENRY HARPENDING ● Anthropology Department, University of New Mexico, Albuquerque, New Mexico 87131.

in population genetics by Fisher, Wright, Haldane, and others who used mathematics to study selection at the level of the individual. Mathematical understanding led to verbal understanding and a consensus that this particular kind of process was predominant in evolution.

Recently many models of group selection have appeared (for a thorough summary see Uyenoyama 1979), and these will be assimilated and lead to new observations and interpretations of data. The development of models of group selection is motivated by observations that many species exhibit coherent social (i.e. group) adaptations which are difficult to explain by simple individual se-lection. These models are much more complex algebraically than the classical models of selection of individuals; this may account for much of the current polarization and doubt about the importance of group selection in nature.

2. Theory in Sociobiology

Evolutionary theory is population genetics, and it is neither trivial nor always intuitive. It is important to grasp the theory underlying sociobiology, because verbal arguments easily become vague, incorrect, or both. I will out-line what I perceive to be some important insights from population genetics. These will be simplified and bare. Elaboration of this theory in some directions would be useful and interesting, but in others it would destroy the important simplicity of the insights to be gained. For example, I will assume local random mating. I have toyed with these forms by assuming various kinds of nonrandom mating, and I have not yet found anything interesting. The evolution of incest avoidance and mating preference in general is one of the more interesting and exciting areas in sociobiology, but I will avoid the topic here because it would interfere with the ideas which I am trying to handle. More realistic theory is not necessarily, nor even usually, better theory.

The challenge of sociobiology for population genetics is that the theory is concerned with fitness interactions among organisms rather than with fitness as a simple property of individuals; this is the essence of Hamilton's (1964) paper which started so much of the current burst of interest. This extension of classical population genetics leads to an increase in difficulty and complexity in the theory. Classical population genetics was built around the idea of individual fitness which was, in continuous time, an instantaneous rate of reproduction r or, in discrete time, a ratio R of numbers at successive time intervals. Usually

$$R \approx e^r \approx 1 + r$$

It is not conventional but it is helpful here to think of a fitness matrix like this:

$$F_c = \begin{bmatrix} r_{11} & & & & & 0 \\ & r_{22} & & & & \\ & & r_{33} & & & \\ & & & \cdot & & \\ & & & & \cdot & \\ 0 & & & & & r_{nn} \end{bmatrix}$$

where rows and columns correspond to individuals. In the classical theory the only nonzero elements are on the diagonal, so that an individual has only the single property of his individual fitness. Evolution is then studied by averaging individuals by genotype to obtain genotypic fitnesses.

In sociobiology the raw material for theory building is from the start very different. The fitness matrix looks like this:

$$F = \begin{bmatrix} a_{11} & a_{22} & \cdot & \cdot & \cdot & a_{1n} \\ a_{21} & a_{22} & \cdot & \cdot & \cdot & \\ \cdot & & a_{33} & & & \\ \cdot & & & \cdot & & \\ \cdot & & & & \cdot & \\ a_{n1} & & & & & a_{nn} \end{bmatrix}$$

This is no longer only a diagonal matrix because we are considering fitness interactions among individuals. Obviously classical population genetics and its matrix F_c are a very special case of this more general formulation. Just as in the classical theory, we summarize the matrix by averaging genotypes to study the course of gene frequency change. One approach to this summary, due to Hamilton, is discussed below. The point to be made here is that there is a new order of complexity in the population genetics of interactions and that our implicit shared ideas about evolution (for example, that evolution leads to improved adaptation) may fail completely when this new kind of theory is considered. In fact, the conditions under which adaptation in any reasonable sense should increase when there are interactions are very stringent. Insofar as these conditions may be rare in nature, I believe that adaptation as a principle has outlived its heuristic usefulness. Lewontin (1978) makes similar points.

3. Inbreeding and Relationship

Many of us think of relationship in terms of gene identity by descent, and much of the theory in textbooks is written in these terms. This approach has its roots in the theory of animal or plant breeding where either identity by descent from or correlation with respect to the *founding stock* was of great interest (Wright, 1921). In natural populations there is no sensible founding stock, so that ideas like identity by descent or fraction of shared genes between individuals have no useful meaning. Any pedigree extends arbitrarily far into the past, and reckoning from the most recent generations is easy to do but impossible to justify. In evolutionary biology the useful concepts are simple gene identity and gene frequency. In many but not all cases the results of both approaches are the same, but when things become complex reasoning about identity by descent can lead to some terrible muddles. Jacquard (1974) is the best summary of the many meanings associated with inbreeding, kinship, and relationship.

Hamilton's method for summarizing and studying the implications of the fitness matrix F will use the notion of the coefficient of kinship between individuals x and y. The definition of the coefficient is as follows. Pick a gene from the locus to be studied from individual x. Then the (expected) frequency of this same gene in any individual y is

$$p_y = f_{xy} + (1 - f_{xy})p \tag{3.1}$$

where p is the population frequency.

This is not the most general definition of kinship possible, nor is it an adequate specification for complex models of diploids. In systems where interactions are consequent to phenotypic cues, kinship may be different for different genes at the same locus. In diploids it may be of interest to specify genotype–genotype interactions in inbred populations; here kinship is not sufficient to parameterize the system and one must use Gillois' partial identity coefficients (see Jacquard, 1974).

The statement above that kinship specifies a gene frequency in y is shorthand for the idea that the conditional probability that a random gene from y is the same as the one from x is p_y. Conditional now means conditional upon the model one is studying or upon the knowledge one has. The coefficient of kinship between myself and my full sib is approximately one-fourth because the probability of identity of a gene picked from him, given mine, is one-fourth (the probability that they are both copies of the same parental gene) plus three-fourths of the population frequency of the gene (the probability that they are not copies from the parent but are identical by the luck of the draw from the population at large). This assumes random mating. Rearrangement of formula (3.1.) gives

$$f_{xy} = \frac{p_y - p}{1 - p}$$

which is one-fourth in this example. The information here is that x and y are full sibs. In a model of interactions among full sibs we use the fact that the average gene identity among full sibs is $(\frac{1}{4} + \frac{3}{4} p)$, while with a random individual it is simply p. This coefficient of kinship is the device used to reduce the information in the fitness matrix F to a usual form.

Note that there is no necessity that kinship be positive; with respect to the species kinship between members of different racial groups is negative. A potent snare here is p, the frequency of the gene in the total population. Kinship between two individuals changes with the definition of this population. The following example is silly, but it does make the point that kinship depends upon the population under study.

Consider an Italian feeding a Swede. With respect to the gene pool "Europe" they are negatively related, the act has negative "inclusive fitness," and the frequency of Italian genes decreases in Europe. With respect to the human species Italians and Swedes are positively related, the act has positive inclusive fitness, and the frequency, on average, of genes carried by the Italian increases in the world gene pool.

4. Gene Frequency Change

Armed with this specification of the coefficient of kinship we are ready to study gene frequency change by a formalism devised by Hamilton (1964). We must assume that the interaction coefficients a_{ij} in the matrix F are additive fitness increments dispensed by individual x_i to individual x_j. This means that the rate at which individual x_j reproduces is

$$r_j = \sum_i a_{ij}$$

in continuous time, or that the number of offspring of x_j one time unit later is

$$R_j = \sum_i a_{ij}$$

in a discrete-time model. This assumption of additive increments has punch to it, since there are many possible ways in which interactions might be specified.

In discrete time it is easy to see that the relative frequency of an allele G_i after one generation of selection is

$$p_i(t+1) = \frac{\sum\limits_{x} p_{i,x}(t)R_x}{\sum\limits_{x} R_x}$$

where R_x is the number of offspring of individual x and $p_{i,x}$ is the relative frequency of G_i in offspring of x. Now we use the idea that R_x is the sum of the fitness effects received by x, including the effect from x himself:

$$p_i(t+1) = \frac{\sum\limits_{y} a_{yx} p_{i,x}(t)}{\sum\limits_{y} a_{yx}}$$

Now we assume Hardy–Weinberg proportions in diploids to occur before selection takes place. The number of individuals of genotype $G_j G_k$ is $N p_j p_k$. Averaging individuals of the same genotype, $a_{jk,x}$ is the effect of an individual of genotype $G_j G_k$ upon individual x. The formula becomes

$$p_i(t+1) = \frac{N \sum\limits_{j,k,x} a_{jk,x} p_k p_j p_{i,x}}{N \sum\limits_{j,k,x} p_j p_k a_{jk,x}}$$

and there is light at the end of the tunnel, since $p_{i,x}$, recalling the definition of the coefficient of kinship, can be written

$$p_{i,x} = f_x + (1 - f_x)p_i$$

if a gene from individual y (that is, in this formula, from individuals included in the summation over indices j and k) is G_i, while if it is not G_i then

$$p_{i,x} = (1 - f_x)p_i$$

Heterozygotes bearing G_i are split between the two categories since a random gene from one of them will be G_i with probability one-half, to obtain

$$p_i(t+1) = \frac{N\left\{ \sum\limits_{k,x} a_{ik,x} p_i p_k [f_x + (1-f_x)p_i] + \sum\limits_{\substack{j \neq i \\ k,x}} a_{jk,x} p_j p_k [(1-f_x)p_i] \right\}}{N \sum\limits_{j,k,x} p_j p_k a_{jk,x}}$$

This is a terrible mess, but it will now simplify very neatly. Clearly,

$$R = \sum\limits_{j,k,x} a_{jk,x} p_j p_k$$

is the sum of all the fitness increments, so that it is simply the rate of population growth, or mean fitness. Define

$$w_i = \sum\limits_{k,x} p_k a_{ik,x} f_x$$

to be the genic inclusive fitness of G_i. Inclusive fitness of a gene is the weighted average effect of genotypes in which it occurs upon all other individuals x in the population, each effect or increment discounted by the coefficient of kinship f_x. Mean inclusive fitness is the weighted average of the genic inclusive fitnesses

$$w = \sum_j w_j p_j$$

When these are substituted in the mess and some algebraic rearrangement is done, we have

$$p_i(t+1) = p_i(t)\frac{(w_i - w + R)}{R}$$

or, in more conventional format,

$$\Delta p_i(t) = p_i(t+1) - p_i(t) = p_i\frac{(w_i - w)}{R} \tag{4.1}$$

This is exactly the same form as the general expression for gene frequency change in the classical theory, except here the genic inclusive fitnesses rather than genic fitnesses are used. If there are no interactions, the original fitness matrix collapses to a diagonal matrix of self-effects, inclusive fitness becomes identical to simple fitness in the classical theory, and the formula above is then identical to the standard expression. Thus most of standard population genetics is a very special case of Hamilton's theory.

It is now simple to manipulate the above formula to follow the change in mean inclusive fitness w. We know that

$$w(t+1) = \sum_{ij} p_i(t+1)p_j(t+1)w_{ij}$$

$$= w(t) + \sum_{ij} (p_i\Delta p_j w_{ij} + p_j\Delta p_i w_{ij} + \Delta p_i\Delta p_j w_{ij})$$

so that

$$\Delta w = \frac{2\sum_j w_j p_j(w_j - w)}{R} + \delta$$

$$\cong \frac{2 \text{ var } w_j}{R}$$

where δ is a small term in the cross products of gene frequency change which can be ignored. This is an extension of Fisher's fundamental theorem of natural selection; the rate of increase of mean inclusive fitness is positive and equal to twice the variance of genic inclusive fitnesses. This assumes that genotypic inclusive fitnesses are constant in time. In the classical theory Fisher's theorem is a statement of the widely accepted notion that adaptation increases and organisms evolve to exploit their niche more efficiently. Hamilton's extension says that when there are interactions the average *inclusive* fitness increases. What does this mean? It certainly does not mean that adaptation in any conventional sense increases since inclusive fitness increases as much from killing strangers as it does from helping relatives. I do not know what it means, but I suspect that this simple result of Hamilton's theory means that we should not expect to see adaptation and optimization in social evolution in general.

When algebraic manipulation corresponding to the above is applied to R, the change in population number or mean fitness (*not* mean *inclusive* fitness), there results

$$\Delta R = 2 \operatorname{cov}(a_j, w_j) + \delta$$

where a_j is the average effect of genotypes containing G_j. This says that the change in mean fitness is given by the covariance over alleles between average effect and inclusive fitness. If in a population those alleles with higher inclusive fitness are, on average, those with generally detrimental effects (e.g., selfishness, dominance striving, killing strangers), then mean fitness decreases. When we study social organization or other kinds of interindividual interactions there is no general notion to guide us in the way that Fisher's theorem is the (often implicit) background justification for engineering-type studies (as Lewontin, 1978, calls them) showing morphological or behavioral adaptation when there are no or very weak interactions. The evolution of optimal foraging behavior, the shape of the whale, and the like presumably reflect direct individual confrontation between an organism and a (nearly) unchanging environment. In this kind of context adaptation has meaning.

This all has relevance for the study of cultural ecology. It is easy to name a function for any phenomenon, and it is even easier then to call it a cultural adaptation, but this is a distortion of the meaning of the term. Warfare in New Guinea, for example, may be a very fine thing for regulating population but it does not increase mean fitness in any sense that the term is used in evolutionary theory. A real evolutionary approach to cultural ecology would examine strategy choices available to and used by individuals, and it would see social phenomena as the catenation of the choices of individuals. There does not seem to be now any proper theory for a social science *per se.*

5. Hamilton's Inequality

The most familiar aspect of Hamilton's theory is his derivation that an act will be positively selected over the alternative of no action if

$$b/c > 1/2f$$

where b is the benefit to the recipient, c is the cost to the actor, and f is the kinship between actor and recipient (the coefficient of relationship is approximately twice the kinship). This is true, but I think that it is not the most interesting way to look at pairwise interactions. Language is part of the problem; "cost" and "benefit" predispose us to think of altruistic acts at some personal cost, while Hamilton's theory is much more general than that. Figure 1 shows graphically some of the consequences of Hamilton's inequality. The axes are the effects on fitness of a single act on the actor (horizontal axis) and on the recipient (vertical axis), and it is assumed that the recipient is a full sib with f equal to one-fourth. The lines are lines of equal inclusive fitness; anywhere on a line the inclusive fitness of the actor is the same. Hamilton's inequality is the line through the origin, expressing the condition that the alternative is no action at all. If there is an alternative then the inequality no longer holds, but the graphics in Fig. 1 still apply. The arrows to the northeast show the direction of maximum increase in inclusive fitness, and evolution should presumably push things in that direction at any point. In a direction perpendicular to the arrow, change is selectively neutral so that a wide variety of interactions could evolve between pairs of identical relationship. There is an interpretation of Hamilton's inequality that

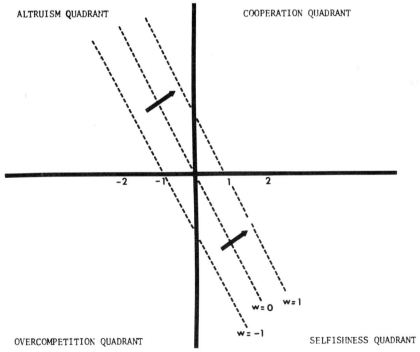

FIGURE 1. Inclusive fitness for an actor of an act directed to a full sib. Horizontal axis is the increment to the actor, the vertical axis the increment to the sib. Isoclines of equal inclusive fitness are shown, while arrows show direction of change due to selection.

relatives will be the objects of altruism in proportion to the relationship, but I cannot see it even in the simplicity of Fig. 1.

6. Nonlinear Relationships between Resources and Fitness

Much of the study of social organization in man is the study of transfer of resources among individuals. These transfers can often be quantified easily, so it is of interest to see how inclusive fitness theory predicts patterns of resource transfer. Consider here transfers only among those positively related, and imagine that an individual controls some fixed amount of resource which he can either retain or distribute. The nature of the resource, that is, the relationship between amount of resource and fitness, is now of importance in deriving optimum apportionment. I will assume that there is a law of diminishing returns, so that the effect on y's fitness of a transfer t_y from x to y is small for some small amount of resource but that it approaches an asymptote a_m for large amounts of resource. A convenient form for the effect on y by x is

$$a_{xy} = a_m(1 - e^{-\alpha t_y})$$

so α measures the rate at which y's fitness is saturated by the resource transfer. For example, a bushman with a dead giraffe is faced with a large α indeed, since a gift to y of 50 pounds of perishable meat is worth no more to y's fitness than a gift of ten pounds. At the other extreme a resource like land, which can feed many people for many generations, would be characterized by a very small α. How do these varying saturation rates affect patterns of allocation which would be selected according to Hamilton's theory?

An allocation by x to various y's (including perhaps x himself) has inclusive fitness

$$w_x = \sum_y f_y a_{xy}$$

$$= \sum_y f_y a_m(1 - e^{-\alpha t_y})$$

and this quantity achieves its maximum when

$$\frac{\partial w_x}{\partial t_y} = \frac{\partial w_x}{\partial t_z} \qquad \text{for all } y, z \qquad \text{(marginal value theorem)}$$

so that

$$f_y e^{-\alpha t_y} = f_z e^{-\alpha t_z} \qquad \text{for all } y, z$$

or

$$\log(f_y/f_z) = \alpha(t_y - t_z)$$

This says that for any pair of relatives y and z, the difference in the amount of resource transferred to each increases with decreasing α. This implies that relatives of varying degree should be given nearly equal portions of the dead giraffe, while a peasant's land should be dispensed very carefully and to the closest possible kinsman. This is, of course, what one sees in ethnographies. The generalized sharing which supposedly characterizes bushmen and other foraging peoples reflects the character of the resources shared. Vegetable foods decay more slowly, so they correspond to a smaller α, and indeed they are never shared so freely. It is interesting that here multiplicative changes in kinship generate

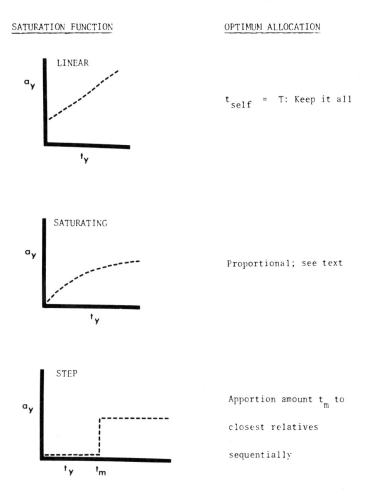

FIGURE 2. Relationship between fitness saturation functions in the left column and resource allocation strategy which maximizes inclusive fitness.

additive changes in allocation. The optimum apportionment, here and in general, is not allocation proportional to kinship. Figure 2 shows some other possible saturation functions and corresponding optimum allocation patterns.

7. Population Structure and Group Selection

This section is related to the foregoing, but the formalism is very different. I want to discuss population structure and group selection. Hamilton's theory could be used here, but it is not the easiest route to follow.

The variety of population breeding structure in man is fascinating, and we have detailed knowledge of it from ethnographic and genetic studies (Morton, 1973; Harrison and Boyce, 1972). Yet a good case could be made for the assertion that, from the perspective of current evolutionary theory, none of this knowledge is very useful nor important for understanding evolution in our species. Drift, after all, is mere noise, especially in a species such as our own where there is not, anywhere, much local isolation in comparative perspective. The kind of process envisioned by Wright where new advantageous combinations may occur via the random exploration of the possibility space in isolated subpopulations is probably of importance, but we don't know much about it.

Weiss and Maruyama (1976) made creative use of knowledge of the population structure of low-energy societies by inquiring how fast advantageous alleles would spread throughout a species of such a structure distributed uniformly over the old world. Population structure interacts in interesting ways with environmental heterogeneity in variable selection models, but most of our knowledge about humans concerns local genetic drift, and it is this phenomenon which seems sometimes to be a marvelous answer looking for a question.

Recent theory has revealed that when interactions and group effects of individuals occur, local structure and drift are crucially important. I want to outline here one example of this recent kind of model. I will call a trait social if its evolution is specified by an effect both upon the individual fitness of its bearers and its effect on all the members of the group in which its bearers occur. The two polar cases are altruism, where the effects are negative on bearers and positive for the group, and selfishness, where the effects are the opposite.

Consider a very large number of groups all of equal size N. This constant size is maintained by ecological conditions in the face of a reproductive excess each generation. This excess emigrates to die without reproducing or, possibly, to enter and reproduce in some group. The rate at which groups accept immigrants is constant, but those groups with higher proportions of altruists among their members have a greater reproductive excess each generation. This means that the pool of potential immigrants comes disproportionately from colonies with more altruists. This indirect selection for altruists opposes simple natural selection within each colony against altruists. The startling (to me) property of this process is that altruism disappears in any deterministic model, but the introduction of population structure and genetic drift can reverse this outcome and lead either to polymorphism or fixation of the altruistic type. This finding is not at all intuitive to me; yet analogous results come up in a number of related models (Eshel, 1972; Uyenoyama, 1979). I believe that in several years the kind of phenomenon described below will enter the popular culture or intuition of behavioral biology and will be widely regarded as obvious. This is an example of theorizing preceding intuition, I believe, as discussed in the introduction to this chapter.

The reproductive excess from each group is, for simplicity, a linear function of the frequency of altruists. Thus

$$e_i = a + bp_i \qquad a, b > 0$$

where e_i is the excess from group i and p_i is the relative frequency of altruists in the group. The model will be of haploids, or it would apply to a codominant locus in diploids. The advantage of haploid models is that they are simple and they are not really specific to genetic transmission at all.

The excess from all colonies mixes to form the pool of potential immigrants. The frequency of altruists in this pool is

$$p_p = \frac{\sum_j e_j p_j}{\sum_j e_j}$$

$$= \frac{\sum_j p_j(a + bp_j)}{\sum_j (a + bp_j)}$$

$$= p + \frac{bV}{a + bp}$$

where p is the mean frequency of altruists in all colonies and V is the variance. It is clear that the greater the variation among colony frequencies the greater will be the difference between the average colony frequency and the average frequency in the reproductive excess.

Within each colony selection and migration occur each generation according to standard models. If immediately after reproduction the frequency of altruists in colony i is p_i, then selection and migration transform it to

$$p_i' = p_i(1 - m) + mp_p - cp_i(1 - p_i) \qquad c, m > 0 \qquad (7.1)$$

This says that a fraction m of the colony is replaced by individuals from the excess pool among whom the frequency of altruists is p_p. The last term is selection against altruists with coefficient c. This formula is an approximation since properly a term close to one (the mean fitness) should divide the right-hand side and there should be some term in the cross product of selection and migration. Simulation indicates that the above is good enough, and there are worse approximations to follow.

Before this cycle of selection and migration occurred the variance of colony gene frequencies was V. The magnitude of the change is obtained by using a standard approximation from probability theory that the variance of a function G of a random variable p_i is

$$\text{var}\,[G(p_i)] \;\cong\; \left(\frac{dG}{dp_i}\right)^2 \; \text{var}\,(p_i)$$

Applying this to the transformation above gives

$$\text{var}\,(p_i') \cong \text{var}\,(p_i)[1 - 2m - 2c(1 - 2p_i)] + \text{higher-order terms}$$

so that both the migration and the selection decrease the variance when the frequency of altruists is low, while when the frequency of altruists is greater than one-half selection increases the variance as it drives the frequency down.

After selection and migration reproduction occurs in each colony. The new generation is assumed to be a binomial sample from the parental gamete pool, where the frequency was p_i'. The gene frequency after reproduction can be written

$$p_i'' = p_i' + \epsilon_i$$

Where ϵ_i is the change due to genetic drift. This change is a random variable with mean 0 and variance

$$\text{var}\,(\epsilon_i) = \frac{p_i'(1 - p_i')}{N}$$

Assuming now that the gene frequency after selection and migration is not too different from the frequency p_i before these occurred (this will be roughly true any time and a very good approximation close to equilibrium), the variance of the colony gene frequency after migration, selection, and drift is [writing $p_i(t + 1)$ for p_i'']

$$\text{var}\,[p_i(t + 1)] = \text{var}\,[p_i(t)]\,[1 - 2m - 2c(1 - 2p_i)] + \frac{p_i(t)[1 - p_i(t)]}{N}$$

Now we average this equation for the variance and Eq. (7.1) above for the mean over all colonies to obtain our model for the evolution of the mean frequency of altruists in the array of colonies:

$$p(t + 1) = p(t) - cp(t)[1 - p(t)] + cV(t) + \frac{mbV(t)}{a + bp(t)} \qquad (7.2)$$

$$V(t + 1) = V(t)\{1 - 2m - 2c[1 - 2p(t)]\} + \frac{p(t)[1 - p(t)] - V(t)}{N}$$

This pair of equations may have several equilibrium solutions for p between 0 and 1. In addition $p = 0$ and $p = 1$ are equilibrium solutions. The relevant question is whether these are stable equilibria, that is, whether a nudge away from the equilibrium leads to a return or to the system evolving to some other equilibrium. Here I will only look at the point where altruism is absent and there is no variance, so that p and V are both zero. Standard methods for stability analysis of systems of difference equations (Roughgarden, 1979: Appendix 3) show that this point will be unstable when the following matrix has an eigen-value outside the unit circle in the complex plane;

$$S = \begin{bmatrix} 1 - c & 1/N \\ (mb/a) + c & 1 - 2c - 2m - (1/N) \end{bmatrix}$$

Instability will ensue, that is, altruism will increase in frequency when it is rare, whenever

$$N < \frac{mb}{2ac(c + m)}$$

Evolution of altruists is thus facilitated by small a and large b, that is, a small reproductive excess from selfish colonies and a large effect of altruists on colony excess, and by small c, that is, by weak selection in colonies against altruists. A small local effective size N facilitates the evolution of altruists, and, surprisingly, a large migration rate m is necessary for instability. This goes against my intuition and against some of the literature on group selection.

The corresponding deterministic model is identical to this model, except that the last term in Eq. (7.2) is absent. This equivalent to letting N be infinite, and the above shows that in this case altruism cannot evolve. Drift or some other source of randomness is necessary.

I think that the preceding model is both simple and likely to reflect fairly well evolutionary events which occur in social species. The algebra is unpleasant, but this should not obscure the underlying simplicity of the model. Further, the same kind of model could represent as well learning and cultural transmission, where an "altruistic trait" would be one which would disappear in an isolated group but which increases group propagation rate, or even the rate at which the group transmits culture to other groups. In these situations randomness of trans-mission and the structure of migration and breeding are crucial determinants of the course of evolution.

Figure 3 shows the results of a Monte Carlo simulation of this kind of process. There are 25 colonies each of effective size $N = 20$. The selection against altruists within colonies occurs with intensity $c = 0.05$, while the repro-ductive excess from each colony is $0.2 + p_i$, that is, $a = 0.2$ and $b = 1$. The migration rate is 0.2 per generation. The solid line shows the population mean gene frequency as a function of time when colony reproduction is random

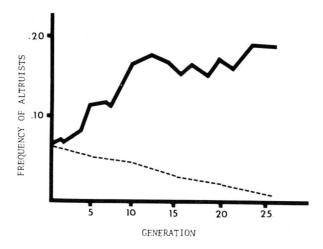

FIGURE 3. Monte Carlo simulation of social selection model as described in text. Solid line is stochastic model; dashed line is deterministic model.

(binomial sampling), while the dotted line shows gene frequency change when no randomness is introduced.

8. Population Genetics and Culture

It is necessary to ask how the foregoing can help understand human culture. There is no consensus among anthropologists and biologists about the proper sphere of applicability of evolutionary theory to the behavior of complex organisms.

None of the models discussed in this chapter are tied to genetics; they apply to the evolution of the relative proportions of anything which reproduces according to the simple underlying assumptions. For example, if some practice Z_i is growing (or declining) at rate w_i while other practices are growing at other rates, then the change in the proportion which are Z_i follows Eq. (4.1). The rate of appearance of new variance in the model of group selection reflects genetic assumptions, and other traits might have some different source of new variance, such as transmission error for a cultural trait. The general form of the model would be the same.

Feldman and Cavalli-Sforza (1976) have been studying models specifically of cultural transmission interacting with genetic transmission. Their papers are very interesting but the complexity of their models make them difficult to read. A more direct application of genetic theory to behavior, through a more sophisticated theory of learning (Hamburg, 1963), will be as fruitful for understanding the evolution of social behavior.

8.1. Ease of Learning

Different organisms prefer to learn different things and this learning propensity evolves. Anyone who has had either a baby or a pet monkey knows that primates are not interested in being toilet trained, while a cat learns about cat litter without effort. There is something wired into the cat brain which makes this learning task very congenial. The difference between the cat and the baby surely reflects the evolutionary past of the two species. Those concerned with the political implications of sociobiology should note that the relative human difficulty with toilet training implies neither that man can not nor that man should not be toilet trained.

Evolutionary theory predicts that there will be selection for careful discrimination of kin. Everywhere humans recognize biological relatedness between individuals; the manifestation of selection for kin recognition is a universal human interest in and affinity for learning kinship structures rather than any inflexibile system coded in the genome.

An important advantage of dependence upon learning is the flexible ability to adapt to a complex and rapidly changing environment; a disadvantage is the susceptibility of any particular individual to being taught things by others which are contrary to that individual's genetic interest. For example, in many warring exogamous patrilineal systems a male's sisters and their offspring, members of a different lineage, are enemies. There is no reason to expect that interacting selfish individuals will produce a system of taught and learned behavior genetically optimal for anyone.

The above examples refer to human universals, but the real use of evolutionary theory will be its ability to explain how people differ, not how they are alike. I want to discuss here some ideas being developed by Patricia Draper and myself. These are preliminary and tentative, and I discuss them only to exemplify a way in which evolutionary theory can illuminate seemingly complex data on differences among individuals and among groups.

8.2. Father Absence

Human societies, in comparison with the social groups formed by other mammals, are unusual in a particularly important respect. Mammalian groups usually have either persistent and structured multimale social groups, or else persistent pair bonds or harems. Humans manage simultaneously both forms of social organization, and we have probably had this bifocal structure for many millenia. Further, the specific details of this system vary widely from group to group and they have always been capable of rapid transformation in time. This variable social environment is precisely the context where phenotypic plasticity (i.e., learning) should be selected over any fixed alternative (Cavalli-Sforza, 1974).

I would ascribe much of the evolution of human intelligence to this complex social environment since it requires the individual to operate in two rather different social systems requiring reasonably distinct kinds of behavior for successful operation in each.

An important dimension on which the optimum individual behavior varies from one society to another is that of mating and reproductive behavior (Trivers, 1974; Dawkins, 1976). Males may commit time and resources to obtaining sexual access to a large number of females, on the one hand, or to providing for the offspring of a stable pair bond on the other. The appropriate abilities in the two contexts are those leading to success in competition with other males in the former and success in manipulating technology and the physical and biological environment in the latter. The corresponding female strategy "choice" is between reproducing fast and early in the context of a social environment populated with competing males, on the one hand, and careful choice of a male who will provide resources for the offspring of a pair bond on the other.

During the long period between birth and maturity humans expend much energy practicing skills and abilities which will make them successful adults. Different immature humans have different learning and activity preferences. It is common for little boys to practice dominance behavior more than little girls and for little girls to practice parental behavior more than do little boys. These behaviors do not have to be taught. But the extent to which children of both sexes vary in these propensities and others may reflect evolved early sensing of the social environment setting preferences and predispositions for what is practiced later in development. The advantage of early critical period learning is that it enables adaptation to a changing environment on the part of individuals, while allowing appropriate tracking of learning activities through the long development period.

Numerous studies have shown certain cognitive and behavioral outcomes, particularly for boys, of being reared in infancy in households without an influential masculine figure. Such males exhibit at adolescence excessively masculine and aggressive postures which psychological theory has attributed to "underlying insecurity" about masculine identity. Such males are revealed in later retrospectives of their life careers to form weak transient pair bonds and to devote proportionately a greater amount of time and energy to their roles in male hierarchies (Burton and Whiting, 1961; Biller, 1970; Rohrer and Edmonson, 1960). Studies of father-absent females are rare, but one careful controlled study (Hetherington, 1972) of adolescent girls showed a remarkably consistent pattern of greater sexual precocity on the part of girls whose early years had been spent in father-absent households due to divorce and desertion. Girls from father-present households and daughters of widows showed much greater sexual conservatism and reticence.

An evolutionary interpretation of these data is that humans have evolved the ability to sense household structure in infancy. This sets preferences for later development leading to practice of, and interest in, abilities leading to reproductive success in the particular kind of social situation characterized by the household structure. Thus the interest in violence, competition, and hierarchies of males from father-absent households reflects developmental adaptation for participation in a social organization where access to females is regulated by interaction with other males. Males from father-absent households also show consistently greater "verbal" than "quantitative" ability on psychological cognitive tests. This pattern is characteristic of females, and this has led to the interpretation that these males are somehow "feminized." We hypothesize that these males are not feminized in any way but are simply more interested in people and interpersonal phenomena as an adaptation to competition and that this preference is reflected in greater verbal competence. Males from father-present homes, according to our hypothesis, are more interested in the impersonal environment, less interested in interpersonal interaction and competition, and show less verbal competence.

Our interpretation of the data about father-absent females follows the same general logic. Daughters of divorced parents show an earlier interest in and practice of sexuality, while daughters of widows and intact families show patterns of sexuality appropriate to finding, with care, a male who will be a stable and reliable mate and to delaying reproduction until this pair bond is established.

9. Concluding Remarks

The examples given here having to do with human plasticity begin with the idea that the individual's genetic makeup predisposes him or her to learning within certain restricted ranges of behavior. Comparative social science, on the other hand, has for many decades taken the extreme environmentalist position that the individual can or does learn whatever arbitrary message is presented. The thrust of the latter part of this chapter has been that individuals are organized to learn easily or readily certain classes of behavior and that learning of this type goes on without any necessary regard for culturally sanctioned practice. I have suggested that reproductive strategy (as described above) is an example of a behavior complex which is learned at an early critical period and that the only way to make sense out of the otherwise disparate body of data on father absence is through understanding its evolutionary biology. Anthropologists often think of learning and socialization as one-way effects of teachers upon the taught; it is more fruitful, I think, to study what organisms are willing to learn and how this evolved willingness constrains the variety of human cultures.

References

Biller, H. (1970), Father absence and the personality development of the male child, *Dev. Psychol.* **2**:181–201.

Burton, R., and Whiting, J. (1961), The absent father and cross sex identity, *Merrill-Palmer.* **7**:85–95.

Dawkins, R. (1976), *The Selfish Gene*, Oxford University Press, London.

Cavalli-Sforza, L. (1974), The role of plasticity in biological and cultural evolution, *Ann. N.Y. Acad. Sci.* **231**:43–59.

Eshel, I. (1972), On the neighbor effect and the evolution of altruistic traits, *Theor. Popul. Biol.* **3**:258–277.

Feldman, M., and Cavalli-Sforza, L. (1976), Cultural and biological evolutionary processes, selection for a trait under complex transmission, *Theor. Popul. Biol.* **9**:238–259.

Hamburg, D. (1963), Emotions in the perspective of human evolution, in *Expression of the Emotions in Man* (P. Knapp, ed.), International Universities Press, New York.

Hamilton, W. (1964), The genetical evolution of social behavior, I, II. *J. Theor. Biol.* **7**: 1–52.

Harrison, G., and Boyce, A. (eds.) (1972), *The Structure of Human Populations*, Oxford University Press, London.

Hetherington, E. M. (1972), Effects of father absence on personality development in adolescent daughters, *Dev. Psychol.* **7**:313–326.

Jacquard, A. (1974), *The Genetic Structure of Populations*, Springer-Verlag, Berlin.

Lewontin, R. (1978), Adaptation, *Sci. Am.* **239**:212–230.

Morton, N. (ed.) (1973), *Genetic Structure of Populations*, University of Hawaii Press, Honolulu.

Rohrer, J., and Edmonson, M. (1960), *The Eighth Generation*, Harper, New York.

Roughgarden, J. (1979), *Theory of Population Genetics and Ecology: An Introduction*, Macmillan, New York.

Trivers, R. (1974), Parent-offspring conflict, *Am. Zool.* **14**:249–264.

Uyenoyama, M. (1979), Evolution of altruism under group selection in large and small populations in fluctuating environments, *Theor. Popul. Biol.* **15**:58–85.

Weiss, K., and Maruyama, T. (1976), Archeology, population genetics, and studies of human racial ancestry, *Am. J. Phys. Anthropol.* **44**(1):31–50.

Williams, G. (1966), *Adaptation and Natural Selection*, Princeton University Press, Princeton, New Jersey.

Wright, S. (1921). Systems of mating, *Genetics* **6**:111–178.

4

The Anthropological Usefulness of Highly Polymorphic Systems

HLA and Immunoglobulin Allotypes

MOSES S. SCHANFIELD

1. Introduction

In 1919 Hirszfeld and Hirszfeld published the first studies of human populations using the newly discovered ABO blood groups. Since that time an extensive array of hereditary markers have been defined on erythrocytes, leukocytes, plasma proteins, and erythrocyte and leukocyte enzymes. Some are of no anthropological use because only rare variants occur, while others are highly polymorphic. For working purposes, we will call a trait polymorphic if the frequency of at least one allele is greater than 1% and highly polymorphic if one or more alleles have frequency(ies) of 10% or more. Some genetic polymorphisms are of limited anthropological usefulness because the polymorphic allele only occurs in a single population, e.g., K, Js^a, and Di^a are limited to Caucasians, Black Africans, and Orientals, respectively (Mourant, Kopec, and Domaniewska-Sobczak, 1976).

Finally, genetic systems such as the ABO, Rh, and MNS systems are polymorphic in many populations and can be used to characterize various human populations. Other systems which have been used to characterize human populations are the immunoglobulin allotypes (Gm) and the human leukocyte

MOSES S. SCHANFIELD • American Red Cross, Blood Services, Washington, D.C. 20006. Author's work was supported in part by Grant HL 23654-01.

antigens or the HLA system. Both systems have been compared to other polymorphic systems for the ability of single systems to discriminate human populations. Schanfield (1971) compared the contribution of the Gm, Km, ABO, Rh, and MN systems to measures of genetic distance in eastern Asia and Oceania, and found that Gm was the single largest contributor to genetic distance between populations which are widely separated or among closely related villages. Stevenson (1978) investigated the relationships of Teutons, Slavs, and Jews in European populations. Using Gm, Km, ABO, Rh, MN, Rh, Kell, Duffy, haptoglobin, and Gc, she found that Gm and Km accounted for 75.1% of the variance in the first factor analysis, while all of the systems accounted for 78.6% of the variance – a negligible increase. Part of this may have been amplified by the use of indices. Menozzi, Piazza, and Cavalli-Sforza, (1978) using a total of ten loci and 38 "independent" alleles examined European and near eastern populations by principal components analysis (PCA). The first three principal components for all 38 alleles accounted for 56.4% of the variance, while HLA alone accounted for 54.9% of the variance. In comparison, the first three factors in Stevenson's analysis included 56.5% of the variance, while the immunoglogulins (Gm, plus Km) accounted for 75.1% of the variance. The results of these two studies have provided the first opportunity to compare the anthropological usefulness of these two systems. On the surface, there appear to be few differences as determined by this measure of genetic variability. It was decided that a direct comparison of these two systems on the same populations would be desirable to evaluate the anthropological usefulness of these two highly polymorphic systems.

Before proceeding, a definition of the term anthropological usefulness is in order. Genetic markers can be characterized by their ability to differentiate the major populations of the world and can be said to have macrodifferentiation usefulness. Markers which are able to differentiate villages within a single population can be said to have microdifferentiation usefulness. Unfortunately, although data are available to study this latter level of microdifferentiation for immunoglobulin allotypes and many other systems (ABO, Rh, MNS, haptoglobin, Gc, etc.), they are not available for the HLA system, thus precluding analysis at this level of microdifferentiation. An intermediate step between the macro- and microdifferentiation previously defined is the study of major subdivisions within a major population, such as the various countries of Europe. Extensive data are available for European populations.

Another measure of anthropological usefulness for a genetic system would be its ability to detect or measure admixture. This depends on the presence of markers with racially limited populations of origin. Examples of this are K in Caucasians, Js^a in black Africans, and Di^a in Orientals.

Finally, in evaluating the anthropological usefulness of a system, the cost, difficulty of specimen collection, stability of the marker, and ease of testing must be taken into account.

2. Materials and Methods

In order to study the anthropological usefulness of HLA antigens and Gm haplotypes, data were collected on as many populations as possible. At the same time, data on other genetic systems were collected on the same populations. In some cases, the population to be studied covered large geographical areas or genetic heterogeneity was known to exist. In those cases, with known or suspected heterogeneity, the weighted mean gene frequencies were calculated. The weighting, in all cases, was based on the proportion of the subdivisions tested for HLA. For example, among the Austronesian (AN) speakers from Coastal Papua New Guinea, 50% of the specimens were from the Central District near Port Moresby; therefore, all other genetic data were weighted so that the reported results were proportionally representative of the Central District.

Data were collected on the following independent markers: HLA- (A1, 2, 3, 9, 10, 11, 28; B5, 7, 8, 12, 13, 14, 15, w16, 17, 18, w21, w22, 27, w35 and 40); Gm(z,a;g-z,a,x;g-f;b-f,a;b-z,a;b,s,t-z,a,;b [including z,a;b (Oceania), z,a;b (Asia), and z,a;b (Africa)] z,a;b,c3,5-z,a;b,c3-z,a;b,s-z,x;g, and f;b,c5,s); Km (Km^1); ABO (A^1, B, O); Rh $(R^z, R^1, R^2, R^o, r', r)$; MNS (MS, Ms, NS); Kell (K); Duffy (Fy^a); Kidd (Jk^a); Lewis (Le); Lutheran (Lu^a); P (P^1); Diego (Di^a); haptoglobin (Hp^1); vitamin D binding protein (Gc^1); phosphoglucomutase (PGM^1); acid phosphatase (P^A, P^B); phosphogluconate dehydrogenase (PGD^A); and adenylate kinase (AK^1).

Data on HLA and Gm systems were available for 54 populations. All other systems have incomplete data sets. The references for all data sources are listed in Appendix A. The data include all major human populations with the following breakdown: Caucasians (non-Jewish) $(N = 19)$ including Basques and India; Caucasians (Jewish) $(N = 5)$; Orientals $(N = 9)$, including Amboenese, Filipino, and Ainu; Austral-Oceania including Australian Aborigines $(N = 3)$, New Guinea $(N = 2)$, Fiji and Samoa; Africans including Bantu, Bushman, and Afro-Americans; and Amerindians including Eskimos $(N = 3)$, North American $(N = 2)$ and South American Indians $(N = 2)$. Also included are Finnish Lapps. The summary data for these populations are presented in Table 1.

Principle components analysis was done using BMDP program P4M (factor analysis) (Frane and Jennrich, 1977) on the George Washington University computer. The F_{st} statistic was calculated using the unweighted means and variances generated by the BMDP–P4M program or by manually calculating the arithmetic mean and the variance from the data for those markers not subjected to computer analysis (Cavalli-Sforza and Bodmer, 1971).

Though many readers are familiar with the details of blood group serology and the determination of electrophoretic variants of polymorphic enzyme systems, it is useful to review the typing procedures and the overall data for HLA and Gm systems.

The human leukocyte antigens (HLA) are serologically defined antigens

Table 1. Summary of Genetic Data by Population

POPULATION	A1	A2	A3	A9	A10	A11	A28	B5	B7	B8
Australia										
Aborigines	0.000	0.134	0.000	0.290	0.169[a]	0.035	0.000	0.001	0.000	0.000
New Guinea										
Papuans	0.000	0.000	0.000	0.742	0.032	0.060	0.013	0.000	0.000	0.000
Austronesians	0.000	0.000	0.000	0.525	0.156	0.143	0.100	0.004	0.008	0.000
Melanesian	0.001	0.073	0.000	0.587	0.206	0.134	0.000	0.005	0.000	0.000
Polynesians	0.009	0.227	0.017	0.220	0.052	0.120	0.018	0.004	0.020	0.002
Orientals										
S.E. Asian	0.019	0.296	0.008	0.140	0.028	0.303	0.010	0.062	0.043	0.001
N.E. Asian	0.015	0.269	0.023	0.268	0.080	0.112	0.037	0.189	0.028	0.008
Amerindians										
Eskimos	0.014	0.200	0.013	0.649	0.010	0.004	0.090	0.143	0.058	0.015
N. American	0.000	0.511	0.002	0.337	0.005	0.008	0.017	0.069	0.005	0.005
S. American	0.007	0.461	0.015	0.130	0.000	0.000	0.052	0.192	0.000	0.000
Indo-Europeans										
Teutons	0.143	0.281	0.131	0.119	0.093	0.058	0.031	0.060	0.104	0.088
Slavs	0.122	0.270	0.108	0.130	0.071	0.064	0.021	0.103	0.087	0.060
Jews										
Ashkanazi	0.148	0.175	0.081	0.118	0.104	0.063	0.053	0.053	0.045	0.042
Asian	0.158	0.134	0.093	0.189	0.030	0.049	0.042	0.158	0.058	0.013
African	0.256	0.162	0.141	0.070	0.083	0.011	0.025	0.105	0.074	0.047
Indian	0.102	0.194	0.101	0.211	0.022	0.126	0.041	0.122	0.106	0.036
Africans										
Afro-American	0.058	0.174	0.076	0.146	0.050	0.019	0.102	0.046	0.101	0.038
Bantu	0.021	0.146	0.046	0.108	0.059	0.000	0.089	0.012	0.101	0.027
Bushman	0.025	0.210	0.117	0.148	0.073	0.000	0.052	0.057	0.135	0.082
Ainu	0.005	0.329	0.020	0.314	0.194	0.041	0.041	0.134	0.010	0.005
Lapps	0.023	0.355	0.350	0.113	0.040	0.073	0.031	0.107	0.285	0.006
Sardinia	0.064	0.301	0.027	0.101	0.032	0.084	0.021	0.096	0.015	0.015
mean	0.076	0.242	0.076	0.213	0.066	0.072	0.037	0.077	0.072	0.040
s.d.	0.077	0.113	0.075	0.166	0.067	0.075	0.031	0.061	0.068	0.048

POPULATION	B12	B13	B14	B15	B17	B27	B22	B35	B40	B18
Australia										
Aborigines	0.000	0.101	0.000	0.130	0.000	0.000	0.271	0.001	0.371	0.000
New Guinea										
Papuans	0.000	0.071	0.000	0.310	0.000	0.055	0.231	0.000	0.224	0.000
Austronesians	0.000	0.161	0.000	0.079	0.016	0.064	0.175	0.023	0.184	n.t.[b]
Melanesians	0.000	0.036	0.000	0.188	0.106	0.061	0.352	0.000	0.206	0.041
Polynesians	0.008	0.040	0.000	0.019	0.010	0.013	0.211	0.011	0.313	n.t.
Oriental										
S.E. Asian	0.036	0.074	0.002	0.160	0.059	0.028	0.048	0.051	0.141	0.019
N.E. Asian	0.054	0.023	0.009	0.106	0.037	0.029	0.081	0.072	0.143	0.002
Amerindians										
Eskimos	0.006	0.000	0.001	0.112[a]	0.004	0.098	0.052	0.042	0.416	0.002
N. American	0.007	0.000	0.000	0.028	0.008	0.068	0.003	0.222	0.216	0.002
S. American	0.000	0.000	0.000	0.215	0.000	0.003	0.000	0.067	0.289	0.000
Indo-Europeans										
Teutons	0.100	0.051	0.044	0.034	0.040	0.049	0.018	0.079	0.089	0.034
Slavs	0.153	0.018	0.036	0.039	0.056	0.061	0.023	0.101	0.059	0.051
Jews										
Ashkanazi	0.062	0.031	0.114	0.025	0.089	0.025	0.023	0.190	0.022	0.037
Asian	0.147	0.023	0.043	0.017	0.037	0.018	0.017	0.155	0.047	0.051
African	0.133	0.121	0.047	0.029	0.018	0.036	0.029	0.113	0.036	0.021
Indian	0.116	0.036	0.000	0.073	0.069	0.009	0.041	0.064	0.111	0.027
Africans										
Afro-American	0.098	0.006	0.033	0.016	0.128	0.017	0.033	0.182	0.035	0.035
Bantu	0.187	0.009	0.046	0.028	0.165	0.000	0.000	n.t.	0.030	0.040
Bushman	0.062	0.010	0.015	0.030	0.332	0.000	0.007	0.028	0.125	0.028
Ainu	0.041	0.005	0.000	0.279	0.010	0.036	0.020	0.000	0.122	0.015
Lapps	0.003	0.003	0.000	0.350	0.000	0.023	0.003	0.159	0.037	0.020
Sardinia	0.030	0.018	0.079	0.020	0.126	0.025	0.029	0.081	0.019	0.303
mean	0.073	0.035	0.025	0.097	0.055	0.033	0.057	0.086	0.124	0.037
s.d.	0.064	0.043	0.033	0.097	0.072	0.024	0.088	0.069	0.098	0.047

Table 1. (continued)

POPULATION	B16	B21	za g	zax g	f b	fa b	za bst	za b(Oc)	za b(As)	za b(Af)
Australia										
Aborigines	0.015	n.t.	0.705	0.235	0.001	0.000	0.000	0.059[a]	0.000	0.000
New Guinea										
Papuans	0.005	n.t.	0.659	0.043	0.000	0.055	0.000	0.241	0.000	0.000
Austronesians	n.t.	n.t.	0.070	0.003	0.000	0.718	0.000	0.170	0.000	0.000
Melanesians	0.106	0.000	0.620	0.129	0.000	0.242	0.000	0.009	0.000	0.000
Polynesians	0.014	n.t.	0.178	0.063	0.000	0.759	0.000	0.000	0.000	0.000
Orientals										
S.E. Asian	0.044	0.005	0.118	0.055	0.000	0.798	0.022	?	?	?
N.E. Asian	0.058	0.003	0.511	0.156	0.000	0.110	0.222	0.000	0.000	0.000
Amerindians										
Eskimos	0.005	n.t.	0.754	0.003	0.072	0.000	0.167	0.000	0.000	0.000
N. American	0.123[a]	0.110	0.905	0.041	0.031	0.000	0.021	0.000	0.000	0.000
S. American	0.051[a]	0.000	0.823	0.142	0.027	0.000	0.002	0.000	0.000	0.000
Indo-Europeans										
Teutons	0.021	0.015	0.217	0.124	0.650	0.001	0.000	?	?	?
Slavs	0.050	0.026	0.144	0.065	0.775	0.003	0.007	?	?	?
Jews Ashkanazi	0.133	0.046	0.150	0.035	0.795	0.005	0.008	?	?	?
Asian	0.046	0.097	0.182	0.022	0.707	0.007	0.037	?	?	?
African	0.058	0.070	0.183	0.023	0.720	0.000	0.032	?	?	?
Indian	0.005	0.027	0.259	0.088	0.498	0.017	0.003	0.000	0.136	0.000
Africans										
Afro-American	0.008	0.047	0.038	0.020	0.135	0.000	0.000	0.000	0.000	0.544
Bantu	0.018	0.028	0.000	0.000	0.000	0.000	0.000	0.000	0.000	0.644
Bushmen	0.002	0.007	0.112	0.000	0.000	0.000	0.000	0.000	0.000	0.271
Ainu	0.151	0.015	0.548	0.088	0.000	0.038	0.258	0.000	0.000	0.000
Lapps	0.009	0.000	0.241	0.022	0.697	0.000	0.039	0.000	0.000	0.000
Sardinia	0.021	0.076	0.111	0.007	0.827	0.000	0.002	?	?	?
mean	0.052	0.029	0.325	0.076	0.333	0.119	0.034	0.012	0.003	0.041
s.d.	0.046	0.032	0.269	0.063	0.346	0.266	0.138	0.047	0.019	0.135

POPULATION	za b	za bc3,5	za bc3	za bs	zx g	f bc5s	Km^1	A^1	B	O
Australia Aborigines	0.059[a]	0.000	0.000	0.000	0.000	0.000	0.229	0.310	0.000	0.690
New Guinea Papuans	0.241	0.000	0.000	0.000	0.000	0.000	0.015	0.218	0.113	0.668
Austronesians	0.170	0.000	0.000	0.000	0.000	0.000	0.185	0.155	0.120	0.725
Melanesians	0.009	0.000	0.000	0.000	0.000	0.000	0.165	0.251	0.102	0.647
Polynesians	0.000	0.000	0.000	0.000	0.000	0.000	0.256	0.239	0.131	0.630
Orientals S.E. Asian	0.003	0.000	0.000	0.000	0.000	0.000	0.243	0.153	0.181	0.659
N.E. Asian	0.000	0.000	0.000	0.000	0.000	0.000	0.300	0.229	0.193	0.578
Amerindians Eskimos	0.000	0.000	0.000	0.000	0.000	0.000	0.200	0.287	0.069	0.630
N. American	0.000	0.000	0.001	0.000	0.000	0.000	0.324	0.039	0.027	0.932
S. American	0.000	0.005	0.000	0.000	0.000	0.000	0.350	0.015	0.000	0.985
Indo-Europeans Teutons	0.008	0.000	0.000	0.000	0.000	0.000	0.065	0.210	0.077	0.640
Slavs	0.004	0.000	0.000	0.000	0.000	0.000	0.070	0.235	0.148	0.557
Jews Ashkanazi	0.006	0.000	0.000	0.000	0.000	0.000	0.043	0.214	0.133	0.592
Asian	0.043	0.002	0.000	0.000	0.000	0.000	0.081	0.194	0.126	0.611
African	0.040	0.002	0.000	0.000	0.000	0.000	0.089	0.172	0.216	0.588
Indian	0.136	0.000	0.000	0.000	0.000	0.000	0.071	0.160	0.257	0.554
Africans Afro-American	0.544	0.173	0.039	0.034	0.000	0.000	0.355	0.114	0.119	0.710
Bantu	0.644	0.213	0.098	0.044	0.000	0.000	0.330	0.102	0.157	0.661
Bushman	0.271	0.017	0.034	0.585	0.000	0.000	0.391	0.189	0.025	0.736
Ainu	0.000	0.000	0.000	0.000	0.068	0.000	0.195	0.250	0.174	0.574
Lapps	0.000	0.000	0.000	0.000	0.000	0.000	0.224	0.226	0.175	0.406
Sardinians	0.023	0.000	0.000	0.000	0.000	0.030	0.090	0.156	0.063	0.732
mean	0.064	0.009	0.007	0.030	0.001	0.001	0.180	0.184	0.109	0.649
s.d.	0.138	0.038	0.028	0.120	0.001	0.004	0.115	0.078	0.066	0.148

Table 1. (continued)

POPULATION	R^z	R^1	R^2	R^o	r	r'	K	Fy^a	MS	Ms
Australia										
Aborigines	0.061	0.592	0.299	0.048	0.000	0.000	0.001	1.000	0.000	0.292
New Guinea										
Papuans	0.000	0.907	0.061	0.032	0.000	0.000	0.000	1.000	0.001	0.040
Austronesians	0.010	0.901	0.081	0.009	0.000	0.000	0.000	1.000	0.003	0.238
Melanesians	0.011	0.753	0.126	0.106	0.002	0.002	0.000	1.000	0.013	0.348
Polynesians	0.012	0.572	0.332	0.040	0.000	0.000	0.000	0.901	0.020	0.643
Orientals										
S.E. Asian	0.007	0.762	0.164	0.053	0.009	0.006	0.000	0.933	0.041	0.594
N.E. Asian	0.016	0.602	0.282	0.049	0.026	0.003	0.001	0.897	0.071	0.478
Amerindians										
Eskimos	0.003	0.601	0.313	0.009	0.062	0.012	0.005	0.821	0.183	0.686
N. American	0.025	0.688	0.271	0.015	0.000	0.000	0.000	0.802	0.285	0.485
S. American	0.054	0.633	0.307	0.005	0.000	0.000	0.010^a	0.779	0.155	0.563
Indo-Europeans										
Teutons	0.003	0.428	0.154	0.017	0.385	0.008	0.040	0.419	0.233	0.311
Slavs	0.005	0.414	0.139	0.024	0.400	0.011	0.049	0.441	0.248	0.324
Jews										
Ashkanazi	0.000	0.497	0.127	0.072	0.289	0.017	0.063	0.473	0.256	0.308
Asian	0.004	0.540	0.131	0.054	0.247	0.019	0.037	0.343	0.271	0.394
African	0.019	0.550	0.096	0.105	0.225	0.000	0.071	0.288	0.265	0.365
Indian	0.013	0.592	0.097	0.040	0.241	0.014	0.001	0.422	0.217	0.385
Africans										
Afro-American	0.000	0.148	0.085	0.490	0.250	0.010	0.008	0.091	0.097	0.351
Bantu	0.000	0.036	0.086	0.721	0.144	0.013	0.000	0.009	0.103	0.414
Bushman	0.000	0.034	0.005	0.891	0.083	0.000	0.003	0.298	0.092	0.429
Ainu	0.000	0.551	0.264	0.001	0.026	0.004	0.000	0.941	0.022	0.398
Lapps	0.000	0.648	0.177	0.062	0.099	0.014	0.013	0.728	0.370	0.310
Sardinia	0.009	0.624	0.078	0.027	0.198	0.020	0.027	0.347	0.361	0.408
mean	0.013	0.518	0.163	0.111	0.168	0.008	0.020	0.595	0.161	0.382
s.d.	0.023	0.217	0.103	0.222	0.165	0.010	0.023	0.298	0.114	0.133

POPULATION	NS	P^1	Jk^a	Lu^a	Le	Di^a	Hp^1
Australia							
Aborigines	0.000	0.243	0.655	0.000	0.699	0.000	0.243
New Guinea							
Papuans	0.051	0.206	0.618	0.000	0.533	0.000	0.677
Austronesians	0.115	0.274	0.657	n.t.	n.t.	n.t.	0.654
Melanesians	0.023	0.382	0.564	0.000	n.t.	n.t.	0.480
Polynesians	0.000	0.242	0.355	n.t.	n.t.	n.t.	0.540
Orientals							
S.E. Asian	0.011	0.180	0.404	0.004	0.757	0.022	0.307
N.E. Asian	0.039	0.204	0.327	0.000	0.739	0.044	0.259
Amerindians							
Eskimos	0.005	0.164	0.695	0.003	0.807	n.t.	0.305^a
N. American	0.050	0.559	0.329	0.000	0.436	0.042	0.560^a
S. American	0.014	0.564	0.512	0.000	0.480	0.040	0.716^a
Indo-Europeans							
Teutons	0.067	0.521	0.502	0.039	0.797	n.t.	0.391
Slavs	0.089	0.498	0.473	0.038	n.t.	n.t.	0.382
Jews							
Ashkanazi	0.105^a	0.488	0.582^a	n.t.	n.t.	n.t.	0.313
Asian	0.098^a	0.448^a	0.520^a	0.006	n.t.	0.000	0.295
African	0.082	0.510	0.403	n.t.	n.t.	n.t.	0.283
Indian	0.097	0.423	n.t.	0.012	0.732	n.t.	0.178
Africans							
Afro-American	0.058	0.765	0.720	0.028	0.537	0.001	0.554
Bantu	0.073	0.651	0.810	0.031	0.267	n.t.	n.t.
Bushman	0.024	0.639	0.891	n.t.	0.530	n.t.	0.319
Ainu	0.206	0.127	0.304	0.000	0.575	0.025	0.162
Lapps	0.040	0.300	0.258	0.067	0.440	0.000	0.439
Sardinia	0.033	0.493	0.462	0.019	0.372	n.t.	0.404
mean	0.058	0.402	0.513	0.015	0.611	0.017	0.383
s.d.	0.044	0.167	0.170	0.015	0.192	0.022	0.144

Table 1. (continued)

POPULATION	Gc^1	PGM_1^1	p^A	p^B	PGD^A	AK^1
Australia						
Aborigines	0.902	0.945	0.003	0.997	0.981	1.000
New Guinea						
Papuans	0.491	0.980	0.256	0.744	0.875	1.000
Austronesians	0.532	n.t.	0.200	0.793	n.t.	n.t.
Melanesians	n.t.	0.635	0.175	0.800	0.820	1.000
Polynesians	n.t.	0.673	0.213	0.787	0.867	1.000
Orientals						
S.E. Asian	0.805	0.753	0.261	0.738	0.950	0.997
N.E. Asian	0.726	0.802	0.223	0.777	0.917	0.978
Amerindians						
Eskimos	0.674	0.736	0.450	0.537	n.t.	0.978
N. American	0.846	0.830	0.208	0.792	n.t.	n.t.
S. American	0.801	0.944	0.008	0.992	1.000	1.000
Indo-Europeans						
Teutons	0.728	0.784	0.361	0.578	0.978	0.962
Slavs	0.694	n.t.	0.345	0.575	n.t.	n.t.
Jews						
Ashkanazi	n.t.	0.722	0.272[a]	0.687[a]	0.985	0.935
Asian	0.782	0.718	0.222[a]	0.734[a]	0.961	0.956
African	0.714	0.599	0.222	0.735	0.928	0.969
Indian	0.689	0.706	0.316	0.681	0.979	0.908
Africans						
Afro-American	0.892	0.810	0.213	0.757	0.961	0.992
Bantu	n.t.	0.814	n.t.	n.t.	0.939	0.998
Bushman	n.t.	0.951	0.203	0.573	0.998	0.949
Ainu	0.750	0.858	0.242	0.758	0.930	1.000
Lapps	0.813	0.699	0.254	0.643	0.970	0.997
Sardinia	n.t.	0.738	0.217	0.686	n.t.	0.987
mean	0.745	0.789	0.240	0.682	0.958	0.970
s.d.	0.088	0.095	0.132	0.160	0.044	0.025

[a] average of markedly different values.
[b] n.t. not tested.

found on the surface of all nucleated human cells. The genes determining these antigens have been mapped to the short arm of chromosome 6.

The serologically defined antigens of the HLA system map to three loci, which are closely, but not absolutely, linked. They are called A, B, and C. For the purposes of this report, only the A and B loci will be discussed. The A and B loci have a recombination rate of about 0.8%. The maximum number of antigens an individual can normally express is four. These are inherited in groups called haplotypes. Due to the occurrence of recombinants between the two loci, the haplotypes are normally random combinations of A locus and B locus antigens. However, within populations, certain haplotypes may occur with significant linkage disequilibrium. Since these normally occur in low frequency and the percentage of haplotypes in disequilibrium is low when compared to the total number of haplotypes present, these will not be considered in any further detail.

For the purpose of this presentation, seven A locus antigens and 15 B locus antigens were included in the analysis. However, there are only complete or nearly complete data for 12 B locus antigens. The antigen A19 was not included because it includes five specificities (A29, 30, 31, 32, and 33), and many populations were not tested with the antisera required to define all of the specificities.

The test system to detect the HLA antigens consists of purified lymphocytes from the person to be tested, antisera to HLA antigens, a source of complement, and an indicator of cellular cytotoxicity. See Perkins (1978) for greater details of the test system. The test is considered to be positive if a specified proportion of the cells tested are killed, and negative if a value below a threshold value is observed. Testing is very time consuming when compared with red blood cell serology, enzyme electrophoresis, or immunoglobulin allotyping.

The genetic markers on human immunoglobulins are called allotypes. They are found on the heavy chains of IgG(Gm), IgA(Am), and on the kappa light chains (Km). The allotypes located on the heavy chains of human immunoglobulins are closely linked and no recombinants have been observed, although the products of recombinational events have been found in population surveys. The genes for immunoglobulin heavy chains have not been conclusively mapped to a human autosome. Heavy-chain allotypes have been found on the IgG1, IgG2, IgG3, and IgA2 subclasses of immunoglobulins. Thus far there are 4 IgG1 markers, 1 IgG2 marker, 12 IgG3 markers, and 2 IgA2 markers. For the majority of this report, only IgG1 and IgG3 allotypes will be included. The immunoglobulin allotypes are inherited in groups called "haplotypes," which vary in frequency and occurrence among human populations (Table 1).

Testing for the immunoglobulin allotypes is done by passive hemagglutination inhibition. The indicator for the test is red blood cells coated with the antigen to be tested, usually by means of nonagglutinating antibodies to red blood cell antigens. The test system consists of diluted test serum or plasma, allotype specific antisera, and the coated red blood cells. If a serum is positive for the factor tested, it blocks the agglutination of the coated red blood cells. If the serum is negative for that factor, agglutination occurs (Schanfield, 1978).

The haplotypes presented only include allotypic markes on IgG1 and IgG3. However, this produces some misleading data. The haplotype $Gm^{za;b}$ which occurs in Africa, New Guinea, Australia, and India would be lumped together. However, on the basis of more extensive testing, the African haplotype, which is usually $Gm^{za;\cdots;b}Am^2$, is different from the Papuan haplotype, which is usually $Gm^{za;n;b}Am^1$, and the Asian haplotype, which is usually $Gm^{za;\cdots;b}Am^1$. In Europeans, the haplotype found is usually $Gm^{za;\cdots;b}Am^1$; however, it is not possible, in most cases, to trace the origin of that haplotype. Therefore, two analyses were done – one with a $Gm^{za;b}$ haplotype and one using three different haplotypes (African, Asian, and Oceanic). However, only those populations tested for all antigens needed to define the three different haplotypes were included in the latter analysis.

The allotypic marker Km^1 is found on the kappa light chains of all immunoglubulins. It is polymorphic in most human populations. It is tested in the same manner as Gm allotypes (Schanfield, 1978). The details of the other polymorphic systems reported can be found in Mourant, Kopec, and Domaniewska-Sobczak (1976).

3. Results and Discussion

One criterion of anthropological usefulness is the ability of a marker to serve as a unique population marker. Examples of population-restricted markers are the antigens K and Js^a of the Kell blood group system, which only occur in Caucasian or black African populations, and the marker Di^a, which is limited to Oriental populations or their derivatives. However, these markers are of low frequency and thus subject to large errors in frequency and variance estimates. Table 1 condenses of all the data collected into groups which related to known groups.

Among the HLA antigens presented, none of the antigens occur in only a single population; though HLA-A1 had its highest incidence in Caucasians, it also occurs in Orientals, Bantu, and Bushmen which should be free of Caucasian admixture. Most HLA antigens appear to occur in Caucasian and African populations. Recently, a new HLA antigen was defined which is largely restricted to Orientals; however, it could not be included because few populations have been tested for it (Perkins, 1978).

In contrast to the HLA system, most Gm haplotypes are largely population limited. The haplotype $Gm^{f;b}$ appears to be restricted to Caucasian populations. Similarly, $Gm^{fa;b}$ is limited to populations originating in Southeast Asia or having contact with them, while $Gm^{za;bst}$ appears to have its origins in Northeast Asia. African populations are characterized by the haplotypes $Gm^{za;b}$

(African), $Gm^{za;bc3,5}$, $Gm^{za;bc3}$, and $Gm^{za;bs}$. Within Africa, the distribution of these haplotypes is not uniform, such that Bantu have all four haplotypes — Pygmies (not included in this report due to a lack of HLA data) only have $Gm^{za;b}$ and $Gm^{za;bc3,5}$, while Bushmen have the highest frequency of $Gm^{za;bs}$ and low frequencies of the other haplotypes. In Oceania, Papuans and northern Australian Aborigines are characterized by the presence of $Gm^{za;b}$ (Oceania). Similarly, in Central Asia a haplotype, or series of haplotypes, defined as $Gm^{za;b}$ (Asia), which may have been the evolutionary precursor of $Gm^{za;bst}$ and $Gm^{fa;b}$, are found. Finally, of the populations studied, two have unique haplotypes; $Gm^{f;bc5s}$ has only been found polymorphically in Sardinia, while $Gm^{zx,g}$ has only been found polymorphically among the Ainu of Japan. Thus, with the exception of $Gm^{za;g}$ and $Gm^{zax;g}$, which are generally polymorphic in all human populations except Africans, most Gm haplotypes are largely limited to specific populations.

Among the other polymorphisms studied, few possess the dramatic differences observed in the Gm system. The ABO distribution of phenotypes can be used to characterize many populations. For example, Australian Aborigines are characterized by the presence of the A^1 and O genes, and no B, while pure South American Indians only have the O gene. In the Rh system, the gene R^o is predominant in African populations, while r is found in highest frequency in Caucasian populations. The antigens K, Di^a, Js^a have been previously mentioned, and no other red cell antigens have their degree of exclusivity. The antigen Lu^a appears to be limited to Caucasians and Africans. The marker with the greatest range appears to be Fy^a, which occurs in very low frequencies in Africans and near fixation in many Oceanic populations.

From a purely operation definition, on the basis of the largest number of haplotypes restricted to specific populations, the Gm system would be a candidate for the most useful single system.

As stated above, the concept of anthropological usefulness is at best operationally defined. As previously stated, it is possible to look at macro-differentiation and microdifferentiation. To look at macrodifferentiation 22 populations from all over the world were selected to represent historically established groups in equal numbers. To look at microdifferentiation, data from 20 Indo-European populations were used. The results of the factor analysis with regard to the number of variables generated and the proportion of variance explained are presented in Table 2. No significant differences are observed between the HLA system and Gm system with regard to the percent of variance. One method to represent factor analysis data is a plot of the standardized factor scores ($F_1/\lambda^{1/2}$) (Harpending and Jenkins, 1973). However, to adequately present the data generated would require excessive space (a total of 12 figures).

A total of 22 worldwide populations were used as source data for Gm and HLA systems for factor analysis. These included distinct groups such as Amerindians (3), Africans (2), Orientals [Northern (2) and Southern (2)], Australian

Table 2. Principle Components Analysis Results

	Number populations	Number alleles	Components	% variance
HLA				
Europeans	20	19	5	82.6
World	22	17	5	75.8
Gm				
Europeans	20	10	3	82.4
World	22	11	4	79.1

Aborigines (2), Papuans (1), Oceanics [Malayo-polynesian speakers (3)], Indo-Europeans (4), and populations of indeterminate origins (Lapps, Ainu, and Afro-Americans). Using the 19 populations which are part of distinct groups, it is possible to see which fell together in clusters as defined by the three possible plots of the first three components. Clusters were defined using the locations of the members of a group. For the purposes of this report, they are Australian Aborigines-Papuans (3), Amerindians (3), Indo-Europeans (4), Northern Orientals (2), Southern Orientals (2), Malayo-Polynesian speakers (3), and Africans (2) (total of 19).

For the Gm system 13 of 19 fell into distinct groups while for the HLA system 10 of 19 fell into distinct groups, suggesting that Gm may be slightly better at classifying than HLA on a worldwide basis.

For comparison, the plots of the first three components for HLA and Gm were performed for Indo-Europeans. Using seven defined populations of the 22, four were classified as Teutons (Norway, Denmark, Germany, and Holland), while three were classified as slavic (Poland, Czeckoslovakia, and Russia). Gm completely separated these two groups (7/7), while the HLA system readily clustered three of the Teuton populations but could only clearly separate one of the slavic populations.

Another method of looking at variation among populations independent of preconceived ideas of relationships is the F_{st} statistic of Wright (Cavalli-Sforza and Bodmer, 1971), which examines the ratio of the observed variance in gene frequency to the theoretical variance. For the statistic to be unbiased, it is necessary to remove any sampling bias by correcting for heterogeneity in sample size by weighting the frequency and variance estimates. This was a tedious procedure, and it was found that using unweighted values did not significantly alter the conclusions, in the few cases tested. Therefore, it was decided to use unweighted data for the analysis of F_{st}. The mean and standard deviations for all of the genetic markers included are found at the bottom of Table 1 and are based on the total sample and not just the data presented in Table 1. Statistical testing of F_{st} can be done using chi-square to test either among loci heterogeneity, or within locus heterogeneity in multiallelic systems.

However, since the statistical test is related to F_{st} by the factor $2N$, and the sample sizes are quite large, all differences except the very smallest will always be highly significant. For example, the HLA data presented represent the typing of about 26,000 individuals. Multiplying any F_{st} by $2N$ will always yield significant results, even with 22 degrees of freedom. Therefore, no attempts have been made to test for statistical significance. It is assumed that any appreciable differences are probably significant.

Unlike the factor analysis, which requires multiple alleles, F_{st} can be calculated for any genetic system with data on at least one allele. The data on F_{st} for HLA, Gm, and the polymorphic systems are presented in Table 3. The F_{st} values for systems other than HLA and Gm are based on all data available and reflect maximal values. If increased values of F_{st} indicate those systems which on the average have the greatest variation among populations, and therefore useful anthropologically, then on a worldwide basis Duffy should be the single, most useful system followed by the Gm, Rh, P_1, and Kidd, and Acid Phosphatase systems, with the HLA system falling in the middle of the range. These results are not unexpected on a worldwide basis, due to the nature of the F_{st} statistic. The mean frequency of Fy^a is 0.595 with a range of 0.009–1.000.

Table 3. F_{st} Analysis of Genetic Systems

System	Number alleles	Number cases	Mean F_{st}	Range
HLA				
World	17	22	0.090	0.028–0.186
Indo-Europeans	19	20	0.022	0.008–0.088
Gm				
World	10	22	0.338	0.068–0.661
Indo-Europeans	11	20	0.026	0.004–0.083
ABO	3	50	0.061	0.040–0.097
Rh	6	50	0.061	0.014–0.499
MNS	3	48	0.068	0.035–0.096
Ad. Phosph.	2	41	0.105	0.092–0.118
Km	1	51	0.089	
Kell	1	50	0.027	
Duffy	1	50	0.368	
P_1	1	50	0.177	
Kidd	1	38	0.116	
Lutheran	1	32	0.018	
Lewis	1	25	0.156	
Diego	1	23	0.030	
Haptoglobin	1	50	0.088	
Gc	1	39	0.040	
PGM_1^1	1	42	0.055	
PGD	1	30	0.048	
AK	1	36	0.022	

The seven Gm haplotypes with the highest F_{st} (values greater 0.10) have a mean of 0.414 with a total range of 0.068–0.661. In contrast the seven highest F_{st} values for the HLA system (values greater than 0.10) have a mean of 0.130, and a total range of 0.028–0.186. Thus, the ability of F_{st} to detect differences is to some extent dependent on the nature of the distribution. If F_{st} were the sole criteria for the evaluation of anthropological usefulness, then the Gm system would be more useful than the HLA system though perhaps not as useful as the Duffy system (Table 3).

The F_{st} values for Indo-Europeans are less than those observed for both the Gm and HLA systems observed worldwide. Unlike the marked differences in haplotypes observed in a worldwide basis for the Gm system among Indo-Europeans, both systems are similar to each other in the degree of variability indicated by these markers (Table 3).

If testing with only a single system, using a limited sample size to produce the genetic and geographical relationships of the population studied, is the objective then the HLA system may be more useful anthropologically. The Gm system could not differentiate Australian Aborigines from the Central and Western Deserts of Australia from South American Indians. However, the HLA system is extremely expensive to use; specimens must be specifically collected and transported rapidly from the field site to the test site. Further only a few specimens can be tested at a time, necessitating collection of small groups of specimens. Finally, it has several distinct disadvantages: the estimation of admixture rates and genetic distance, though informative, is hampered by the low frequency of most antigens. Also, unless large samples are tested, the low frequency for most antigens (mean for all HLA antigens is 0.077), makes estimates of gene frequencies susceptible to large errors. One of the greatest difficulties with HLA technology is in the scarcity of reagents. Although miniscule amounts of reagent are used per test (1–2 microliters), monospecific reagents are almost unheard of. Therefore, testing is done with multiple reagents, which hopefully have been well characterized. Also, many of the reagents that are useful in detecting informative new markers are not readily available. Thus, care must be used in selecting laboratories to do HLA typing. One of the greatest difficulties with HLA typing as a tool for anthropologists is the fact that the interest in HLA typing is largely clinically oriented, originally in the area of transplantation. The majority of the anthropological studies done in the past have been associated with international workshops on HLA. Very few new population studies on nonwestern countries have been published since the 1971 workshop. In conclusion, the HLA system may be one of the most useful tools for anthropological investigation; however, its practicality is in question.

The preceeding reservations concerning the HLA system lead logically to a closer examination of the Gm system and immunoglobulin allotyping. As an anthropological tool, the immunoglobulin allotypes are excellent. The antigens can be detected in specimens collected under the most adverse conditions.

Typing of large numbers of specimens can be done at a convenient time and place with storage of serum or plasma a matter of simple freezing. The difficulties of the system lie in the availability of informative reagents. At the present time, there are only four laboratories doing extensive allotyping. Of these, two will be less active in the future. In addition, informative reagents are rare, and the future supply may be in question. However, the interests of the individuals working extensively with allotypes have usually been genetic or anthropological and not clinical; thus the accessability of these laboratories to individuals interested in having specimens tested has not been a problem and should not pose a problem in the near future. Even in the absence of the more esoteric reagents, typing of specimens from most parts of the world with a limited number of specificities is often very useful in detecting the majority of the haplotypes of interest. In conclusion, the Gm allotypes probably offer a more practical anthropological tool than the HLA system, since the informative haplotypes are usually in high frequency, making admixture estimates and more importantly gene frequency estimates, possible with small sample sizes and more readily adaptable to the routine collection of blood specimens in less than ideal field situations.

ACKNOWLEDGMENTS

The author would like to thank Dr. B. Bonne-Tamir for sharing her submitted manuscript with me — the data contained were invaluable; Mr. Len Stark of the George Washington University Center for Computational Analysis for his assistance in mastering the system; the many collaborators over the years who have provided specimens for immunoglobulin typing; and Dr. H. Perkins, who allowed me to participate in two international HLA workshops with him to learn about the HLA system; and Ms. S. Schoeppner for aid in manuscript preparation.

References

Cavalli-Sforza, L. L., and Bodmer, W. F. (1971), *The Genetics of Human Populations*, Freeman, San Francisco.

Frane, J., and Jennrich, R. (1977), Factor analysis, in *BMDP Biomedical Computer Programs, P Series*, pp. 656–684, University of California Press, Los Angeles.

Harpending, H., and Jenkins, T. (1973), Genetic distance among Southern African populations, in *Methods and Theories of Anthropological Genetics*, (M. H. Crawford and P. L. Workman, eds.), University of New Mexico, Albuquerque.

Hirszfeld, L., and Hirszfeld, H. (1919), Serological differences between the blood of different races. The results of research on the Macedonian front, *Lancet* ii:675–679.

Menozzi, P., Piazza, A., and Cavalli-Sforza, L. (1978), Synthetic maps of human gene frequencies in Europeans, *Science* 201:786–792.

Mourant, A. E., Kopec, A. C., and Domaniewska-Sobczak, K. (1976), *The Distribution of Human Blood Groups and Other Polymorphisms*, Oxford University Press, London.

Perkins, H. A. (1978), The human histocompatability complex (MHC), in *Basic and Clinical Immunology*, 2nd ed. (H. H. Fudenberg, D. P. Stites, J. L. Caldwell, and J. V. Wells, eds.), pp. 165–174, Lange, Los Altos, California.

Schanfield, M. S. (1971), Population studies on the Gm and Inv antigens in Asia and Oceania, Ph. D. thesis, University of Michigan, Ann Arbor.

Schanfield, M. S. (1978), Genetic markers of human immunoglobulins, in *Basic and Clinical Immunology*, 2nd ed. (H. H. Fudenberg, D. P. Stites, J. L. Caldwell, and J. V. Wells, eds.) pp. 59–65, Lange, Los Altos, California.

Stevenson, J. C. (1978), Immunoglobulin haplotype distribution in Europe as support for historically based hypotheses, Ph. D. thesis, University of Wisconsin, Milwaukee.

Additional References

The data used for this report was obtained from one or more of the following references.

Bjarnessen, V., Edwards, J. H., Fredrickson, S., Magnuson, M., Mourant, A. E., and Tills, D. (1973), The blood groups of Icelanders, *Ann. Hum. Genet.* **36**:425–458.

Bonne-Tamir, B., Ashbel, S., and Bar-Shani, S. (1978), Ethnic communities in Israel: The genetic blood markers of the Babylonian Jews, *Am. J. Phys. Anthropol.* **49**:457–464.

Bonne-Tamir, B., Ashbel, S., and Bar-Shani, S. (1978), The ethnic communities in Isreal: The genetic blood markers of the Moroccan Jews, *Am. J. Phys. Anthropol.* **49**:465–471.

Bonne-Tamir, B., Ashbel, S., and Kennett, R. (1979), Genetic markers: benign and normal traits of Ashkenazi Jews, in *Genetic Diseases Among Ashkenazi Jews* (Goodman, R. M., Motulsky, A. G., eds.) Raven Press, New York.

Bonne-Tamir, B., Bodmer, J. G., and Modai, J. (1978), HLA polymorphism in Israel. 3. Ashkanazi Jews of German descent, *Tiss. Antigens* **11**:206–212.

Booth, P. B., Faoagali, J. L., Kirk, R. L., and Blake, N. M. (1977), HLA types, blood groups, serum proteins and red cell enzyme types among Samoans in New Zealand, *Hum. Hered.* **27**:412–423.

Brautbar, C., Zamir, R., Efter, T., and Gazit, E. (1978), HLA polymorphism in Israel. 2. Israeli Jews orginating from Russia, *Tiss. Antigens* **11**:210–205.

Campillo, F., Gallardo, L. E., and Senra, A. (1973), Distribution of Kell blood groups in the Spanish population, *Hum. Hered.* **23**:499–500.

Colina, F., and Campillo, F. (1975), Distribucion del sistema saguino MNSs on lo populacion espanola, *Sangra* **22**:421–425.

Curtain, C. C. (1974), Blood markers in Melanesia, *Yearb. Phys. Anthropol.* **18**:246–284.

Dausset, J., and Colombani, J. (1973), *Histocompatability Testing 1972*, Munksgaard, Copenhagen.

Fujita, Y., Tanimura, M., and Tanaka, K. (1978), The distribution of the ABO blood groups in Japan, *Jpn. J. Hum. Genet.* **23**:63–109.

Fraser, G. R., Volkers, W. S., Bernini, L. F., *et al.* (1974), Gene frequencies in a Dutch population, *Hum. Hered.* **24**:435–448.

Gazit, E., Brautbar, C., Efter, T., Cohen, K., Yehoshua, H., and Zamir, R. (1978), HLA polymorphism in Israel. 1. Jews of Polish Extraction, *Tiss. Antigens* **11**:195–200.

Gazit, E., Brautbar, Mizrachi, Y., Cohen, R., Yehoshua, H., and Zamir, R. (1978), HLA Polymorphism in Israel. 7. The Babylonian Jews, *Tiss. Antigens* **11**:226–229.

Gazit, E., Zamir, R., Efter, T., Zfat, Z., and Brautbar, C. (1978), HLA polymorphism in Israel. 5. The Moroccan Jews. *Tiss. Antigens* **11**:217–220.

Gershowitz, H., and Neel, J. V. (1978), The immunoglobulin allotypes (Gm and Km) of twelve indian tribes of Central and South America, *Am. J. Phys. Anthropol.* **49**:289–302.

Goedde, H. W., Hirth, L., Benkmann, H. G., Pellicer, A., Pellicer, T., Stahn, M., and Singh, S. (1972), Population genetic studies of red cell enzyme polymorphisms in four Spanish populations, *Hum. Hered.* **22**:556–560.

Goedde, H. W., Hirth, L., Benkmann, H. G., Pellicer, A., Pellicer, T., Stahn, M., and Singh, S. (1973), Population genetic studies of serum protein polymorphisms in four Spanish populations, *Hum. Hered.* **23**:135–146.

Greiner, J., Schleiermacher, E., Lenhard, V., Kulapongs, P., and Vogel, F. (1978), HLA antigen, gene and haplotype frequencies in Thailand, *Hum. Genet.* **41**:73–87.

Jenkins, T., Harpending, H., and Nurse, G. T. (1978), Genetic distances among certain southern African populations, in *Evolutionary Models and Studies in Human Diversity* (R. J. Meier, C. M. Otten, and F. Abdel-Hameed, eds.), pp. 227–243, Mouton, The Hague.

Jenkins, T., and Nurse, G. T. (1976), Biomedical studies of the desert dwelling hunter–gatherers of southern Africa, *Prog. Med. Genet.* **1**:211–286.

Jenkins, T., Zoutendyk, A., and Steinberg, A. G. (1970), Gammoglobulin groups (Gm and Inv) in various southern African populations, *Am. J. Phys. Anthropol.* **32**:197–218.

Kirk, R. L., Blake, N. M., Moodies, P. M., and Tibbs, G. J. (1971), Population genetic studies in Australian Aborigines of the Northern Territory: The distribution of some serum proteins and enzyme groups among populations at various localities in the Northern Territory of Australia, *Hum. Biol. Ocean.* **1**:53–76.

Layrisse, A., Layrisse, M., Mulave, I., Terasaki, P., Ward, R. H., and Neel, J. V. (1973), Histocompatibility antigens in a genetically isolated American Indian tribe, *Am. J. Hum. Genet.* **25**:493–509.

Lie, H., and Teisbert, P. (1973), Red cell acid phosphatase polymorphism in Norway, *Hum. Hered.* **23**:257–262.

Matsumoto, H., and Miyazaki, T. (1972), Gm and Inv allotypes of the Ainu in Hidaka area Hokkaido, *Jpn. J. Hum. Genet.* **17**:20–26.

Mayajima, T., Hasegawa, T., Itakura, K., Juji, T., Mori, T., Nomoto, K., Naito, S., Ohkochi, K., Saito, S., Sekiguchi, S., Tsuji, K., and Yoshida, T. (1977), The joint report of the 3rd Japan HLA workshop, *Tiss. Antigens* **10**:39–44.

Morris, P. J., Ting, A., Alpers, M. P., and Simons, M. (1971), Leukocyte antigens in a New Guinea population. *Tiss. Antigens* **1**:49–52.

Mourant, A. E., Kopec, A. C., and Domaniewska-Sobczak, K. (1976), *The Distribution of Human Blood Groups and other Polymorphisms*, Oxford University Press, London.

Nakajima, H., and Abe, T. (1977), Gm and Km allotypes of the Japanese in Aomori and Fukishima, Northeastern part of Japan, *J. Anthropol. Soc. Nippon* **85**:245–247.

Nakajima, H., Sato, Y., Sato, K., and Takeda, K. (1977), The Diego blood groups of the Japanese in Aomori and Fukushima Prefectures, Northeastern Japan, *J. Anthropol. Soc. Nippon* **85**:155–158.

Nevanlina, H. R. (1972), The Finnish population structure, *Heridital* **71**:195–236.

Nielson, J. C., Martensson, L., Gurtler, H., Gilberg, A., and Tingsgard, P. (1971), Gm types in Greenland Eskimos, *Hum. Hered.* **21**:405–419.

Omoto, K. (1974), Polymorphic traits in peoples of eastern Asia and the Pacific, in *Genetic Polymorphisms and Diseases in Man* (R. Ramot, ed.), pp. 69–89, Academic Press, New York.

Payne, R., Feldman, M., Cann, H., and Bodmer, J. G. (1977), A comparison of HLA data of the North American Black, with African Black and North American Caucasoid populations, *Tiss. Antigens* **9**:135–147.

Piazza, A., Von Loghem, E., de Lange, G., Curtoni, E. S., Ulizzi, L., and Terrenato, L. (1976), Immunoglobulin allotypes in Sardinia, *Am. J. Hum. Genet.* **28**:77–86.

Ryder, L. P., Anderson, E., and Svejgard, A. (1978), An HLA map of Europe, *Hum. Hered.* **28**:171–200.

Schanfield, M. S., unpublished data.

Schanfield, M. S. (1977), Population affinities of the Australian Aborigines as reflected by genetic markers of immunoglobulins, *J. Human. Evol.* **6**:341–352.

Schanfield, M. S., and Carbonell, F., unpublished data.

Schanfield, M. S., Gergely, J., and Fudenberg, H. H. (1975), Immunoglobulin allotypes in European populations. I. Gm and Km(Inv) allotypic markers in Hungarians, *Hum. Hered.* **25**:370–377.

Schanfield, M. S., and Gershowitz, H. (1973), Nonrandom distribution of Gm haplotypes in East Asia, *Am. J. Hum. Genet.* **25**:567–574.

Schanfield, M. S., Gershowitz, H., and Ohkura, K. (1972), Studies on immunoglobulin allotypes of Asiatic populations. IV. Gm and Inv allotypes in three Japanese prefectures and Okinawa, *Hum. Hered.* **22**:496–502.

Schanfield, M. S., Herzog, P., and Fudenberg, H. H. (1975), Immunoglobulin allotypes of European populations. II. Gm. Am and Km(Inv) allotypic markers in Czeckoslovakians, *Hum. Hered.* **25**:382–392.

Schanfield, M. S., and Kirk, R. L., in preparation.

Schanfield, M. S., and Nevo, S., unpublished data.

Schanfield, M. S., and Stutz, D., unpublished data.

Schanfield, M. S., and Ward, R. H., unpublished data.

Schanfield, M. S., Watterson, C. W., and Boettcher, B., unpublished data.

Simmons, R. T., and Booth, P. B. (1971), A compendium of Melanesian genetic data, Commonwealth Serum Laboratories, Parkville.

Simmons, R. T., and Graydon, J. J. (1971), Population genetic studies in Australian Aborigines of the Northern Territory: Blood group genetic studies on populations samples at 16 localities including Arnhem Land and Groote Eylandt, *Hum. Biol. Ocean.* **1**:23–53.

Simmons, R. T., Graydon, J. J., Gajdusek, D. C., Alpers, M. P., and Hornabrook, R. W. (1972), Genetic studies in relation to Kuru. II. Blood group patterns in Kuru patients and populations of the Eastern Highlands of New Guinea, *Am. J. Hum. Genet.* **24** (supplement):S39–S71.

Singh, S. (1974), Distribution of certain polymorphic traits in populations of the Indian peninsula and South Asia, in *Genetic Polymorphisms and Diseases in Man* (B. Ramot, ed.), pp. 99–11, Academic Press, New York.

Steinberg, A. G., and Kageyama, S. (1970), Further data in the Gm and Inv allotypes of the Ainu: Confirmation of the presence of a $Gm^{2,17,21}$ phenogroup, *Am. J. Hum. Genet.* **22**:319–325.

Steinberg, A. G., Tiilikainen, A., Eskola, M. R., and Ericksson, A. W. (1974), Gammaglobulin allotypes in Finnish Lapps, Finns, Aland Islanders, Maris (Cheremis) and Greenland Eskimos, *Am. J. Human. Genet.* **26**:223–243.

Stevenson, J. (1978), Immunoglobulin haplotype distributions in Europe as support for historically based hypothesis, Ph. D., thesis, University of Wisconsin, Milwaukee.

Stevenson, J. S., and Duquesnoy, R. J. (1979), Distribution of HLA antigens in Polish and German populations in Milwaukee, Wisconsin, *Am. J. Phys. Anthropol.* **50**:19–22.

Tills, D., Teesdale, P., and Mourant, A. E. (1977), Blood groups of the Irish, *Ann. Hum. Bio.* **4**:35–42.

Tills, D., Warlow, A., Mourant, A. E., Kopec, A. C., Edholm, D. G., and Garrard, G (1977), The blood groups and other hereditary blood factors of Yemenite and Kurdish Jews, *Ann. Hum. Biol.* **4**:259–274.

Ting, A., James, M., Woodfield, D. G., and Morris, P. J. (1972), The distribution of HL-A antigens in the coastal populations of Papua New Guinea, *Tiss. Antigens* **2**:409–414.

Tran, M. H., Daveau, M., Dumitresco, S. M., and Rivat, L. (1978), Immunoglobulin Gm and Km genetic markers in Vietnamese, *Hum. Hered.* **28**:435–444.

Tran, M. H., Hors, J., Busson, M., and Degas, L. (1978), HL-A markers in the Vietnamese population, *Tiss. Antigens* **11**:139–143.

van Loghem, E., Chandanayingyang, D., and Douglas, R. (1975), Immunoglobulin genetic markers in the Thai population, *J. Immunogenet.* **2**:141–154.

Ward, R. H., unpublished data.

Ward, R. H., Gershowitz, H., Layrisse, M., and Neel, J. V. (1975), The genetic structure of a tribal population, the Yanomama Indians. XI. Gene frequencies for 10 blood groups and the ABH-Le secretor traits, in the Yanomama and their neighbors; the uniqueness of the tribe, *Am. J. Hum. Genet.* **27**:1–30.

Weitkamp, L. R., Arends, T., Gallengo, M. L., Neel, J. V., Schultz J., and Shreffler, D. C (1972), The genetic structure of a tribal population, the Yanomama Indians. III. Seven serum protein systems, *Ann. Hum. Genet.* **35**:271–279.

Weitkamp, L. R., and Neel, J. V. (1972), The genetic structure of a tribal population, the Yanomama Indians. IV. Eleven erythrocyte enzymes and a summary of protein variants, *Ann. Hum. Genet.* **35**:433–444.

Workman, P. L., Lucarelli, P., Agostino, R., Scarabino, R., Scacchi, R., Carapella, E., Palmarino, R., and Bottini, E. (1974), Genetic differentiation among Sardinian villages, *Am. J. Phys. Anthropol.* **43**:165–176.

Workman, P. L., Niswander, J. D., Brown, K. S., and Leyshon, W. C. (1975), Population studies on Southwestern Indian tribes. IV. The Zuni, *Am. J. Phys. Anthropol.* **41**: 119–132.

Yamaguchi, H., Okubo, Y., Seno, T., Yoshimura, K., Tanaka, M., and Yokota, T. (1978), A study of the blood group Duffy in Japanese, *Jpn. J. Hum. Genet.* **23**:267.

Yasuda, N., Tsuji, K., Aizawa, M., Itakura, K., Inou, T., Matsukura, M., Yoshida, T., Fukunishi, T., Orita, K., Nomoto K., and Ito, M (1976), HLA antigens in Japanese populations, *Am. J. Hum. Genet.* **28**:390–399).

5

Natural Selection and Random Variation in Human Evolution

Frank B. Livingstone

1. Variation and Selection

Ever since science or its predecessor, philosophy, have considered the problem of human variation, there have been two opposing explanations. One can be termed deterministic or causal in that it attempts to relate human variation to some environmental determinant. Today, this kind of interpretation would most likely fall under the rubric of natural selection or adaptation. The other explanation tends to be nondeterministic in the sense that it relies on historical factors or happenstance. Today, this alternative would be concerned with or based on some form of random genetic drift, but generally drift is used as a more sophisticated model to justify the old practice of taxonomy. Hence the old nonadaptive traits and survivals are now marker genes and neutral amino acid substitutions.

As the recent furor about Darwinian explanations of social behavior or sociobiology has emphasized, the concept of natural selection was not the first implication of the Darwinian paradigm to be taken up by the scientific community. Instead, the idea that evolution had occurred or that all animals or life were related to one another led to the diligent pursuit of phylogenetic relationships. The Linnean taxonomy, which had preceded Darwin by 100 years, suddenly took on new evolutionary meaning, and the major task became to find out who was related to whom and how closely. Thus, the central problem was to find

FRANK B. LIVINGSTONE • Department of Anthropology, University of Michigan, Ann Arbor, Michigan 48109.

which traits were taxonomically useful or had phylogenetic significance, and the concepts of homology and analogy were introduced to distinguish between similarities. Analogies such as bird and bat wings were obviously due to adaptation to a common environment or similar ecological niche, but homologies between bat wings and other mammalian forelimbs could show phylogenetic proximity.

The study of human variation was concerned with the same problem of the discovery of phylogenetic relationships through taxonomic classification. And these studies made the assumption that racial traits were nonadaptive; as Howells (1950) said, racial traits "had not been strained through the sieve of natural selection." Such traits as ear shape or dermatoglyphics do seem to have very small selective differences associated with them, but others such as skin color, stature, body shape, hair form, or various facial features seem to have clear adaptive significance. It is of course very difficult to measure the selective effect of these traits given the apparent magnitude of the effect that would be expected and that could have evolutionary significance — it would only have to be about 1% — but the correlation of these traits with climatic and cultural variation seems to be convincing evidence for selection, at least to this old Darwinian.

Although the nonadaptive nature of racial traits was beginning to be questioned by Coon, Garn, and Birdsell (1950) in their landmark book, at the same time newer traits that had a known genetic basis were being studied and used in the same old taxonomic way. Boyd (1950) developed a new racial taxonomy based on blood group frequencies, and Lehmann and Raper (1949) were advancing a hypothesis on the ethnological significance of the sickle cell trait. And again the same assumption of the nonadaptive nature of these loci was made. As Dobzhansky (1950) said, "environmental selection is neither proved or disproved. Fortunately, other evolutionary factors exist and can bring about race so selection conjectures are unnecessary."

Fortunately, this was a short-lived effort and should have been shorter since the data were already present to show that the blood groups were not nonadaptive. With the discovery in the 1930's of maternal—fetal incompatibility, Haldane (1940) had speculated as to why the *cde* or *r* gene was so frequent in Europe. Given the selection due to incompatibility the most frequent gene should become fixed and the less frequent one disappear. Since this has not happened, Haldane and later Boyd hypothesized an early European race with very high frequencies of *r*. The evidence that seemed to convince the scientific profession that selection was acting on the blood groups was the association of the ABO blood groups with peptic ulcer and stomach cancer, but these diseases have little selective effect. Cavalli-Sforza and Bodmer (1971) compute it to be an average of 10^{-5}. On the other hand, data showing selection by infectious disease had existed since the 1920's (Livingstone, 1960), and now there is much more convincing evidence (Vogel, 1975). Although this evidence is much harder to measure, it is undoubtedly more important in determining the differences in frequencies of blood groups.

Despite the fact that selection has been demonstrated for the blood groups, most recent attempts to reconstruct phylogenetic trees for the human species still use blood group data for this purpose (Nei and Roychoudhury, 1974). The blood groups are only a small part of the great number of newly discovered loci that are polymorphic in human populations and vary significantly among them. But this enormous amount of newly discovered human variation has still been forced into the same phylogenetic straitjacket. Loci as variable as the HLA antigens and the red cell enzymes have been used to construct tree diagrams which in many cases are quite contradictory. For example, Bodmer's (1973) tree for the HLA antigens has the African populations clustering together, which seems reasonable, but has the Eskimos most closely related to the New Guineans and the Lapps closest to the Koreans; these seem to be not only unreasonable but absurd. Admittedly, the genetic variation in many newly discovered loci such as the Ig or HLA types or many red cell enzymes is complex and bewildering. It seems to have no simple relationship to anything. But the analysis of this variation surely requires more than simple-minded statements as to how they show ancestral connections. It is almost a scientific counterpart of the quest for various pre-Columbian evidence of Hebrews in Iowa or Druids in New Hampshire.

Implicit in much of this phylogenetic reconstruction is the assumption made explicit by Sarich in his work on albumin that the change in these non-adaptive traits is constant, so that their changes are an evolutionary clock. However, it now doesn't seem to run on time. Sarich and Wilson (1967) have used antigenic variation in albumin, but the neutralist position uses most known polymorphic loci, makes the same assumptions, and draws similar conclusions. Given the similarity of many amino acids and the redundancy of the genetic code, it seems plausible that many substitutions in evolution would be neutral or very close to it. How close is, of course, a very important matter, but comparable to Howells's sieve of natural selection, King and Jukes (1969) in their classic defense of non-Darwinian evolution stated that natural selection is the editor and not the composer and could not detect changes that had no meaning — meaning being differential function.

So after 100 years and hordes of new data we are still trying to do the same thing. I do not mean to imply that phylogenetic reconstruction, or in other words the reconstruction of the population history of the human species, is not a very crucial problem; in fact, it has to be a major priority and will be of major significance in solving the problems of the explanation of how human variation has evolved. I can cite my own work in the sickle cell gene in West Africa that shows how the history of populations, their movements, and their ecological niches are essential to understanding the genetic variation in hemoglobins and their relationship to malaria (Livingstone, 1958). But the assumption of neutral variation uses gene frequency differences to reconstruct the population history. In terms of the basic theoretical model of population genetics this is a backward approach. Mutation, natural selection, and population structure, which includes the usual parameters of gene drift, gene flow, and inbreeding, that depend on the size, dispersal, and mating patterns of the population, respectively, are considered to be the determinants of gene frequency change and to assume that one of these forces, in this case natural selection, doesn't exist seems to be a misuse of the theory.

The neutralist—selectionist controversy has had all kinds of evidence produced by both sides to support their position. It would be impossible to review it all here, but there are certain aspects of the controversy relevant to human genetic variation. I will state categorically that the gene frequency distributions among major human populations seem to provide no evidence for the neutralist position despite many papers to the contrary. At first this position averred that evolution of protein differences occurred at a constant rate whether it was Kimura's (1968) or King and Jukes' (1969) constant for amino acid substitutions or Sarich's constant for immunological differences. This position was so obviously false, and as Stebbins and Lewontin (1972) pointed out, confused a constant with an average, that Sarich (1977) has more recently proposed that there are fast and slowly evolving proteins and hence two evolutionary "clocks." The exact composition of these two groups is not known, but why two? To think that all genetic change is divided into two specific sets contradicts the overwhelming evidence that natural selection operates on each locus, individually. A good example is again the hemoglobin loci. Two clocks, or what is really two averages, seems as simplistic and unrealistic as one.

Albumin has been used to develop the evolutionary clock, but the assumption that this protein has changed by neutral evolution seems to me as false as the previous assumption of a generation ago that skin color and other morphological traits were nonadaptive. Albumin is known to have vital biochemical functions in the binding and transport of fatty acids, bilirubin, and other complex chemical substances, and its osmotic effect is important in maintaining fluid balance. Walter and Schobel (1975) have shown that the level of albumin varies with latitude apparently due to the necessity in the tropics of higher albumin levels to maintain fluid balance in heat stress. How can anyone deny that the structure of this protein does not attain its most adaptive shape for a particular niche? The antigenic differences are obviously related to shape differences, so that variations among populations are undoubtedly related to differential functions according to climate or perhaps diet or nutrition.

As with most gene frequency distributions among human populations, the albumin variants do not accord with expectations of neutral evolution. Although most neutralists' measures of heterozygote frequency have included such loci as the ABO blood groups that are clearly not neutral but are highly polymorphic or heterozygous, there is still a marked deficiency of frequencies between 0.05 and 0.50. Too many loci have several rare variants and a few polymorphic ones that range around 0.05 with most of the population being homozygous for the normal allele. If neutral variants were gradually replacing one another, this would not be expected, but it is true for human albumin, as well as many other loci. For albumin over 50 variants are now known (Weitkamp, Salzano, Neel, Porta, Geerdink, and Tarnoky, 1973a; Weitkamp, McDermid, Neel, Fine, Petrini, Bonazzi, Ortali, Porta, Tanis, Harris, Peters, Ruffini, and Johnston, 1973b) but very few attain polymorphic frequencies (Weitkamp, 1973; Weitkamp *et al.*, 1973b), and these are very low frequencies with Naskapi albumin at a frequency of about 0.125 in the Naskapi being the highest. Most polymorphisms for albumin are found in the American Indians in both North and South America with albumins Naskapi and Mexico being widely distributed in North America. But there are some possible polymorphisms in New Guinea and Afghanistan. Thus, both the gene frequencies and the known functions of this protein seem to be strong evidence against neutral evolution. The same can be said for most of the enzyme polymorphisms that have been discovered in recent years when there is any knowledge of their function.

On the other hand, the arguments against phylogenetic reconstruction do not mean that the concept of marker gene is not useful within certain time frameworks or that population history and structure are not major determinants of present gene frequency differences at some loci. In particular, in the last 500 to 1000 years there have been a great many massive migrations and other minimigrations, some of extremely endogamous isolates. Thus, the populations in the Americas that have African ancestry can be detected by many genetic variants which do not occur in European or American Indian populations. And the Chamorros of Guam can be shown to have gene frequencies very close to the Filipinos (Plato, Rucknagel, and Kurland, 1966). There are many other cases where gene flow or population migration can be measured, but the major question is how far in the past can these relationships be detected. This of course depends on the magnitude of the other forces of gene frequency change at the particular locus involved. However, suggestions that the Ashkenazic Jews have Bushmen ancestry (Steinberg, 1973) or that central American Indians have Ainu ancestry (Mourant, Kopec, and Domaniewska-Sobczak, 1976) are utterly unconvincing.

That the last 1000 or 2000 years of human population history is still reflected in many gene frequency differences is only indicative of the rate of change due to other factors and to the nature of the human species. It is one of the most widespread and most numerous of any large mammalian population. Thus, for a gene to spread throughout the populations of this species far more time is required than for most species, especially when the long generation time is considered. Equilibrium for many genes may be attained in a restricted number of human populations in about 20 generations or 500 years for the sickle cell gene that changes most rapidly to perhaps 2000 years for the lactose tolerance allele in herding and milk drinking populations. One can estimate that since the development of agriculture or civilization there has not been enough time for widespread gene dispersal. Coupled with the very slow rate of change due to natural selection, the large human population and its partition into many isolates are the reasons some gene frequencies reflect the previous 1000 or more years of population history. But, as Lewontin (1974:269) colorfully put it, "equilibria annihilate history." This is why sickle cell gene frequencies in much of Africa do not reflect history, and it is also the reason why long-term genetic differences, although they may seem to be plausible indicators of phylogeny, can be seriously changed by equilibria.

Given the range and large number of isolates of the human species, it is obvious that most loci are not in equilibrium for all the alleles present in any isolate. There will then be marker genes or some with restricted geographical distributions, and this is true even for genes with large selective advantage. The best example is again the sickle cell gene. Although humans have probably been the host of malaria parasites for a long time, the great amount of selection by this disease seems to be much more recent — after the human population has attained large densities due to agriculture. Thus, as malaria selection spread throughout the tropical regions of the Old World, it began to select for a bewildering variety of abnormal hemoglobin genes. It seems that most deviations from normal red cell structure and metabolism were selected for, although very slightly in most cases, because the malaria parasites adapt themselves to their normal environment, the normal red blood cells.

Some of these abnormalities were distinguished by their morphological or biochemical effects; these are primarily the thalassemias. But because the actual gene product is not detected as for the structural abnormalities of the α- and β-hemoglobin chains, similarities between populations do not necessarily mean that the same genetic mutation is involved. Thus, thalassemia is found in New Guinea, China, India, Africa, and Europe, but these alleles are not evidence for gene flow among these diverse populations.

However, there are alleles such as hemoglobins S, C, and E which are single mutations and have spread from a single source. The Hb S gene is very widespread in the Old World, from Africa through the tropics to Greece and India, and now to southern Russia (Nazarli and Abdullaev, 1974). Since the homozygote is lethal or close to it, the heterozygote must have a very high fitness; in fact, compared to the normal fitness in malaria regions it probably has the highest relative fitness of any known human allele. I have argued for years (Livingstone, 1964, 1976) that the Hb S gene is a very "predatory" gene that will replace most other abnormal alleles at the β locus. This accounts for its rapid diffusion in the last 2000 years. It also seems to be a rare mutant given the base pair substitution involved — an internal A to U — and I know of no instance of a Hb S gene that cannot be more probably derived by gene flow from these populations in the central areas of the Old World than postulated as a new mutant. Hb S can then be considered a marker gene in that it indicates ancestry from this region.

Recent data from Arabia (Perrine, Pembrey, Perrine, and Shoup, 1978) and southern India (Brittenham, Lozoff, Harris, and Narasimhan, 1977) demonstrate quite conclusively that homozygosity for the Hb S gene is not as severe in these populations as it is in African and European ones. Much of the clinical data on sickle cell anemia comes from the United States and Africa where it is almost lethal, but the data from India seems to show that there has been further genetic evolution to offset the severity of sickle cell anemia. This may alter the conclusions stated above, i.e., there may be more than one Hb S allele or it could be a different mutant. On the other hand there may be modifiers for the Hb S allele that have increased significantly in Arabian and Indian populations and others (Brittenham, 1977). But this seems dubious to me since it would be difficult for modifiers to evolve in the time that malaria has been an important selective factor (Livingstone, 1977). To evolve they could not be simply modifiers but must have a selective advantage when heterozygous.

The α-thalassemias seem to fulfill the requirements of modifiers since they are found in polymorphic frequencies in many populations in the Mediterranean, the Middle East, and India where malaria has been a selective factor. There now seem to be differences among human populations in the number of α loci with the aforementioned populations plus most other European and Asian populations having two α loci, while those of Africa and Melanesia have just one. Rucknagel and Rising (1975) have shown that the most probable interpretation of the amounts of Hb G Philadelphia in American Blacks is that some have only two α alleles; others, three, and still others, four. This appears to be the result of admixture primarily with European populations. This new development has enormously complicated the genetics of hemoglobin production, but it does show that genetic variation may influence the spread of marker genes.

Hemoglobins C and E seem comparable to Hb S in that they have restricted almost contiguous geographical distributions, but there are differences. Both their homozygotes have a much higher fitness than classical sickle cell anemia, and their amino acid substitutions, which are the same but at different locations, are more frequent mutants than Hb S. The highest frequencies of Hb C are found in West Africa, and there is gradual diffusion from the peak in Northern Ghana. The occurrences of Hb C in Morocco, Spain, Italy, Egypt, and the Sudan are undoubtedly marker genes or indicate gene flow, but the isolated high frequency in an Israeli Arab population (Rachmilewitz, Levi, and Huisman, 1974) may be a separate mutation. Similarly, Hb E occurs throughout Southeast Asia in very high frequencies where there is a high incidence of malaria, and its diffusion has been due to the great selective advantage associated with the heterozygote. But there are other isolated occurrences in Europe and a very high frequency in the Eti-Turks, who have a high incidence of malaria, that seem to be more probably due to separate mutations. Thus, selection does increase the diffusion rate of marker genes but it can also lead to the increase in frequency of separate mutations.

The albumin polymorphisms in the North American Indians are other examples of marker genes, and their distributions seem comparable to those of the abnormal hemoglobins, although there is no evidence that selection is involved. Albumin Naskapi is found in the Northeastern Indians and in the Athabaskans in the Southwest and in Western Canada, but it is also absent in other tribes in between these occurrences (Schell, Agarwal, Blumberg, Levy, Bennett, Laughlin, and Martin, 1978). Albumin Mexico is found in the Southwest and in Mexico in a much more contiguous distribution. These distributions certainly qualify as marker genes, but the question arises, is it possible for this diffusion to occur without a selective advantage? If one uses a model of constant populations with stable numbers, then when a gene is begun in one population and diffuses from it to others, it is simply overwhelmed after diffusing through a few populations. Given the large number of tribes and isolates of North American Indians such diffusion without selection would seem impossible. However, large-scale population movements or expansions would tend to detract from the applicability of this model, but the linguistic differences among Indian tribes and their cultural variations do not indicate any migrations to explain the distributions of these polymorphisms.

These examples lead to the paradoxical conclusion that the detection of gene flow after 1000 or more years is dependent on selection and that if a gene were truly neutral it probably would not diffuse very far and thus would be of little value for phylogenetic reconstruction. In addition, if a gene qualifies as a marker then it is not in equilibrium for the whole species, since if it were, its distribution would indicate the fitness differences associated with it and not the history of the populations that have the gene. These conclusions, it must be stressed, would seem to apply to the detection of gene flow or the reconstruction of population history more than 1000 years ago. Of course 1000 years is an arbitrary dividing line, and one could think of several cases, such as some Jewish populations where the separation is more than that, which still show evidence of relationship. However, even for these very endogamous groups, it appears that even after 1000 years with little gene flow, the isolate is not distinguishable from the surrounding population: for example, the Black Jews of the Cochin coast in India resemble the neighboring Indians, and their gene frequencies seem to be similar to the South Indians (Mourant et al., 1976).

On the other hand, the last 1000 years of human history have been marked by great numbers of population movements and differential population growth. Most human populations during this time, and particularly those that have evolved culturally, have expanded enormously in numbers, while many indigenous and underdeveloped groups have become extinct or decreased. This expansion of some populations has not been a continuous linear growth but marked by wide swings in population size. Again a Jewish population, that of Eastern Europe, is a good example (Fraikor, 1977) of the wide swings in population growth, but most of Europe's populations exhibited comparable oscillations.

These recent population expansions and large-scale migrations have obviously had considerable effect on the present distribution of gene frequencies, and their magnitude is so great as to effect the approach to equilibrium for most gene loci. Selection takes at least 20 generations or a minimum of 500 years to attain equilibrium, and this low estimate is for the sickle cell gene, which probably has the highest fitness differences associated with its genotypes of any gene. Thus, many populations that have undergone these movements in the last 1000 years are undoubtedly not close to equilibrium for many loci.

This does not imply that the assumption of equilibrium is not an important element in population analysis. The recognition of selection as an important force in human evolution resulted from the fact that the frequencies of the sickle cell gene in Africa seemed to be far from equilibrium for a recessive lethal. Explanations involving genetic drift, admixture, and even the absence of selection against homozygotes were advanced, but selection in favor of heterozygotes for this gene soon became the only reasonable possibility. The discovery of the selective advantage for sickle cell heterozygotes was one of the major factors in the rediscovery in the 1950's of selection as an important evolutionary force. But as with every major development in human affairs including science, it went too far. Most genetic polymorphisms were quickly assumed to be due to heterozygote advantage, and these ranged from the blood groups and other common polymorphisms, to the several deleterious genes found in polymorphic frequencies, to such traits as schizophrenia that are due to both genetic and environmental factors. More recently it is being recognized that other kinds of selection are possible and that other forces may be responsible for polymorphic frequencies. In fact, with all the genetic research in the last 20 years, there is not other convincing example of heterozygote advantage except for the hemoglobin variants and G6PD deficiency that are selected by malaria. As Lewontin (1974) has said, he is "tired of sickle cell anemia."

Several lethal or severely deleterious alleles in large populations did seem to require a selective advantage since their frequencies were at least one order of magnitude above the equilibrium expected for a balance of mutation and selection. These were principally the Tay Sachs gene in Eastern European Jews and cystic fibrosis in some European populations, but phenylketonuria or the protease inhibitor in other European populations seem to be comparable.

Some evidence has been published to show that the high frequencies of both Tay Sachs disease and cystic fibrosis are due to heterozygote advantage. Myrianthopoulos and Aronson (1966) showed that Tay Sachs sibships were larger than the controls, and Knudson, Wayne, and Hallett (1967) and Conneally, Merritt, and Yu (1973) in the United States and Danks, Allan, and Anderson (1965) in Australia have shown that cystic fibrosis families have a greater fertility. Despite the fact that many of these data attain statistical significance, I am not convinced because they imply that the heterozygous genotypes involved have an advantage wherever they live and in whatever environment. This is an implicit assumption of much genetical theorizing and is quite obviously wrong. It assumes that the fitness of any genotype is a property of the genotype *per se*, and thus one can measure this fitness in Australia, America, or anywhere else with no reference to the causes of mortality or fertility differences. Shaw and Smith (1969) took at face value the increased fertility of Tay-Sachs-diseased grandparents found by Myrianthopoulos and Aronson (1966), which was on the order of 6%, and mathematically demonstrated that the gene was still increasing in Jewish populations. With no regard for the enormous changes in the environment of Jewish populations and everybody else in the last 100 years, they seem to think the selective advantage is a property of the gene and of the population. Given the racial mixture of modern America, if they are right, the gene should also be increasing in Blacks, Whites, Orientals, Indians, Southerners, and everybody else, but these possibilities are not discussed.

Other evidence for the selective advantage for these genes has been concerned with the specific effect that confers it. For cystic fibrosis Stuart and Burdon (1974) suggested its resistance to typhus, and Crawfurd (1975) has presented some evidence for a resistance to tuberculosis. On the other hand cystic fibrosis probably has a marked selective disadvantage even in heterozygotes in desert or very dry conditions (Super, 1977). Tuberculosis has also been suggested as the disease responsible for the selective advantage of Tay Sachs heterozygotes (Myrianthopoulos, 1972), although indirect evidence of cholera interacting with specific gangliosides may be more persuasive (Fishman and Brady, 1976).

The evidence for a resistance to tuberculosis of heterozygotes for Tay Sachs disease is that the areas in Eastern Europe with higher frequencies of Tay Sachs disease have lower frequencies of tuberculosis than those with lower Tay Sachs frequencies. But the logic of this association is absolutely backward. The high frequencies of the sickle cell gene are obviously found in areas with high malaria incidence because malaria is the factor which confers their advantage. Myrianthopoulos (1972) seems to claim that this so-called evidence is due to the resistance of Tay Sachs carriers who thus lower the incidence of tuberculosis. The frequency of carriers is only 2%–3% so it is difficult to imagine how such a low frequency would affect the epidemiology of the disease. But there seems to be a great desire to show such "feedback" among geneticists. Wiesenfeld (1967) tried to show that the sickle cell gene decreased the transmission of malaria, but there is no evidence to support it, and some to suggest the opposite. Sickle cell trait carriers have more gametocytes and could be better transmitters of malaria.

The absence of evidence for these loci being polymorphisms raises the question of whether these frequencies are at equilibrium, and if not what other evolutionary forces could account for them. This in turn suggests the founder effect and the population history of the groups involved. In the last 1000 years European populations have expanded enormously although there were periods of decrease as during the plagues, and the Eastern European Jewish populations have undergone even larger expansions (Fraikor, 1977). The Tay Sachs gene is found in comparable frequencies in a Berks County, Pennsylvania, religious isolate and in a population in French Canada (Kelly, Chase, Kaback, Komur, and McKusick, 1975; Andermann *et al.*, 1975), and a similar cerebromacular degenerative gene occurs at a comparable frequency in Newfoundlanders (Andermann, Jacob, Carpenter, Karpati, Wolfe, and Andermann, 1974). Cystic fibrosis has been found in polymorphic frequencies in the Boers of South West Africa (Super, 1975) and in the district of Plouzevede in Brittany (Bois, Feingold, Demenais, Runavot, Jehanne, and Tondic, 1978). Thus, such frequencies can occur due to the founder effect.

Two recent attempts to provide analytical solutions to the problem have resulted in conflicting conclusions (Chakravarti and Chakraborty, 1978; Wagener, Cavalli-Sforza, and Barakat, 1978). Both apply steady state gene distribution theory as developed by Sewall Wright. The basic parameter is N, the effective population size, and the first paper estimates N as 5000 for the Ashkenazim in the last 1000 years and concludes that drift is unlikely for Tay Sachs disease since the probability of such a high frequency is 0.007. The second paper uses an average N of 100 and concludes that drift is a possible explanation, although they state the probability to be 0.031. Ewens (1978) comments on the inapplicability of this type of probability statement. But it seems to me that equilibrium theory is obviously inappropriate to this historical case. In about 40 generations the East European Jewish population has increased from 20,000 to 10,000,000 with enormous fluctuations through the years, as Wagener *et al.* (1978) point out.

2. Simulation

Most theoretical models such as the steady state one just discussed assume the simplest model of genetic reproduction, that is, random union of gametes to produce the next generation. This simplifying assumption makes the equations tractable and a general solution possible, but the simulations reported here seem to show that the solutions do not estimate the founder effect very well.

The problem is how many deleterious genes in polymorphic frequencies would be expected in a large population that resulted from rapid growth from a few founders. Among human populations, growth rates close to a doubling of the population every generation are common when the population size is far below carrying capacity. This is equivalent to a growth rate of 2.8% per year, which is still found in many underdeveloped countries. This has been programmed to be the expected growth rate by setting the mean number of offspring per female at 4.0. In most primitive societies, and it would be especially true among those that are doubling every generation, almost all females are married. Competition among males over females is quite common and frequently marriage is an alliance or contract between lineages so that women are very valuable as exchange items. Polygyny is also common in most underdeveloped societies, but its effect on reproduction is still controversial.

In order to simulate this mating pattern, each female is randomly mated every generation to one of the males. Since random mating of each female is done independently more than one can be mated to the same male, and some males may not mate at all. A family size is randomly determined for each mating and the offspring generated. Each offspring is then either selected out randomly according to some set of selective coefficients or stored to form the next generation. Family size in human populations seems to approximate the negative binomial distribution (Kojima and Kelleher, 1962; Cavalli-Sforza and Bodmer, 1971), and this has been programmed with a mean offspring number per female of 4.0 and a variance of 8.0, which is close to the median value for the human populations reported by Spuhler (1976). Of course, some matings produce no offspring – with this distribution it is 6%, and the variance for males would be somewhat larger.

The simulations were run until the population was expected to attain a size of over 1500 although as would be expected with a variance of 8.0 in off-spring number, there was great variation. For example, beginning with 24 founders equally divided among the sexes after six generations the expected population size is 1536, but for 100 runs the mean size was 1391 ± 505, while starting with 12 founders after seven generations the expected number is the same but the mean was 1382 ± 723. These large standard deviations are due in large part to the many populations that attained sizes over 2500. After a population reaches 1000 or more and the deleterious gene has attained a frequency of about 0.05, then the deterministic changes begin to predominate, but the change due to selection is only -0.0025. For a population of 1000 the standard deviation for drift adjusted for family size (Cavalli-Sforza and Bodmer, 1971:421) is about 0.0054, and this would decrease rapidly with a continued doubling of the population. Thus, it will take several generations to reduce the frequency of a lethal below the polymorphic level of 0.01. For founder populations of 24 and 50, the distributions for successive generations are shown on Table 1. The changes are present but small.

Figures 1 and 2 show the differences between our model and a simpler simulation of the random union of gametes. With no family size and random mating, the low frequencies of 0.01–0.03 are high, while the frequency of extinction is lower, and very high frequencies are rare or almost nonexistent (Fig. 1). Introducing family size greatly increases the rare but very high frequencies (Fig. 2). Figures 3 and 4 show the same contrasts with 12 founders. Even with greater numbers of founders, there are still polymorphic frequencies present at an appreciable frequency. Figures 5 and 6 show the results with 50 and 100 founders, respectively. Most human founder populations would very likely include close relatives who would be likely to have the same lethal. Figure

Table 1. Simulation of the Founder Effect

Number of founders	Number of carriers	Number of runs	Generations run	Frequency extinct	Frequency > 0.01	Frequency > 0.02	Frequency > 0.04	Selection		
								S_{11}	S_{12}	S_{22}
6M + 6F	1F	3000	7	0.4003	0.5342	0.4562	0.3022	0	0	1.00
	1M	1000	7	0.554	0.401	0.351	0.260	0	0	1.00
(random)[a]	1F	1000	7	0.168	0.741	0.618	0.344	0	0	1.00
	1F	1000	7	0.369	0.555	0.476	0.356	0	0	0
	1M	1000	7	0.528	0.446	0.403	0.321	0	0	0
12M + 12F	1F	2000	6	0.377	0.486	0.351	0.1435	0	0	1.00
	1F	1000	5	0.383	0.487	0.357	0.159	0	0	1.00
	1F	1000	4	0.369	0.498	0.362	0.169	0	0	1.00
	1M	1000	6	0.529	0.392	0.311	0.165	0	0	1.00
	1F	1000	6	0.197	0.609	0.397	0.104	0	0	1.00
(random)	2F	1000	6	0.133	0.745	0.608	0.340	0	0	1.00
	1M	1000	11	0.695	0.255	0.201	0.098	0.25	0.25	1.00
	1F	1000	6	0.582	0.361	0.291	0.180	0.25	0.25	1.00
	1M	1000	6	0.549	0.388	0.322	0.205	0	0	0
	1F	1000	6	0.389	0.491	0.376	0.192	0	0	0
25M + 25F	1F	2000	6	0.4085	0.3415	0.1635	0.0295	0	0	1.00
	1F	2000	5	0.398	0.3385	0.1655	0.031	0	0	1.00
	1M	1000	5	0.519	0.325	0.194	0.039	0	0	1.00
	2F	1000	5	0.158	0.607	0.364	0.121	0	0	1.00
	1M	1000	8	0.654	0.264	0.177	0.073	0.25	0.25	1.00
	1F	1000	8	0.594	0.278	0.186	0.065	0.25	0.25	1.00
	1F	1000	5	0.575	0.276	0.153	0.054	0.25	0.25	1.00
	1F	1000	5	0.373	0.355	0.191	0.049	0	0	0
(random)	1F	1000	5	0.217	0.467	0.135	0.008	0	0	1.00
50M + 50F	1F	1000	4	0.396	0.175	0.038	0.001	0	0	1.00
	2F	1000	4	0.146	0.386	0.119	0.006	0	0	1.00
100M + 100F	1F	1000	3	0.342	0.029	0.001	0.000	0	0	1.00

[a] Those simulations with no family size but just random union of gametes are indicated by (random).

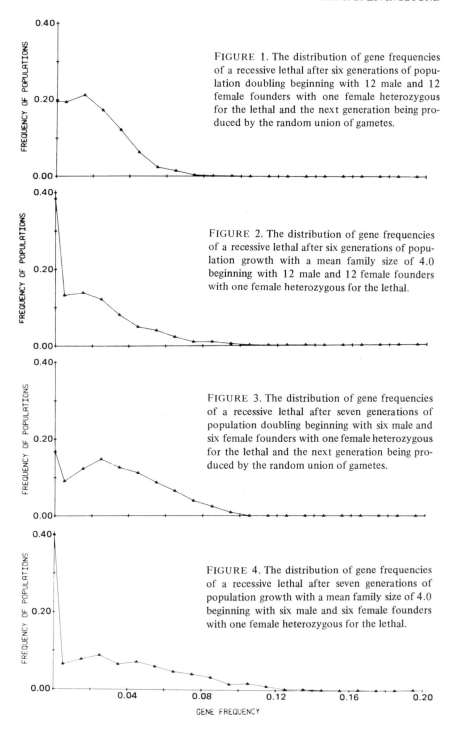

FIGURE 1. The distribution of gene frequencies of a recessive lethal after six generations of population doubling beginning with 12 male and 12 female founders with one female heterozygous for the lethal and the next generation being produced by the random union of gametes.

FIGURE 2. The distribution of gene frequencies of a recessive lethal after six generations of population growth with a mean family size of 4.0 beginning with 12 male and 12 female founders with one female heterozygous for the lethal.

FIGURE 3. The distribution of gene frequencies of a recessive lethal after seven generations of population doubling beginning with six male and six female founders with one female heterozygous for the lethal and the next generation being produced by the random union of gametes.

FIGURE 4. The distribution of gene frequencies of a recessive lethal after seven generations of population growth with a mean family size of 4.0 beginning with six male and six female founders with one female heterozygous for the lethal.

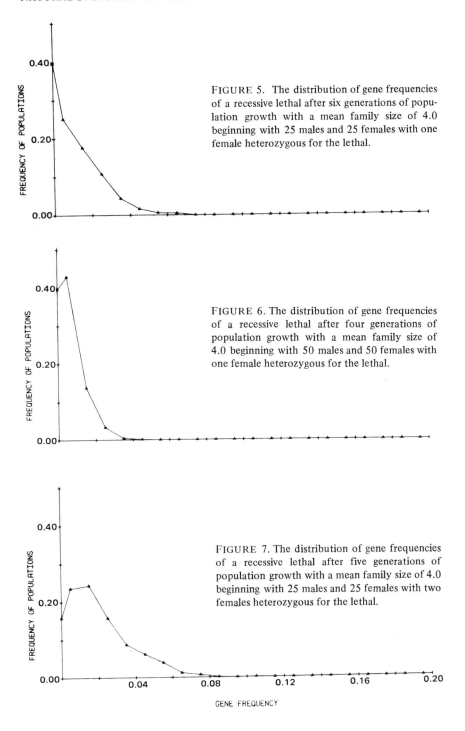

FIGURE 5. The distribution of gene frequencies of a recessive lethal after six generations of population growth with a mean family size of 4.0 beginning with 25 males and 25 females with one female heterozygous for the lethal.

FIGURE 6. The distribution of gene frequencies of a recessive lethal after four generations of population growth with a mean family size of 4.0 beginning with 50 males and 50 females with one female heterozygous for the lethal.

FIGURE 7. The distribution of gene frequencies of a recessive lethal after five generations of population growth with a mean family size of 4.0 beginning with 25 males and 25 females with two females heterozygous for the lethal.

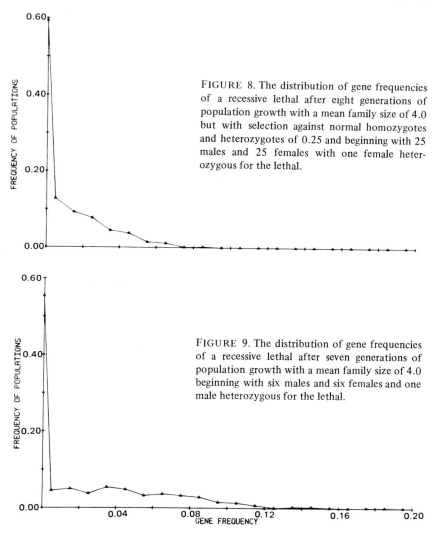

FIGURE 8. The distribution of gene frequencies of a recessive lethal after eight generations of population growth with a mean family size of 4.0 but with selection against normal homozygotes and heterozygotes of 0.25 and beginning with 25 males and 25 females with one female heterozygous for the lethal.

FIGURE 9. The distribution of gene frequencies of a recessive lethal after seven generations of population growth with a mean family size of 4.0 beginning with six males and six females and one male heterozygous for the lethal.

7 shows that with two females as carriers of a lethal gene it is found in polymorphic frequencies in most of the descendant populations. Finally, changing the rate of growth of the population or assuming the lethal occurs in one male would presumably have effects on the distribution. Figure 8 shows that decreasing the growth rate to 1.5 times per generation, which was done by increasing the selection against normal homozygotes and heterozygotes equally, does not decrease the number of times polymorphic frequencies of lethals would be expected. Figure 9 shows that with one male carrier, the frequency of extinction is increased as would be expected, but the rest of the distribution seems relatively unchanged. These differences between beginning with a male or a

female carrier occur in the first generation since the gene would be expected to be equally prevalent in the sexes in the second generation.

The results of most of the simulations are shown on Table 1. In addition to simulating a lethal gene, there are also several runs with a neutral gene. It can be seen that for various founder sizes, the neutral gene attains a frequency of greater than 0.04 more often than the lethal gene, 0.192 vs. 0.1435 for a founder size of 24 with a female carrier. It should also be noted that the neutral gene attained frequencies of greater than 0.25 and in these cases seemed to have a chance of fixation, while the lethal gene never got this high. Neel and his associates (Neel and Thompson, 1978; Thompson and Neel, 1978) have analyzed the distribution of "private" polymorphisms among South American Indian tribes using a similar model although their simulation is much more complex and specifically related to the populations they studied. Comparison is difficult, but generally their results show lower frequencies of polymorphisms, which seems to be due primarily to the low growth rates used in their study, although low growth rates were supposed to increase the amount of drift (Cavalli-Sforza and Bodmer, 1971:417).

Although the estimates derived from these simulations of the number of polymorphic lethals seem high, some data on human populations seem to accord with them. For the average human population, the average number of lethal equivalents is close to 2.0 (Cavalli-Sforza and Bodmer, 1971). Thus, with 12 founders one would expect $(0.26)(12) + (0.3022)(12)$, or 6.7 lethals in frequencies greater than 0.04. Allowing for some dilution by in-migration when the population got large, this would be close to the number expected in some highly inbred human populations. For 24 founders the number expected would be 7.4, while for 50 founders, it would be 3.4; and less for greater founder size. The Brandywine isolate of southern Maryland has one of the highest frequencies of the sickle cell gene in North America and also has high frequencies of dentinogenesis imperfecta, albinism, polycystic kidneys, congenital heart disease, congenital deafness, hypertelorism, and cortical hyperostosis (Witkop, Maclean, Schmidt, and Henry, 1966). Some of these traits are dominant, and the inheritance of others is not known in detail, and most are not lethal. Nevertheless the number of deleterious genes seems to approximate the results of the simulation with either 12 or 24 founders. The Brandywine isolate resulted from the imposition of a law against miscegenation in Maryland in 1710; there are six or seven original surnames associated with the founding of the group and another eight surnames have entered it later. Another triracial isolate, the Haliwa Indians of North Carolina, have a similar demographic history and also have a comparable number of genetic disorders. Recent studies on Welsh Gypsies who seem to originate from just two founders estimate a frequency of phenylketonuria of 0.157, and there are two other genetic disorders in high frequency (Mair Williams and Harper, 1977).

On the other hand, the Eastern European Jews have polymorphic frequencies of a much greater number of deleterious genes in addition to Tay Sachs disease. Chakravarti and Chakraborty (1978), citing McKusick (1975), state that the Ashkenazim have 22 genetic disorders in elevated frequencies. From this they conclude, "Hence, if there had been any founder effect, the early ancestors of Ashkenazic Jews must have been carrying several detrimental genes all in heterozygous form. This is again a low probability event making founder effect an untenable explanation." (Chakravarti and Chakraborty, 1978: 259). Since most humans have detrimental genes in heterozygous form, some would be expected in high frequencies with rapid population growth. In fact, the demographic history of the Ashkenazim is fairly well known (Fraikor, 1977) and accords with this pattern. Their populations were highly endogamous, isolated, and with practically no in-migration during the period of rapid population growth from a few founders. After attaining an appreciable size in Eastern Europe, migration between districts and isolates undoubtedly increased and spread the deleterious genes that began in one isolate throughout the area. These genes are still concentrated within specific populations or areas (Meals, 1971). Tay Sachs disease centers on the northern area around Vilno, while dysautonomia is found in higher frequencies in the south. If the Ashkenazim originated from a limited number, perhaps 5 to 10, of isolates with 12 to 50 founders each, then 22 detrimental genes in polymorphic frequencies would be expectable with the model developed here.

Cystic fibrosis, the other deleterious gene found in polymorphic frequencies in Europe, has a much more widespread distribution in northern Europe. It would be difficult to attribute all of the polymorphic frequencies of this gene to a single founder effect, but the same could be said for the frequencies of phenylketonuria found in Europe that are higher than the rest of the world and are polymorphic in some small isolates. However, for both these conditions there is now considerable evidence for genetic heterogeneity, so that their frequencies are due to several mutations. Most European populations exhibited rapid population growth comparable to the Ashkenazim but with much less endogamy, so that founder effect cannot be ruled out. And the high frequencies of cystic fibrosis in a small isolate in France (Bois et al., 1978) and among Southwest African Boers (Super, 1975) show that since this gene is commonly present as a low frequency mutant it can very often be one of the deleterious genes increased to high frequencies by the founder effect.

The demographic history of European populations in the last 1000 years has thus led to gene frequency change. Hence history has not yet been "annihilated" by genetic equilibria. This seems to be most evident for deleterious genes, but the same founder effect and population growth can result in change at loci with small fitness differences. Not only population growth but also the family structure of human populations leads to much more chance variation or genetic drift than would be expected with simple models. Thus, any analysis of the interaction of drift with the other forces of evolution will have to consider this

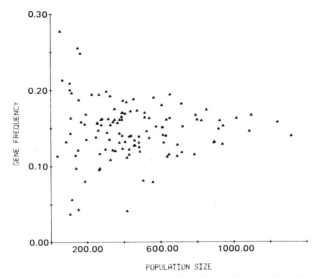

FIGURE 10. The gene frequencies and sizes of 119 populations after 20 generations beginning with 25 males and 25 females with a mean family size of 4.0 and selection coefficients, $S_{11} = 0.45$, $S_{12} = 0.32$, and $S_{22} = 1.0$.

large increase in drift; even when it is adjusted for family size the formula seems to underestimate it.

To show this increase in drift, the simulation was run for 20 generations beginning with a gene frequency of 0.08 and selective coefficients, $S_{11} = 0.45$, $S_{12} = 0.32$, $S_{22} = 1.00$, which lead to a balanced polymorphism with an equilibrium frequency of 0.16. The gene frequency was begun lower than equilibrium but after 20 generations, it could achieve equilibrium. The expected number of generations to equilibrium is closer to ten, and after ten generations there is no correlation between frequencies so the population "forgets" in this time. Figure 10 shows the variations in final gene frequencies and population sizes. It can be seen that some populations increased to over 1000 while others became extinct (these are not shown). For a population size of 400 one would expect a drift variance of 0.000145 when corrected for a variance of 8.0 in family size. This is a standard deviation of 0.014, so most populations should have gene frequencies within 0.028 of the equilibrium value of 0.16. On Figure 10 the variation seems to be four to five times larger. Similarly for a population size of 200, they should be within 0.036 of the mean, but the actual variation is about four times larger.

At genetic equilibrium the rate of increase in population would be about 0.14, and somewhat lower for populations not at equilibrium; at a frequency of 0.06, the rate would be about 0.12 and the decrease would decrease equally as one moves away from the equilibrium. Thus, after 20 generations the population size would be expected to be between 600 and 800, but few populations attain this size. More significantly there is no correlation between population size and final gene frequency ($r = -0.006$). This seems to contradict the general view that genes are important for survival or that genetic change is the process by which a population "survives." Of course, the populations with the greatest numbers are at genetic equilibrium, which has the highest growth rate; nevertheless random factors seem to be more important in determining the survival of the population. Only after the population has survived does it approach genetic equilibrium.

3. Conclusions

In conclusion, I hope that the results reported here show that the issue of drift vs. selection in the interpretation of human genetic variation is still a lively one. While the assumption of neutrality does not seem to be in accord with the world-wide gene frequency distributions for most human loci, the fact that selection is operating at any particular locus does not mean that the frequencies are close to equilibrium in most populations. In the last 1000 years the unstable demographic history of the human species has contributed substantially to the distribution of most gene frequencies, and the many cases of rapid growth have increased the frequencies of detrimental genes far above their mutational balance. Nevertheless, the analysis of human genetic variation must begin with the concept of equilibrium that assumes fitness variation among the genotypes. Although for most human loci equilibrium has not been attained and historical factors are still important, to extend this conclusion to the millennia of primate evolution is hazardous.

References

Andermann, E., Jacob, J. C., Carpenter, S., Karpati, G., Wolfe, L., and Andermann, F. (1974), Cerebromacular Degeneration in Quebec and Newfoundland: Genetic, Neurochemical and Demographic Observations (abstract), *Am. J. Hum. Genet.* **26**(6):10A.

Andermann, E., Scriver, C. R., Gold, R., Wolfe, L., Patry, G., Lafontaine, R., Geoffroy, G., and Andermann, F. (1975), Tay Sachs Screening in a French Canadian Deme: Suggestive Evidence for Polymorphism. *Am. J. Hum. Genet.* **27**(6):12A.

Bodmer, W. F. (1973), The HL-A System and Natural Selection, *Isr. J. Med. Sci.* **9**:1503–1532.

Bois, E., Feingold, J., Demenais, F., Runavot, Y., Jehanne, M., and Tondic, L. (1978), Cluster of Cystic Fibrosis Cases in a Limited Area of Brittany (France). *Clinical Genetics* **14**:73–76.

Boyd, W. C. (1950), *Genetics and the Races of Man*, Little, Brown, Boston.

Brittenham, G. (1977), Genetic Model for Observed Distributions of Proportions of Haemoglobin in Sickle-Cell Trait, *Nature* **268**:635–636.

Brittenham, G., Lozoff, B., Harris, J. W., and Narasimhan, S. (1977), Sickle Cell Anemia and Trait in a Population of Southern India, *Am. J. Hematol.* **2**:25–32.

Cavalli-Sforza, L. L., and Bodmer, W. F. (1971), *The Genetics of Human Populations*, W. H. Freeman, San Francisco.

Chakravarti, A., and Chakraborty, R. (1978), Elevated Frequency of Tay-Sachs Disease among Ashkenazic Jews Unlikely by Genetic Drift Alone, *Am. J. Hum. Genet.* **30**: 256–261.

Conneally, P. M., Merritt, A. D., and Yu, P-I. (1973), Cystic Fibrosis: Population Genetics, *Tex. Rep. Biol. Med.* **31**:639–650.

Coon, C. S., Garn, S. M., and Birdsell, J. B. (1950), *Races: A Study in Adaptation*, C C Thomas, Springfield, Illinois.

Crawfurd, M.d'A. (1975), Frequency of Cystic-Fibrosis Gene, *Lancet* **1**:167.

Danks, D. M., Allan, J., and Anderson, C. M. (1965), A Genetic Study of Fibrocystic Disease of the Pancreas, *Ann. Hum. Genet.* **28**:323–334.

Dobzhansky, T. (1950), The Genetic Nature of Differences Among Men, in *Evolutionary Thought in America* (S. Persons, ed.), pp. 86–155, Yale University Press, New Haven.

Ewens, W. J. (1978), Tay-Sachs Disease and Theoretical Population Genetics, *Am. J. Hum. Genet.* **30**:328–329.

Fishman, P. H., and Brady, R. O. (1976), Biosynthesis and Function of Gangliosides, *Science* **194**:906–914.

Fraikor, A. L. (1977), Tay-Sachs Disease: Genetic Drift among Ashkenazim Jews, *Soc. Biol.* **24**:117–134.

Haldane, J. B. S. (1940), The Blood-Group Frequencies of European Peoples and Racial Origins, *Hum. Biol.* **12**:457–480.

Howells, W. W. (1950), Physical Determination of Race, in *This Is Race* (E. W. Count, ed.), pp. 654–665, H. Schuman, New York.

Kelly, T. E., Chase, G. A., Kaback, M. M., Komur, K. K., and McKusick, V. A. (1975), Tay-Sachs Disease: High Gene Frequency in a Non-Jewish Population, *Am. J. Hum. Genet.* **27**:287–291.

Kimura, M. (1968), Evolutionary Rate at the Molecular Level, *Nature* **217**:624–626.

King, J. L., and Jukes, T. H. (1969), Non-Darwinian Evolution, *Science* **164**:788–798.

Knudsen, A. G., Wayne, L., and Hallett, W. Y. (1967), On the Selective Advantage of Cystic Fibrosis Heterozygotes, *Am. J. Hum. Genet.* **19**:388–392.

Kojima, K-I., and Kelleher, T. M. (1962), Survival of Mutant Genes, *Am. Nat.* **96**:329–346.

Lehmann, H., and Raper, A. B. (1949), Distribution of the Sickle-Cell Trait in Uganda, and its Ethnological Significance, *Nature* **164**:494–495.

Lewontin, R. C. (1974), *The Genetic Basis of Evolutionary Change*, Columbia University Press, New York.

Livingstone, F. B. (1958), Anthropological Implications of Sickle Cell Gene Distribution in West Africa, *Am. Anthropol.* **60**:533–562.

Livingstone, F. B. (1960), Natural Selection, Disease, and Ongoing Evolution, as Illustrated by the ABO Blood Groups. in *The Processes of Ongoing Evolution* (G. W. Lasker, ed.), pp. 17–27, Wayne State University Press, Detroit, Michigan.

Livingstone, F. B. (1964), Aspects of the Population Dynamics of the Abnormal Hemoglobin and Glucose-6-Phosphate Dehydrogenase Deficiency Genes, *Am. J. Hum. Genet.* **16**:435–450.

Livingstone, F. B. (1969), The Founder Effect and Deleterious Genes, *Am. J. Phys. Anthropol.* **30**:55–60.

Livingstone, F. B. (1976), Hemoglobin History in West Africa, *Human Biology* **48**:487–500.

Livingstone, F. B. (1977), The Evolution of Modifiers for Sickle Cell Anemia, *Arq. Anat. Antropol.* **2**:11–12.

Mair Williams, E., and Harper, P. S. (1977), Genetic Study of Welsh Gypsies, *J. Med. Genet.* **14**:172–176.

McKusick, V. A. (1975), Mendelian Inheritance in Man: Catalog of Autosomal Dominant, Autosomal Recessive, and X-linked Phenotypes, 4th ed., Johns Hopkins Press, Baltimore.

Meals, R. A. (1971), Paradoxical Frequencies of Recessive Disorders in Ashkenazic Jews, *J. Chronic Dis.* **23**:547–558.

Mourant, A. E., Kopec, A. C., and Domaniewska-Sobczak, K. (1976), *The Distribution of the Human Blood Groups*, Oxford University Press, London.

Myrianthopoulos, N. C. (1972), Population Dynamics of Tay-Sachs Disease. II. What Confers the Selective Advantage upon the Jewish Heterozygote? in *Sphingolipids, Sphingolipidosis, and Allied Disorders. Advances in Experimental Medicine and Biology*, (B. W. Volk and S. M. Aronson, eds.), pp. 561–569, Plenum, New York.

Myrianthopoulos, N. C., and Aronson, S. M. (1966), Population Dynamics of Tay-Sachs Disease. I. Reproductive Fitness and Selection, *Am. J. Hum. Genet.* **18**:313–327.

Nazarli, A. G., and Abdullaev, A. R. (1974), Sickle-Cell Anemia and its Variant in Azerbaijan (in Russian), *Probl. Gematol.* **19**:22–26.

Neel, J. V., and Thompson, E. A. (1978), Founder Effect and Number of Private Polymorphisms Observed in Amerindian Tribes, *Proc. Nat. Acad. Sci.* **75**:1904–1908.

Nei, M., and Roychoudhury, A. K. (1974), Genic Variation Within and Between the Three Major Races of Man: Caucasoids, Negroids, and Mongoloids, *Am. J. Hum. Genet.* **26**:421–443.

Perrine, R. P., Pembrey, M. E., Perrine, J. S., and Shoup, F. (1978), Natural History of Sickle Cell Anemia in Saudi Arabia, *Ann. Intern. Med.* **88**:1–6.

Plato, C. C., Rucknagel, D. L., and Kurland, L. T. (1966), Blood Group Investigations on the Carolinians and Chamorros of Saipan, *Am. J. Phys. Anthropol.* **24**:147–154.

Rachmilewitz, E. A., Levi, S., and Huisman, T. H. J. (1974), High Frequency of Hemoglobin C in an Israel Bedouin Tribe, *Isr. J. Med. Sci.* **10**:219–224.

Rucknagel, D. L., and Rising, J. A. (1975), A Heterozygote for Hb_β^S, Hb_β^C, and Hb_β^G Philadelphia in a Family Presenting Evidence for Heterogeneity of Hemoglobin Alpha Chain Loci, *Am. J. Med.* **59**:53–60.

Sarich, V. M. (1977), Rates, Sample Sizes and the Neutrality Hypothesis for Electrophoresis in Evolutionary Studies, *Nature* **265**:24–28.

Sarich, V. M., and Wilson, A. C. (1967), Immunological Time Scale for Hominid Evolution, *Science* **158**:1200–1202.

Schell, L. M., Agarwal, S. W., Blumberg, B. S., Levy, H., Bennett, P. H., Laughlin, W. S., and Martin, J. P. (1978), Distribution of Albumin Variants Naskapi and Mexico among Aleuts, Frobisher Bay Eskimos, and Micmac, Naskapi, Mohawk, Omaha and Apache Indians, *Am. J. Phys. Anthropol.* **49**:111–118.

Shaw, R. F., and Smith, A. P. (1969), Is Tay-Sachs Disease Increasing? *Nature* **224**:1214–1215.

Spuhler, J. N. (1976), The Maximum Opportunity for Natural Selection in Some Human Populations, in *Demographic Anthropology: Quantitative Approaches* (E. B. W. Zubrow, ed.), pp. 185–226, University of New Mexico Press, Albuquerque.

Stebbins, G. L., and Lewontin, R. C. (1972), Comparative Evolution at the Levels of Molecules, Organisms and Populations, *Proc. Berkeley Symp. Math. Stat. Probab.* **5**:23–42.

Steinberg, A. G. (1973), The Gm and Inv Allotypes of Some Ashkenazic Jews Living in Northern U.S.A., *Am. J. Phys. Anthropol.* **39**:409–412.

Stuart, A. B., and Burdon, M. G. (1974), Frequency of Cystic-Fibrosis Gene, *Lancet* **2**:1521.

Super, M. (1975), Cystic Fibrosis in the South West African Afrikaner, *S. Afr. Med. J.* **49**:818–820.

Super, M. (1977), Heterozygote Disadvantage in Cystic Fibrosis, *Lancet* **2**:1288.

Thompson, E. A., and Neel, J. V. (1978), Probability of Founder Effect in a Tribal Population, *Proc. Natl. Acad. Sci.* **75**:1442–1445.

Vogel, F. (1975), ABO Blood Groups, the HL-A System and Diseases. in *The Role of Natural Selection in Human Evolution* (F. M. Salzano, ed.), pp. 247–270, Elsevier, New York.

Wagener, D., Cavalli-Sforza, L. L., and Barakat, R. (1978), Ethnic Variation of Genetic Disease: Roles of Drift for Recessive Lethal Genes, *Am. J. Hum. Genet.* **30**:262–270.

Walter, H., and Schobel, B. (1975), Climate Associated Variations in the Human Serum Albumin Level, *Humangenetik* **30**:331–335.

Weitkamp, L. R. (1973), The Contribution of Variations in Serum Albumin to the Characterization of Human Populations, *Isr. J. Med. Sci.* **9**:1238–1248.

Weitkamp, L. R., Salzano, F. M., Neel, J. V., Porta, F., Geerdink, R. A., and Tarnoky, A. L. (1973a), Human Serum Albumin: Twenty-Three Genetic Variants and Their Population Distribution, *Ann. Hum. Genet.* **36**:381–392.

Weitkamp, L. R., McDermid, E. M., Neel, J. V., Fine, J. M., Petrini, C., Bonazzi, L., Ortali, V., Porta, F., Tanis, R., Harris, D. J., Peters, T., Ruffini, G., and Johnston, E. (1973b), Additional Data on the Population Distribution of Human Serum Albumin Genes: Three New Variants, *Ann. Hum. Genet.* **37**:219–226.

Wiesenfeld, S. L. (1967), Sickle-Cell Trait in Human Biological and Cultural Evolution, *Science* **157**:1134–1140.

Witkop, C. J., MacLean, C. J., Schmidt, P. J., and Henry, J. L. (1966), Medical and Dental Findings in the Brandywine Isolate, *Ala. J. Med. Sci.* **3**:382–403.

6

The Simulation of Human Fertility

Strategies in Demographic Modeling

JEAN WALTERS MACCLUER

1. Introduction

Within the past ten years, computer simulation has become a common tool in anthropology, genetics, and demography. The kinds of problems for which simulation is most useful involve studies of the effects of interaction of two or more population processes on the growth, structure and evolution of populations. For example, an anthropologist might model the joint effects of mating rules and migration patterns on the size and geographical distribution of a population; a geneticist might be interested in the combined effects of genetically determined, age-specific differential fertility and mortality on the maintenance of a polymorphism; and a demographer might wish to investigate models in which population growth depends upon fertility and mortality characteristics of both males and females.

Simulation models of population structure may be used (1) to generate distributions which cannot be obtained analytically, (2) to determine the accuracy of estimation procedures, the power of statistical tests, etc., (3) to examine the extent to which the assumptions of simple models invalidate their conclusions, (4) to generate completely ascertained data for use in estimating population parameters, and (5) to test the user's knowledge of a social system.

JEAN WALTERS MACCLUER ● Department of Biology, The Pennsylvania State University, University Park, Pennsylvania 16802.

Examples of these uses in demography, genetics, and anthropology are discussed in the review by MacCluer (1973) and in the volume edited by Dyke and MacCluer (1974).

The problems for which simulation is ordinarily used are those for which no totally satisfactory analytical solutions have been proposed. It is generally believed that simulation is a sort of "last resort", and that if an appropriate analytical model can be developed, the analytical approach is preferable. (In fact, some people consider the use of computer simulation to be unjustified whenever an analytical solution appears even remotely possible, no matter how long the problem has defied solution, nor how useful the simulation results might be.) However, for some purposes, computer simulation models may even have advantages over mathematical ones: their results are understandable to a larger number of people; they are invaluable for helping the modeler to understand the complexities of the system being modeled; and they may be developed and used by investigators who are not mathematically sophisticated, but who are knowledgeable about the processes which they wish to model. In any case, there are many important problems in genetics, anthropology, and demography which can best be approached by computer simulation, and thus, an understanding of simulation techniques is essential for anyone concerned with population dynamics.

In this presentation, I will illustrate some of these techniques as they might be (and have been) applied to the modeling of human fertility. I will described several quite different ways in which fertility may be modeled, and mention the advantages and limitations of each approach. Finally, I will discuss in detail some recent experiments with a fertility simulation model and will point out some general strategies which are important in the development and use of any computer simulation model of population structure.

2. Computer Simulation of Fertility

Human fertility is influenced by so many factors, interacting in such complex ways, that there is no one analytical fertility model which is adequate for any but the simplest of problems. Even a complex fertility simulation model must make many simplifying assumptions, and restrict attention to a few variables which are considered to be important for the problem at hand. Demographic fertility models, for example, are most often applied to the evaluation of contraceptive effectiveness. Demographers are not concerned about the effect of genotype on fertility, and they usually ignore the indirect effect on fertility exerted by population size, which influences availability of mates. Geneticists, on the other hand, do not incorporate in their simulation models variables which indicate religion or socioeconomic status, although these factors are known to affect fertility. The several models to be discussed below differ from each other in the assumptions which are made about the reproductive process, and accordingly, each is appropriate for a different kind of problem. However, all of them may include population size and/or genetic structure as variables which influence fertility, and thus, all are potentially useful in genetic and anthropological investigations.

There are several ways of classifying simulation models, based primarily upon the methods by which decisions are made. Although the classification scheme as I will describe it is dichotomous, most simulation models would have to be placed at an intermediate position, combining features of both extremes.

Deterministic vs. Stochastic. A model is said to be stochastic if random variation is allowed in the outcome of a particular event. For example, the age at which a woman has her first child might be chosen from a normal distribution with a specified mean and variance. Thus, in a particular experiment, not all women would have their first child at the same age. In a deterministic model, there is no random variability in the outcome of an event. In the example above, this would correspond to all women having their first child at the same age. A variation on this scheme, which would still be considered to be deterministic, would allow women to differ in age at first birth according to some input distribution (say 1/4 at age 20, 1/2 at age 21, and 1/4 at age 22) as long as the decision as to which women reproduce at which age is not random. Most simulation models combine both deterministic and stochastic decision making; however, if any of the decisions are stochastic, the model itself is generally classified as stochastic.

Macro vs. Micro. Models are classified as macro or micro depending upon the size of the basic unit about which information is recorded and decisions are made. For example, suppose that a population is subdivided by age, sex, genotype, and clan membership, with numbers of individuals in each category stored in a four-dimensional array and with decisions being made for entire groups of individuals simultaneously (e.g., a proportion p of individuals in a particular cell will reproduce). This model would be classified as a macro model by most geneticists, because information is not recorded for each individual. On the other hand, if population data were stored in an array in which a separate record is kept for each person, and decisions were made separately for each individual, the model would be classified as micro. As we shall see, however, some models are more micro than others.

Discrete vs. Continuous. The distinction between discrete and continuous models is based upon the order and timing of decisions. In a discrete model, time is held constant while decisions are made for all members of the population. Time is then advanced by one unit, and the decision-making process is repeated for the entire population. In contrast, in a continuous model, individual members of the population are processed at different rates. A decision is made, for each individual, on the waiting time to the next event, and the individual is essentially ignored until the time for that next event arrives. Continuous models have the advantage that they are more efficient for many types of problems. For example, age at death (in a model with age structure) is decided in one step. In a discrete model, an individual is "at risk" each year until death occurs, so that 65 separate decisions are required for an individual who lives to age 65. However, continuous models cannot conveniently be used for decisions which require interaction among different segments of the population. Thus, the decision concerning age at marriage might depend upon the availability of marriageable members of the opposite sex. Models have been constructed which combine both discrete and continuous decision making, and which thus avoid many of the problems of both continuous and discrete models.

With this background on types of simulation models, let us consider several alternate ways of modeling human fertility. The following examples are taken from several large simulation programs which are being used in my laboratory.

2.1. KINSIM

KINSIM is a discrete-time, stochastic microsimulation model which was developed in collaboration with Anthony J. Boyce. We have been using it to investigate the effect of migration patterns on inbreeding and kinship within and between subdivisions of a population (Boyce and MacCluer, in preparation). In creating KINSIM, our goal was not to simulate "reality," but rather, to construct a model which would allow us to determine the accuracy of the predictions of some of the simple, analytical models of migration, when there are departures from some of their assumptions. In particular, we were interested in the effects of (1) unequal migration rates among individuals on the basis of sex and marital status, (2) nonrandom migration on the basis of relationship, (3) migration rates dependent upon the size of the populations of origin and of destination, or on the distance between populations, and (4) random fluctuations in sizes of local populations. Because age structure was not one of the departures in which we were interested, generations are nonoverlapping in KINSIM; the time unit for decision making is an entire generation. Because there is no age structure, reproduction for each mated pair is accomplished in a single step: the offspring number for each couple is determined by generating a random number from a negative binomial distribution with specified mean and variance. The only additional steps required are those which determine the sex and genotype of each offspring.

It should be noted that even though reproduction is simulated in a very simple way in KINSIM, it is still necessary to keep track of the characteristics of each individual. Because we are interested in studying inbreeding and kinship, we must be able to ascertain how individuals are related to one another, and we wish to have the option of prohibiting mating between close relatives.

We discovered during our preliminary experiments with KINSIM that this model of reproduction generates large fluctuations in population numbers from generation to generation, to the extent that it is difficult to detect the effects of various migration schemes. Because we were not really interested in studying the influence of these large fluctuations on relatedness, we decided to modify the reproductive process in such a way that these oscillations would be damped. We therefore modified the mean number of offspring per couple from one generation to the next according to the equation

$$\mu = 2[1 + r(1 - N/N_{max})(1 + N_{min}/N)]$$

where μ is the mean number of offspring per couple, r the desired intrinsic rate of natural increase, N the total population size in this generation, N_{max} the desired maximum population size, and N_{min} the desired minimum population size. As N approaches N_{max}, the first term in parentheses approaches zero and the mean offspring number approaches two. If N were to exceed N_{max}, the term in parentheses would be negative and the mean offspring number per couple would drop below replacement level. On the other hand, as N approaches N_{min}, mean offspring number increases. This method of fertility control allows for fluctuations in the size of local groups, but restrains the changes in total population size to a fairly narrow range.

It is worth pointing out that this model, unlike some of the others to be discussed, is not restricted to human population studies. In fact, the first large-scale application will involve populations of baboons and rhesus macaques. KINSIM is being used as a first step in a study of the genetic consequences of male migration and incest avoidance in nonhuman primates (Kurland, Dyke, and MacCluer, in preparation).

In summary, the fertility model as represented in KINSIM is the simplest of all those to be discussed here. Fertility is influenced by availability of mates who are not too closely related; by the desired mean and variance in offspring number, as specified by the experimenter; and indirectly, by total population size. Fertility is not affected by the genetic composition of the population, nor by age.

2.2. POPSIM

In contrast to KINSIM, POPSIM was designed to study the effects of age structure and mating patterns on evolution and growth of small populations. The incorporation of age structure entails a logic which is quite different from that used in KINSIM. It also requires that the investigator know much more about the demographic structure of the populations to be simulated, including the rules by which mates are chosen. Fertility in POPSIM is influenced by availability of mates, marital status, age of female (and, to some extent, age of male), and genotype. Availability of mates, in turn, may be affected by age, clan or lineage membership, relationship, village of residence, and political alliances.

Table 1. Characteristics of Newborn Offspring Generated by POPSIM

Males	Females
Birth date	Birth date
Parents	Parents
(Marital status)	(Marital status)
Patronym (or clan)	Patronym (or clan)
Ages of parents at birth	Ages of parents at birth
Birth interval, parity	Birth interval, parity
(Alliance information)	(Reproductive information)
ID	ID
Village	Village
Mother's patronym (clan)	Mother's patronym (clan)
Grandparents	Grandparents
Great-grandparents	Great-grandparents
Migration information	Migration information
Marriage file pointer	Marriage file pointer
Parents' villages of birth	Parents' villages of birth
(Sibship size information)	(Sibship size information)

The time unit for decision making is a single year, and decisions are made in a discrete fashion. Thus, during every year of simulation, a random number is generated for each female to determine whether she will reproduce in that year. If she does, a series of steps is executed to determine the characteristics of her offspring (see Table 1).

In a sense, POPSIM is a much more realistic model than KINSIM, and there are certain types of problems for which it is far superior. It can be (and has been) used to estimate certain age-specific vital rates for small populations, and to investigate the extent to which tribal populations can adhere to their stated rules for choosing mates. However, POPSIM is not suitable for studies of long-term evolutionary change. Whereas it is relatively inexpensive to simulate 150 generations (4000 years) with KINSIM, even 400 years' simulation is expensive with POPSIM.

2.3. CHOREA

Neither KINSIM nor POPSIM were designed with just one problem in mind. In contrast, the third model, CHOREA, was written specifically to study fertility for a late-onset genetic disease, Huntington's chorea. I wish to describe this model here because it uses a method for modeling fertility which is quite different from those used in KINSIM and POPSIM.

Huntington's chorea is a progressive disease of the central nervous system, inherited as an autosomal dominant. The average age at onset is around 30 to 40. The life expectancy after onset of the disease is about 15 years, and most patients die in institutions. Individuals who carry this abnormal gene are thus well into their reproductive periods before they become affected, and they transmit the gene to half of their offspring. Considerable attention has been devoted to measuring the fertility of Huntington's chorea patients and their relatives, in an attempt to discover why this gene is present in such high frequency (approximately 1/10,000). There is some evidence of increased sexual activity in patients after the onset of symptoms, and also some suggestion that sibs (some of whom carry the gene themselves) might alter their fertility when a brother or sister becomes affected.

CHOREA was designed by Barber (1979) to investigate the potential effects on the fitness of the Huntington's chorea gene of various types and magnitudes of modification of reproductive behavior by choreics and their sibs. Like the previous two models, CHOREA is also a discrete-time, stochastic microsimulation model. Like POPSIM, the time unit for decision making is a single year. Unlike either model, the unit which is simulated is not an entire population, but a single family, over a period of several generations. Fitness calculations are based upon the combined histories of several families, and modifications of reproductive behavior are achieved by multiplying the age-specific fertilities by a specified constant as soon as a member of a sibship develops the disease. Availability of mates is not a factor in reproduction; they marry into the family from an infinite external pool, at ages determined from input distributions derived from the demographic literature. The variables which influence fertility are age, marital status, phenotype (choreic or normal), and phenotypes of siblings. Probabilities of marrying, reproducing, and dying as a function of age, sex, and phenotype, and age-specific probabilities of developing the symptoms of the disease, are all required as input to CHOREA. This is a special-purpose model, used for a problem for which KINSIM and POPSIM would be totally unsuitable.

2.4. FERTSIM

Of all the models described here, FERTSIM has the most detailed fertility structure. It was developed especially to study differential fertility, and it is the model which most closely resembles those used by demographers to study the consequences of family planning, although I have used FERTSIM for quite different purposes. Like the other models, FERTSIM is a stochastic microsimulation model. Unlike the others, it is a continuous-time model, i.e., reproductive histories are generated by determining the waiting times between successive events. Whereas KINSIM and POPSIM simulate entire populations, and CHOREA simulates families, FERTSIM generates reproductive histories for cohorts of women. The time unit for decision making is the month (as opposed to the generation or the year). Since there is no interaction among members of a cohort (i.e., the reproductive history of one woman does not influence the reproduction of others), it is possible to generate an entire reproductive history

Table 2. FERTSIM Input Distributions

Age-specific fecundability	Lengths of pregnancies ending in
Age at menarche	spontaneous abortion
Age at marriage	stillbirth
Age at menopause	live birth
Proportions of pregnancies, by age of	Duration of postpartum infecundability
mother, ending in	for pregnancies ending in
spontaneous abortion	spontaneous abortion
stillbirth	stillbirth
live birth	live birth

for one woman before moving on to the next. Moreover, the record created for each woman contains a detailed account of her fertility, including the timing of each conception, the length and outcome of each pregnancy, the length of the sterile period following each pregnancy, etc. The variables which influence fertility in FERTSIM are shown in Table 2. Notice that fertility is not affected by availability of mates; they are drawn from an infinite external pool. Nor is it influenced directly by male age or length of marriage, although these variables do exert an indirect effect through age-specific fecundability. These limitations do not prevent the use of FERTSIM for anthropological problems, but do restrict its use to cohorts of ever-married women.

With respect to the details of the fertility history, FERTSIM is the most "realistic" of all the models described here. However, it is probably worthwhile at this point to ask what is meant by the term "realistic." FERTSIM is well suited for simulating cohorts of ever-married women who survive through the reproductive period; all the women created by FERTSIM eventually marry, and all survive. For the genetic applications which I shall describe shortly, FERTSIM is the only one of the four models which is appropriate. As we shall see later, there are ways of using the results of FERTSIM under slightly less restrictive conditions, e.g., for cohorts in which women (and their husbands) are at risk of dying throughout the reproductive period, and marriages are at risk of divorce. FERTSIM would not be "realistic" if we attempted to use it to simulate the reproductive history of a small, age-structured population, whose composition was constantly changing as a result of births, deaths, and in and out migration.

I made the statement earlier that some models are more micro than others. Both POPSIM and FERTSIM are classified as micro models, but for studies of the biological factors affecting fertility, FERTSIM can be considered "more micro," since it models these factors in some detail. On the other hand, POPSIM includes greater detail with respect to sociocultural factors which can affect fertility.

3. Some Fertility Simulation Experiments

I have recently been interested in the possibility that a significant proportion of the observed genetic variability within and between populations might be maintained by genetically determined differences in fertility. There is a growing literature (reviewed in MacCluer, 1978) which lends support to this idea: (1) Heterozygotes for some single gene defects appear to have a fertility advantage over normal homozygotes; (2) studies of blood groups and fertility have revealed effects of maternal–fetal incompatibility; and (3) sperm are known to carry HLA, H-Y, and other antigens, and some women with reduced fertility have been shown to have sperm-immobilizing antibodies in their vaginal secretions. On the other hand, the conventional wisdom states that small fertility differences are not likely to be detectable unless sample sizes are extremely large. Thus, there has been no major effort devoted to the search for differential fertility in humans.

I began to wonder about the extent to which differences in some of the components of fertility (such as those listed in Table 2) might be capable of producing effects on completed fertility, and thus on Darwinian fitness. It seemed possible, for example, that small genetic differences in the proportion of fetuses lost shortly after conception might have virtually no effect on total reproductive performance, and thus might have little meaning in an evolutionary context. I also wondered about the statement that in order to detect small fertility differences, one needs large samples. Specifically, how large must samples be, to detect what kinds and magnitudes of fertility difference, and with what degree of certainty? It was in order to investigate questions of this sort that FERTSIM was developed.

Because the model has already been described elsewhere (MacCluer, 1978, 1979) I will summarize it only briefly here. The reproductive history created for each woman in a simulated cohort consists of a sequence of digits, one corresponding to each month of the woman's reproductive period. Each digit indicates the woman's status during one month of that period, as shown in Table 3. The

Table 3. The Reproductive Period

State	
0	premenarche
1	postmenarche, never married
2	married, fecundable
3	pregnant
4	postabortion, infecundable
5	poststillbirth, infecundable
6	postlivebirth, infecundable
7	postmenopause

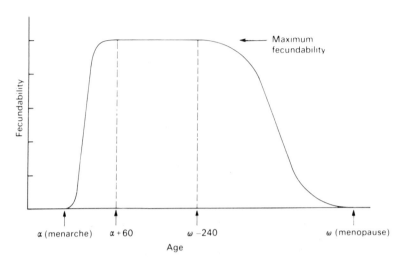

FIGURE 1. The pattern of age-specific fecundability in FERTSIM.

input distributions shown in Table 2 determine the probabilities that a woman
will pass from one state to another in any given month. These probabilities are
a function not only of the age of the woman, but also, in some cases, of the
length of time spent in a previous state. For example, menarche corresponds to
passing from state 0 to state 1. This event happens only once to each woman, at
an age generated from a normal distribution with a specified mean and variance.
The transition from state 1 to state 2 also happens only once, as does passage
into state 7 (postmenopause). State 3 (pregnant) may be entered only from
state 2 (married, fecundable), but that transition may occur numerous times in
the reproductive span of an individual woman. From state 3, a woman enters
one of three states (4, 5, or 6) depending upon the outcome of the pregnancy.

It is possible to get at least crude estimates for the input parameters listed
in Table 2. In some cases, one must make assumptions about the shapes of
distributions. For fecundability (the monthly probability of conception), for
example, I have assumed that the change with female age is as shown in Figure 1.
This curve is similar in shape to one suggested by Henry (1972). Average maximum fecundability is assumed to extend from 60 months after menarche to 240
months before menopause. I have assumed that the shape of the fecundability
curve is the same for each woman in a cohort, with a mean specified as input
and a variance equal to 0.56 times the mean. This relationship between mean
and variance in fecundability has been derived from empirical data analyzed by
Bongaarts (1975). The assumed 20-year decline in fecundability before menopause is also based upon empirical data, and upon some validation experiments
which I will describe later.

Figure 2 illustrates two sample reproductive histories as generated by

```
000000000000  000000000000  001111111111  111111111111  111111111111
111111111111  111111111111  111111111111  111111111111  111111111111
111111111111  111111111111  111111111122  333333333366  666666622222
222222222222  222222222222  222233333333  336666662222  223333333333
666666622222  222233333333  366666662222  222222222222  222222222222
222222222222  222222222222  333333333666  666662222222  233333333666
666622222222  222222222222  222222222333  333333366666  666222222222
222222222222  222222222227  777777777777  777777777777  777777777777
777777777777  777777777777  7
```

```
000000000000  000000000000  000000000011  111111111111  111111111111
111111111111  111111111111  111111111111  111111111111  111111111111
111111111111  111111111111  111111111111  111111111111  111111111111
111111111111  111111222222  222333333333  366666622222  222222223333
333333666666  222222222222  222233333333  366666622233  333333366666
666223333333  333666666666  662222222223  333344422222  222222333333
333355552222  222222233442  222222233333  333366666666  222222333333
333666666662  222222222222  222333333333  666777777777  777777777777
777777777777  777777777777  7
```

FIGURE 2. Sample reproductive histories generated by FERTSIM.

FERTSIM. Each sequence of 12 digits represents one year in the reproductive span of an individual woman, extending from age ten (in the upper left) to age 52. In the first case, menarche (transition from state 0 to state 1) occurs at age 12 (between the second and third month) and marriage (1 to 2) at age 22. This woman has seven pregnancies (sequences of 3's), all of which end in live births (transitions to state 6). The periods of postpartum sterility vary from six to nine months in length. Menopause (transition into state 7) occurs at age 46.

The second reproductive history is atypical, but it was chosen for illustration because this woman has many pregnancies (11) with three different pregnancy outcomes, including two spontaneous abortions (transitions to state 4) and one still birth (transition to state 5). As expected, the period of postpartum sterility after an abortion is not as long as that after a live birth.

These reproductive histories constitute the raw data generated by FERTSIM. There is much more information about the members of one of these artificial cohorts than one can obtain for any real population; the fertility statistics which are routinely computed in actual fertility studies are based upon fairly restricted data. Thus, any attempt to detect differences in fertility will ordinarily have to be based upon relatively crude measures of reproductive performance, such as those listed in Table 4. Because these are the measures which must be used to detect underlying fertility differences between real populations, they are the measures which are used as a basis for comparing artificial cohorts. The strategy

Table 4. FERTSIM *Output Distributions*

Age at marriage	Age at maternity
Reproductive span	first birth
Menarche to menopause	last birth
Marriage to menopause	all births
First to last birth	all women
Marriage to last birth	Number of conceptions
Livebirth interval	Number of detectable
Marriage to first birth	fetal deaths
Births after the first	Completed family size,
Per birth	livebirths
Per woman	Family size by age for
Livebirth interval by parity	ages 20, 25, . . . , 45
and completed family size	

which I used in these experiments with FERTSIM was to generate cohorts which differed in one of the fertility components (Table 2) and to determine the effect upon measurable reproductive performance (the variables in Table 4).

3.1. Experiment 1

The first question which I addressed was the extent to which differences in some fertility components affect Darwinian fitness. I generated two series of cohorts: series I consisted of six cohorts of 4000 women each, differing only in the mean and variance in fecundability; series II included five cohorts of 4000 women each, differing only in the level of fetal loss in the first month after conception. The input characteristics of all these cohorts were chosen to correspond to those of U.S. women in the 1921–1925 birth cohort.

The average maximum fecundabilities in Series I took values of $\phi = 0.10$, $0.12, . . . , 0.20$ with variances of 0.56 times ϕ. The range of probabilities of early fetal loss in Series II is shown in Table 5. The model assumes that in every

Table 5. *Proportions of Pregnancies Ending in Abortion in a Series of Cohorts*

	Probability of fetal loss			
	for women of age 20–24		for all women	
Cohort	in 1st month after conception	Total	in 1st month after conception	Total
7	0.194	0.225	0.354	0.410
8	0.219	0.250	0.399	0.455
9	0.244	0.275	0.447	0.503
10	0.269	0.300	0.495	0.551
11	0.294	0.325	0.544	0.601

*Table 6. Some Fertility Characteristics of Six Cohorts
which Differ in Average Maximum Fecundability*

Fecundability:	0.20	0.18	0.16	0.14	0.12	0.10
Cohort:	1	2	3	4	5	6
Mean age at						
marriage	22.32	22.36	22.41	22.33	22.47	22.25
menarche	13.14	13.12	13.09	13.10	13.11	13.06
menopause	49.90	50.05	50.05	50.05	49.97	49.94
first maternity	23.76	23.92	24.05	24.11	24.32	24.37
last maternity	40.58	40.31	40.09	39.74	39.38	38.70
maternity (all births)	31.23	31.19	31.15	31.04	31.01	30.85
Interval (months) between						
successive live-births	24.19	24.85	25.78	27.11	28.42	30.55
Mean number of						
conceptions	16.80	16.08	15.14	13.99	11.82	11.55
detectable fetal deaths	0.90	0.86	0.81	0.74	0.67	0.62
($\geqslant$ 3rd month)						
livebirths	9.15	8.73	8.29	7.72	7.14	6.39

*Table 7. Some Fertility Characteristics of Five Cohorts which
Differ in Level of Early Fetal Loss*

Proportion of all pregnancies ending in first month after conception:	0.354	0.399	0.447	0.495	0.544
Cohort:	7	8	9	10	11
Mean age at					
marriage	22.31	22.32	22.37	22.37	22.29
menarche	13.07	13.14	13.10	13.08	13.10
menopause	50.01	49.90	50.02	49.94	49.99
first maternity	23.79	23.76	23.80	23.80	23.86
last maternity	41.13	40.58	39.81	38.54	37.34
maternity (all births)	31.53	31.23	30.81	30.25	29.75
Interval (months) between					
successive live births	23.72	24.19	24.39	24.36	24.14
Mean number of					
conceptions	16.31	16.80	17.49	17.89	18.77
detectable fetal deaths	0.86	0.90	0.93	0.96	0.96
($\geqslant$ 3rd month)					
livebirths	9.63	9.15	8.69	8.03	7.49

cohort, the probability of fetal loss is lowest for women of age 20–24, with a rate increasing to approximately three times the minimum value by age 45.

Tables 6 and 7 summarize some of the fertility characteristics of these two series of cohorts. They are presented here primarily to demonstrate that the results of the simulations are intuitively reasonable. A discussion of some of the trends apparent in these tables is given in MacCluer (1978).

The most meaningful measures of fitness in an age-structured population are those which take into account variability in the timing of reproduction. One such measure is

$$W = \sum_{x=\alpha}^{\omega} \frac{l(x)b(x)}{x} \tag{3.1}$$

where $b(x)$ is the number of daughters produced by a woman at age x, $l(x)$ is the probability of surviving to age x, and α and ω are the limits of the reproductive period. This quantity is the number of live-born daughters per live-born female per year. For a population in which there is age-specific variability in probabilities of dying and reproducing, this measure is preferable to one which simply calculates the total number of offspring produced. I used a modification of this formula,

$$W = \sum_{x=\alpha, \alpha+5, \ldots}^{\omega} \left[l(x)\left({}_5b(x) \Big/ \sum_{y=x}^{x+4} y \right) \right] \tag{3.2}$$

where ${}_5b(x)$ is the number of daughters produced by women in the age interval $x \leqslant y < x + 5$. The term in parentheses is thus an estimate of $b(x)/x$.

You will recall that there is no mortality in FERTSIM. Thus, it is possible to calculate directly the effects of differences in fertility components on the $b(x)$'s, but the $l(x)$'s are equal to 1 for all ages, in all cohorts. This presents no difficulties for the calculation of fitnesses, however, since "typical" values for the $l(x)$'s may be chosen from model life tables. But before we turn to these fitness calculations, let us examine the variations in age-specific fertility patterns which are produced by differences in fecundability and early fetal loss.

Values of ${}_5b(x)$ for cohorts which differ in fecundability and in early fetal loss are shown in Figs. 3 and 4, respectively. It is apparent from comparison of these figures that variation in monthly probability of conception has a different effect on age-specific fertility patterns than does variation in amount of early fetal loss. Fecundability differences exert their strongest influence on women in the peak reproductive years, when fecundability is highest. But differences in early fetal loss have their greatest impact toward the end of the reproductive period, since these women have fetal loss rates which approach three times the rates experienced by women of ages 20–24. Obviously, if the differences in fecundability or early fetal loss between two cohorts were not expressed as a

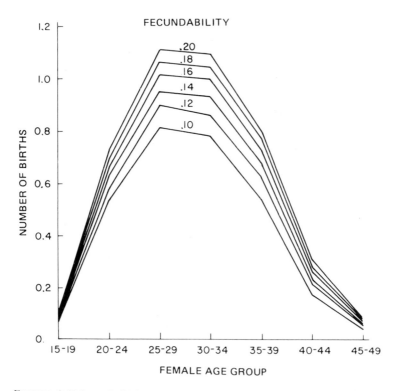

FIGURE 3. Values of $_5b(x)$ computed for six cohorts which differ in fecundability.

constant proportion across all age groups, then these relationships would not necessarily hold.

In order to determine the impact of these differences in fecundability and early fetal loss on Darwinian fitness, I selected values of $l(x)$ corresponding to several different mortality levels, from Coale and Demeny's (1966) model life tables, and substituted them, together with the values of $_5b(x)$ shown in Figs. 3 and 4, into Eq. (3.2). I thus obtained a numerical value for Darwinian fitness for each combination of fertility and mortality levels. The results of these calculations are presented in detail in MacCluer (1979). Of more interest for purposes of this presentation are not the precise values of W for each set of $l(x)$'s and $_5b(x)$'s, but rather, the relative effectiveness of fertility as opposed to mortality changes in altering Darwinian fitness. These relationships are shown in Figs. 5 and 6. Thus (Fig. 5), a 20% reduction in fecundability has approximately the same effect on Darwinian fitness as does the death of 18% of females before and during the reproductive period; and a 20% increase in the proportion of fetuses lost in the first month after conception (Fig. 6) reduces fitness to the same extent as does the death of 16% of females. This amount of mortality is likely

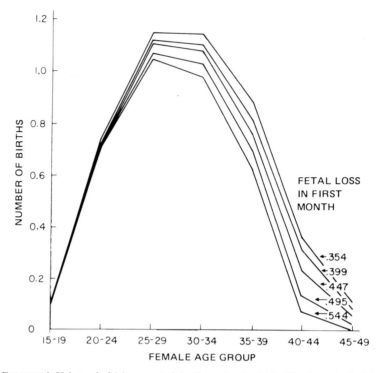

FIGURE 4. Values of $_5b(x)$ computed for five cohorts which differ in early fetal loss.

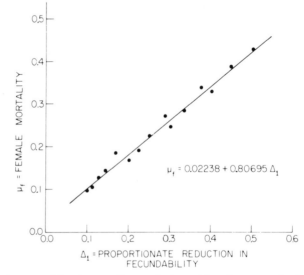

FIGURE 5. Amount of female mortality required to achieve the same reduction in fitness as that produced by a given proportionate reduction in fecundability.

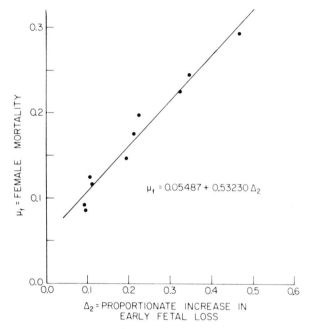

FIGURE 6. Amount of female mortality required to achieve the same reduction in fitness as that produced by a given proportionate increase in early fetal loss.

to impose a significantly greater psychological burden on a population than is a selectively equivalent change in fertility.

3.1. Experiment 2

The next question of interest is whether fertility differences of the magnitude considered here are detectable in samples of one or a few hundred individuals — samples which might reasonably be collected in a genetic study. I will briefly summarize the results of some experiments described in MacCluer (1978).

Each of the cohorts of 4000 women in series I and II was subdivided into 40 cohorts of 100 women each. To determine the probability of detecting the difference between any two fecundability levels (or any two levels of fetal loss), I did analysis of variance on the total number of live births (and several of the other standard fertility measures listed in Table 4) for 40 pairs of small cohorts (one of each pair at one level of fecundability or early fetal loss and one at the other level) and computed the proportion of instances in which the two cohorts differed at the $\alpha = 0.05$ level of significance.

I found that even when I used the most reliable indicator of differences in fecundability (total number of live births), the proportionate reduction in fecundability had to be as high as 0.30 (e.g., from $\phi = 0.20$ to $\phi = 0.14$) before it could be detected in 75% of comparisons. (Thus, in this case, for samples of size 100, the power of analysis of variance was 0.75.) The best indicator of differences in early fetal loss was age at last maternity. But again, pairs of cohorts had to differ by 28% in the level of early fetal loss before the difference could be detected with 75% probability. Therefore, for most genetic purposes, samples of size 100 will not be sufficiently large.

When the analysis was repeated for cohorts of size 200, the results were slightly more encouraging: With probability 0.75, one can detect a 25% reduction in fecundability or a 20% increase in fetal loss in the first month after conception.

An interesting result of this study is that the interval between successive livebirths, which has often been used as an indicator of differences in early fetal loss, is actually one of the worst discriminators of all the fertility measures which were examined. In fact, in comparisons between 400 pairs of cohorts of size 100 which were identical in their underlying fertility components, 12.5% were significantly different in mean interval between successive live births. This departure from the expected 5% (since $\alpha = 0.05$) can probably be attributed to the fact that one or more of the requirements of analysis of variance are not met, in particular, the assumption of normality of the underlying distributions. The inadequacy of livebirth interval as a measure of underlying differences in early fetal loss appears to be a result of the fact that many women who are at increased risk of fetal loss simply stop producing liveborn offspring and therefore do not contribute to the calculation of mean livebirth interval.

This study is currently being extended in several ways:

(1) The shapes of the distributions of the fertility measures listed in Table 4 are being examined. If the distributions are normal, or if a transformation can be used which will make them normal or nearly so, then powers of analysis of variance may be derived for any sample size, using standard statistical methods, without the need for repeated sampling of cohorts.

(2) Other statistical tests are being investigated in order to determine whether any of them might prove to be better discriminators of differences in fertility components.

4. Discussion

The models and results which I have presented here illustrate some general principles which apply to any experiments with simulation models, and in particular to simulations of human populations.

First, simulation experiments may tell the investigator something about the consequences of a postulated set of interactions among variables, or of a postulated range of variation for some component of a complex system; but they say nothing about whether the interactions, or the variation, actually exist. Thus, FERTSIM cannot be used to determine *whether* there is a genetic effect on fecundability, but rather whether small fecundability differences can be detected, and whether, *if* they are genetically determined, they affect fitness appreciably.

Second, the *validation* of a computer model (assuring yourself that the model gives the expected results for certain well-understood cases) is essential before the model is used to study more poorly understood situations. In fact, in the process of validating a simulation model, the investigator may learn that some aspects of the simple test cases were not really so obvious after all. For example, in validating FERTSIM, I attempted to simulate reproductive histories of a natural fertility population, the Hutterites. I discovered that I could not achieve the proper distribution of completed family sizes, spacing of births, and ages at maternity for this population unless I assumed that (1) the length of the postpartum sterile period followed a distribution similar to that for lactating women; (2) the decline in fecundability began at least 20 years before menopause; and (3) the variance in fecundability between women was zero. The requirement for the first of these assumptions was not surprising, and in fact gave me some confidence that the model was sensitive to small differences in the length of the sterile period. The second assumption (a 20-year decline in fecundability) has received some support in fertility studies of other populations, but I was surprised to discover that even for the Hutterite women, who continue to have children well into their 40's, I could not simulate the observed distribution of ages at maternity without imposing this early fecundability decline. Perhaps the most surprising aspect of this validation experiment is the implication that Hutterite women are all nearly identical in their age-specific probabilities of conception. This interesting possibility is one that will be pursued in a future study. However, this result illustrates a third general principle:

The data produced by a simulation model are only as good as the assumptions built into the model. One of the important uses (and misuses) of simulation can be inferred from this statement: If a model produces results which are consistent with observations from the "real world," you are not justified in concluding that the model is correct. But if the results are at odds with reality, then you may be sure that your understanding of the system is incomplete, or that you are introducing an inappropriate simplifying assumption.

The uncertainty generated by the agreement between model and reality is (or should be) a constant source of concern for the modeler. To minimize the possibility of making gross errors in the assumptions underlying a model, it is essential to use as many different prototype systems as possible for validation, always checking for inconsistencies. If the modeler suspects that a particular assumption of the model is producing serious departures from expectation, he or she should alter that assumption in one or more ways and then do additional simulations to determine the sensitivity of the results to the specific nature of that one assumption.

The fourth general principle concerns the nature of the simplifying assumptions included in a model. No simulation model is an exact replica of the real world. The decision of the experimenter as to what simplifications will be made must be based upon the particular set of problems for which the model is intended. FERTSIM, for example, includes the assumptions that there is (1) no reliable contraception or conscious family limitation, (2) no reproductive compensation, (3) no fluctuation in fecundability as a result of prolonged absence of spouses, (4) no divorce, (5) no death of women, their husbands, or their children, and (6) no failure to marry.

Some of these assumptions may be relaxed easily; in fact, I have already indicated how female mortality may be introduced with no modification of FERTSIM. Death of husbands and children, divorce, and failure to marry may be handled in a similar way. However, the first three assumptions are violated in many real populations which are of interest to geneticists, and they may not be relaxed without modifications of FERTSIM (which will be introduced in the next version of the model) and addition of new input parameters. Thus, the results of the current version of FERTSIM are strictly applicable only to natural fertility populations in which spouses are not absent for long periods. In fact, however, lower values of ϕ may be used in FERTSIM to mimic imperfect contraception and frequent, short absences of spouses. In any event, the inclusion of these assumptions was not merely an oversight; it was based upon the fact that if differences in fertility components cannot be detected even in natural fertility populations of the type being simulated, then such differences could certainly not be demonstrated in contracepting populations. At this stage, therefore, FERTSIM is being used to provide guidelines for the most favorable case.

5. Summary and Conclusions

I have used examples of the simulation of human fertility to illustrate (1) the variety of ways in which any system may be modeled; (2) the variety of problems for which simulation models may be used; and (3) the variety of mistakes which may be made in the process of developing and using a simulation model. Some experiments with FERTSIM, a continuous-time, stochastic microsimulation model, have been described. Finally, FERTSIM has been used as a basis for discussing some general principles which are important in the development and use of computer models.

References

Barber, L. J. (1980), Fitness of Huntington's Chorea: A Simulation, Master's thesis, Pennsylvania State University.
Bongaarts, J. (1975), A method for the estimation of fecundability, *Demography* **12**: 645–60.
Boyce, A. J., and MacCluer, J. W., The effects of migration pattern on inbreeding and kinship (in preparation).

Coale, A. J., and Demeny, P. (1966), Regional Model Life Tables and Stable Populations, Princeton University Press, Princeton, New Jersey.

Dyke, B., and MacCluer, J. W. (eds.) (1974), *Computer Simulation in Human Population Studies*, Academic Press, New York.

Henry, L. (1972), *On the Measurement of Human Fertility*, Elsevier, Amsterdam.

Kurland, J. A., Dyke, B., and MacCluer, J. W., Genetic consequences of mating structure in baboons and rhesus macaques (in preparation).

MacCluer, J. W. (1973), Computer simulation in anthropology and human genetics, in *Methods and Theories in Anthropological Genetics* (M. H. Crawford and P. L. Workman, (eds.), pp. 219–248, University of New Mexico Press, Albuquerque.

MacCluer, J. W. (1978), On the probability of demonstrating differential fertility in genetic studies, *Ann. Hum. Genet.* **42**:59–75.

MacCluer, J. W. (1979), Fertility and mortality effects on Darwinian fitness in man, *Hum. Biol.* **51**:391–410.

PART III

ANALYTICAL THEORY

7

The Genetic Structure of Subdivided Human Populations

A Review

LYNN B. JORDE

1. Introduction

Much of the theory of population genetics is based on the assumption that populations are panmictic. While this may be nearly true in some instances, most populations of interest (particularly in man) exhibit some form of subdivision. Most often, spatial subdivision is observable, and population geneticists have studied subdivisions ranging in magnitude from villages to continents. Other types of subdivisions exist as well. Linguistic differences often define barriers to random mating, as do differences in social class, clan or caste membership, and religious affiliation. In addition, various cultural regulations, such as taboos or prescribed mating systems, result in subdivision.

A number of major review papers have been written which deal with population structure (usually emphasizing subdivision): Cannings and Cavalli-Sforza (1973), Cavalli-Sforza (1973), Felsenstein (1976), Goodman (1974) (reviews genetic distance measures), Harpending (1974), Harrison and Boyce (1972) (deals with migration models), Morton (1969), Roberts (1975) (especially concerned with isolates), Schull (1972) (a more historically oriented review), Schull and MacCluer (1968), and Yasuda and Morton (1967). In addition, a number of texts deal to a greater or lesser extent with population structure: Cavalli-Sforza and Bodmer (1971), Crawford and Workman (1973), Crow and

LYNN B. JORDE • Division of Medical Genetics, Department of Pediatrics, University of Utah Medical Center, Salt Lake City, Utah 84132.

Kimura (1970), Eriksson, Forsius, Nevanlinna, and Workman (1980), Harrison (1977), Harrison and Boyce (1972b), Jacquard (1974), Malécot (1948), Maruyama (1977), Moran (1962), Morton (1973), Nei (1975), Salzano (1975), Thompson (1975), Weiner and Huizinga (1972), and Wright (1969, 1978).

Most of these papers and texts emphasize theoretical models and methodology. This review will also cover theory and methodology; additionally, it will summarize the empirical studies thus far carried out in subdivided human populations.

Genetic data from subdivided populations may be analyzed in a number of ways. The simplest is to examine visually the gene frequencies in each subdivision. When the number of alleles and/or subdivisions approaches a moderate number, this method becomes cumbersome. Genetic distance methods can be used to summarize the relationships between pairs of subpopulations. To examine the degree of *overall* differentiation among the subdivisions, measures such as Wright's F_{ST} or a heterogeneity χ^2 provide (under specific assumptions) a convenient comparative statistic. Finally, it may be of interest to examine regular patterns of spatial variation in gene frequencies (clines). The first section of this review will summarize the theories and methods used in these three major approaches to the study of genetic variation in subdividued populations.

Often, data are available on intersubdivision migration patterns. A number of models have been derived to predict the degree of genetic relationship between subdivisions when migration patterns are known. Included among these are island, stepping stone, migration matrix, and continuous isolation by distance models. The theory and underlying assumptions of these models, as well as some empirical applications, will be discussed in the next section.

Once a matrix of predicted or actual genetic correlations is obtained, a number of methods may be employed to provide an easily interpretable two-dimensional display of the intersubdivision relationships. The two principal groups of display techniques, "maps" and "trees," will be discussed in the next section.

Populations can be divided into more than one level of subdivision. For example, there may be several linguistic groups in a population which are in turn composed of counties, districts, or villages. Attempts to deal with *hierarchical* subdivision will next be summarized.

In addition to cross-sectional subdivision, populations can sometimes be subdivided temporally. When sufficient data exist to allow the study of change through time, a number of interesting microevolutionary phenomena can be studied.

In the discussion section of this paper, the concordance of several types of data commonly used to predict genetic structure will be explored. Genetic correlations can be predicted from migration, anthropometrics, isonymy, and pedigree data, as well as from gene frequencies themselves. Empirical correlations among these data types will be tabulated, and theoretical and methodological explanations for the observed degree of congruence will be advanced.

The other topic to be addressed in this section is the set of factors which determine genetic structure itself. Geographic distance is probably the most commonly studied component; in addition, population history, linguistic differences, cultural factors, demographic effects, and random events can each affect the genetic structure of populations.

2. Methods of Genetic Analysis

2.1. Genetic Distance Measures

A multitude of distance measures are currently available. Indeed, it appears that each of the major "schools" of population structure has developed its own favorite distance measure, and a great deal of controversy has been generated over the question of which measure has the most attractive biological and/or mathematical properties. Adding to the confusion is the fact that many of the measures are mathematically similar or identical. This section will summarize the characteristics of the several major groups of distance measures, and the circumstances under which each is most applicable will be indicated.

Several excellent reviews of distance measures are available. Gower (1972) discusses some of the major types of measures (as well as multivariate techniques for their graphic display) and offers some advice on their application to data. Lalouel (this volume) provides an amplified discussion of several of the measures summarized more briefly in this chapter. Goodman (1974) applies a number of distance measures to a set of genetic data for 25 populations from various parts of the world. These results are then subjected to principal coordinates analysis, and a dendrogram of the relationships of the distance measures themselves is obtained by using an unweighted cluster analysis method. This gives a convenient summary of the similarities of different types of measures. Goodman used only three loci in this analysis. It would have been preferable to have used more loci, since, as many workers have noted (Chakraborty and Tateno, 1976; Nei, 1975), the error variance of distance measures becomes very high when only a few loci are used.

Perhaps the simplest possible distance measure is computed by summing the absolute values of the differences in gene frequencies for two populations. This method, used by Livingstone (1963), suffers from at least two liabilities. First, correlations between alleles are not accounted for; thus, a large amount of essentially redundant information is used in computing distance values. Second, the distributional properties of this measure are not known, which means that standard errors of the estimate cannot be calculated, nor can statistical significance be assigned to differences in distance.

A similar measure has been proposed recently by Smith (1977):

$$\delta_i = \bar{X}_i^x - \bar{X}_i^y$$

$$\Delta_{xy} = \left[\sum_i \left(\frac{\delta_i}{\sigma_i} \right) \right]^{1/2} \tag{2.1}$$

where $\bar{X}_i^x$ is the mean value of the ith character in population x, $\bar{X}_i^y$ is the mean value of the ith character in population y, σ_i is the standard deviation of the ith character (assumed equal in X and Y), and Δ_{xy} is then the distance between x and y. This measure has the same drawbacks as the one discussed above.

Perhaps the earliest multivariable measure of distance is Pearson's (1926) Coefficient of Racial Likeness. This measure essentially sums the mean differences in characters, standardizing by the variances of the means. Pearson himself admitted that "the fundamental weakness of the Coefficient of Racial Likeness lies in the fact that it neglects the correlations betwen the characters dealt with" (Pearson, 1926:111).

To correct for this weakness, Mahalanobis (1936) introduced his generalized distance measure:

$$D_{ij}^2 = \sum_k (x_{ik} - x_{jk})' S^{-1} (x_{ik} - x_{jk}) \tag{2.2}$$

where x_{ik} and x_{jk} are the values of the kth character in populations i and j, respectively, S^{-1} is the inverse of the variance–covariance matrix of the variables X. Rao (1952, Chapters 7, 8, 9) gives a further discussion of this measure.

The first major group of distances measures discussed here are derived from Mahalanobis' measure. Sanghvi (1953) adapted the measure for gene frequency data (Sanghvi's G^2). The equation he used to define G^2 can be simplified algebraically to give

$$G^2 = \sum_{i=1}^{n} \sum_{j=1}^{k} \frac{(p_{ij} - p'_{ij})^2}{p_{ij} + p'_{ij}} \tag{2.3}$$

where p_{ij} and p'_{ij} are the frequencies of the jth allele at the ith locus in two different subpopulations. The measure is then summed across loci and divided by the degrees of freedom.

Smith (1977) provides an excellent description of the relationship between Mahalanobis' D^2 and Sanghvi's G^2, and he derives the estimation bias of G^2, giving a correction factor for it. Balakrishnan and Sanghvi (1968) present two other measures, G_c^2 and B^2, that are closely related to G^2.

One of the major problems with all these measures is that they use a single common dispersion matrix. Since variance is dependent on sample size in a multinomial distribution (i.e., the expected distribution for gene frequencies), equal sample sizes are required. A more serious drawback is the fact that the variances and covariances also depend on the gene frequencies. Thus, the common dispersion matrix is strictly valid only when the gene frequencies are equal in all populations! Balakrishnan, Sanghvi, and Kirk (1975) emphasize the robustness of the statistic, maintaining that these assumptions do not cause problems in common practice.

The distance measure of Steinberg, Bleibtreu, Kurczynski, Martin, and Kurczynski (1967) has been shown to be identical to G^2 (Balakrishnan and Sanghvi, 1968). Also Kurczynski's (1970) D_k^2 is very closely related to G^2, although it does not assume equal sample sizes.

Morton's "hybridity" measure, θ, is "nearly proportional" to G^2 (1975a, also Morton, Imaizumi, and Harris 1971). This measure, derived from a matrix Φ of probabilities of identity by descent, is mathematically similar to the Euclidean distance derived from the R matrix of standardized genetic variances and covariances (Harpending and Jenkins, 1973). Conceptually, however, the two measures are quite different: the former deals with probabilities of identity, while the latter treats genetic correlations. Thus, they differ in their assumptions and in a few simple transformations (see Workman, Harpending, Lalouel, Lynch, Niswander, and Singleton, 1973, for a good discussion).

θ can be used as a measure of mean allelic substitutions (Morton, 1974b; Morton and Lalouel, 1973b), assuming that the contemporary mean gene frequencies represent the frequencies of an ancestral founding population. This assumption has been criticized by Nei (1973). Also, Thompson (1976) has carefully analyzed the assumption that identity by descent can be inferred from correlations in contemporary gene frequency data. She points out that identity by descent can be exactly measured only if one analyzes a pedigree which extends from the present subdivided population to the original ancestral population. She demonstrates mathematically that F (probability of identity by descent) and H (allelic correlation) can diverge considerably.

The second major group of distances grew out of the desire of Cavalli-Sforza and his colleagues to use a measure in which the variance of gene frequencies is not dependent on the gene frequencies themselves (as it is in binomial and multinomial distributions). This is because they were using an evolutionary model in which variance measured divergence time and thus would have to be independent of gene frequency. Fisher (1930) first suggested an "angular transformation" of the gene frequency, p, to make the variance of p independent of its value. The transformation was given as $2p = 1 - \cos\theta$. Fisher (1930:205) noted this would make the variance of p "nearly constant" over the range of p, and that, *following* one generation of random mating (a condition often overlooked by contemporary users of the transformation), the distribution of θ will be approximately normal.

Bhattacharyya (1946) applied this transformation to multiallelic loci in order to convert the multinomial gene frequency distribution into a more tractable normal distribution (he appears to have been unaware of Fisher's earlier use of the transformation). Bhattacharyya was the first to use the transformed

gene frequencies in a measure of the distance between two multinomial populations. His equation is of the form

$$D' = \arccos \sum_{i=1}^{k} (p_i p_i')^{1/2} \tag{2.4}$$

where p_i and p_i' are the frequencies of the ith alleles of a k-allelic locus in two
populations.

Edwards and Cavalli-Sforza (1964) reintroduced this transformation, at
the suggestion of Fisher, in their model of evolution as a pure drift Brownian
motion process (further discussion of this model is given below). They inserted
$2/\pi$ on the right side of the equation to force the values of D' to lie between zero
and one. Geometrically, their model represents populations as points on a unit
hypersphere. D' is the arch length between them. Edwards and Cavalli-Sforza
used an approximation to D' in which the chord length, rather than the actual
arc length, is used. Edwards and Cavalli-Sforza (1972) admit that this approximation causes large distances to be underestimated. However, Wright (1978)
found that, in practice, the chord and arc distances give very similar results.

To give the measure more desirable Euclidean properties, Edwards (1971a,
b) introduced the "stereographic projection." This measure retains the inde-
pendent-variance property necessary for the Cavalli-Edwards model of evolution;
it also projects the distance measure onto the Euclidean space in which the
hypersphere is embedded.

The most common criticism of this widely used distance measure is that
its variance-independence property breaks down when p is outside the interval
$0.1 < p < 0.9$ (Balakrishnan, Sanghvi, and Kirk, 1975; Harpending, 1974; Nei,
1973). Cavalli-Sforza (1969) maintains that the measure is useful in the interval
between 0.05 and 0.95, while da Rocha, Spielman, and Neel (1974) conducted
a computer simulation which demonstrated independence in the interval
$0.005 < p < 0.995$. Whatever the allowable range of p may be, there is agreement that the measure is suspect at extreme frequencies. Geometrically, this is
due to the projection of a curved portion of a hypersphere on a flat Euclidean
space.

Using sophisticated techniques from tensor calculus and differential
geometry, Antonelli and co-workers (Antonelli, Chapin, Lathrop, and Morgan,
1977; Antonelli and Strobeck, 1977) have shown that the random drift diffusion
equation only approximates spherical Brownian motion. Due to the existence of
Christoffel velocities, which vanish near the centroid of the gene frequency space,
the approximation to a Brownian motion process becomes worse as gene frequencies approach one or zero.

Another frequently voiced criticism of this distance measure is that it does
not control for correlations among alleles (Sanghvi and Balakrishnan, 1972; Goodman, 1972; Kurczynski, 1970). Edwards (1971a) replies that the transformed

θ values, which are correlated, are "discarded," having been used only to define the desired hyperspace. Thus, the E^2 distance value computed for the Euclidean space is not the product of correlated variables.

A final criticism of this measure, voiced by Gower (1972), is that it is not appropriate for small sample sizes or for data sets in which the sample sizes vary greatly among subdivisions. In fact, Bhattacharyya (1946) himself assumed equal sample sizes.

Masatoshi Nei and his colleagues have long been interested in macro-evolutionary events, such as speciation. The third major group of distance measures, advocated by this school, is well suited for studying macroevolutionary processes and focuses particularly on the length of time since populations have diverged. Nei (1972, 1973a, b) has introduced three distance measures, based on the "gene identity" concept. He defines first the normalized probability of identity of genes from population X and population Y at the jth locus:

$$I_j = \frac{j_{xy}}{(j_x j_y)^{1/2}} \tag{2.5}$$

where $j_{xy} = \Sigma_i x_i y_i$ (x_i and y_i are the frequencies of the ith allele of a locus in X and Y), $j_x = \Sigma_i x_i^2$, $j_y = \Sigma_i y_i^2$, and I_j is summed over all loci to give I. Then, the "standard" genetic distance, D, is given by

$$D = -\ln I \tag{2.6}$$

Nei defines two similar measures, D_m (minimum distance) and D' (maximun distance). For within-species comparisons, these three measures are nearly identical (Nei, 1975; Roychoudhury, 1974). Nei and Roychoudhury (1974a) (see also Mitra, 1975, 1976) have derived the sampling variance of D and advocate the use of 20 or more loci in estimating D in order to reduce the error variance to an acceptable level.

Nei argues that D, since it is linear with evolutionary time, can be used to estimate the number of codon substitutions by which two populations differ. He (1976) and Latter (1973b) demonstrate with simulation that D and Latter's γ (Latter, 1972, 1973a) (which are nearly identical) are linear with time, while a number of other distance measures are not. However, this linearity depends on a constant rate of gene substitution through time. While King and Jukes (1969) and Kimura (1968, 1969) have argued for constancy, evidence has been presented to the contrary (Goodman, Barnabas, and Moore 1974; Langley and Fitch, 1973).

Another assumption made by Nei is that the sample sizes of each population are equal. Chakraborty and Nei (1974) have shown that the measure is quite robust with regard to this assumption, *provided* that there are rather large migration rates between populations. This, of course, diminishes the utility of the measure for species-level comparisons.

In order to estimate effectively the number of codon differences, it is necessary to secure a random sample of the genome, including both mono-morphic and polymorphic loci (Li and Nei, 1975). In human population structure studies, this is often quite difficult.

Slatkin and Maruyama (1975) have shown that a small amount of gene flow ["far too small to be measured" (p.599)] can greatly change Nei's estimate of divergence time. Li (1976) has given a similar demonstration. Therefore, for population comparisons below the species level, the estimation of the divergence times or the number of codon substitutions is questionable. To apply these esti-mates to human populations (e.g., Ward, 1972; Nei and Roychoudhury, 1974b), in which a great deal of gene flow takes place, is nearly always an exercise in futility.

The gene identity approach can also be used in estimating admixture (Chakraborty, 1975). Korey (1978, 1979) provides substantive criticisms of Chakraborty's method.

Hedrick (1971) has taken a rather unique approach by defining a gene identity measure based on genotypes rather than gene frequencies. One reason given for doing this is that "selection operates primarily on the organism in the diploid state" (Hedrick, 1971:277). Nei (1973a) has criticized this measure because it is biased greatly by the mating system of the organism. Also, Cannings and Cavalli-Sforza (1973) have questioned the theoretical appropriateness of this measure. And Morton (1973b) comments that the estimate requires perfect codominance at a locus in order to be useful.

Another way to look at overall genetic distance is in terms of between- and within-groups diversity. Lewontin (1972) adapted the Shannon−Wiener infor-mation index as a genetic distance measure. As the Shannon−Weaver index, this measure is used by ecologists to measure community diversity. It is given by the equation

$$H = -\sum_i p_i \log_2 p_i \qquad (2.7)$$

Lewontin prefers this measure because it yields more "diversity" when there are more alleles at a locus, even if the alleles are of equal frequency. Mitton (1977) criticized this measure because it is insensitive to gene frequency differences of less than 0.5, which certainly invalidates it for use in nearly all human populations. Lewontin's measure has also been attacked on the grounds that it "is not directly related to any genetic entity" (Nei 1973b:3322) (actually, Nei criticizes nearly all distance measures on this basis).

Another rather different approach to genetic distance has been proposed by Carlson and Welch (1977). Their measure calculates the percentage of each population that would have to undergo "genetic death" in order to obtain genetic identity between the populations. Li (1978) gives a simpler version of this measure; his measure requires the estimation of only one parameter (rather than three) and does not require the linear programming procedure used by

Carlson and Welch (see Smith, 1978, for a minor correction of Li's measure). Since selection works faster at intermediate gene frequencies, populations with extreme frequencies will have a greater distance for a given absolute gene frequency difference. This selection model would be inappropriate for most human population structure studies, since many or most markers have no apparent selective advantage. However, in some cases (e.g., the distance between American and African blacks on the Hb_S allele) it would be useful.

Once the genetic distance has been computed for each locus, the issue of a proper weighting for the summation of the loci arises. Many authors prefer not to weight loci (e.g., Nei, 1972; Edwards, 1971a; Sanghvi, 1953). Morton and co-workers (Morton, Yee, Harris, and Lew, 1971a; Morton, Harris, Yee, and Lew, 1971b; and Morton, Roisenberg, Lew, and Yee, 1971c) weight each locus by its information value (i.e., the inverse of its variance among subdivisions). Karlin, Kenett, and Bonné–Tamir (1979) propose a number of functions designed to weight alleles differentially depending on whether they are of high, low, or intermediate frequency. In their analysis of Jewish populations, they find that the results are not affected greatly by the type of weighting function used. When sample sizes are unequal it is sometimes desirable to weight by the sample size at each locus. With distance measures designed to have Euclidean properties, however, any weighting of the loci distorts the Euclidean relations.

With regard to the "best" genetic distance measure, it should be apparent that selection of an appropriate measure depends upon the characteristics of the data and upon one's theoretical perspective. For macroevolutionary (species-level and above) comparisons, Nei's measures are probably the best, since they give the best estimates of divergence time and are related to a well-defined biological process—codon substitution. In microevolutionary studies, divergence times and number of codon substitutions are distorted by ever-present gene flow, and it becomes more important to consider measures that are well defined in a statistical-mathematical sense. Here, one can choose from two basic groups of measures: those of Edwards and Cavalli-Sforza and those related to Sanghvi's G^2. Gower (1972) has recommended that, when sample sizes are approximately equal and the differences in gene frequency are great, Edwards' (1971a) E^2 is preferable. If, on the other hand, sample sizes are quite variable and gene frequencies do not differ greatly (meaning that the dispersion matrices of the populations will be similar), Sanghvi's G^2 or related measures would be most appropriate.

In any event, most measures of genetic distance are highly correlated under most conditions. A large number of studies have reported "high" correlations among different distance measures used on the same set of data (usually in the range of 0.80 to 0.95) (Balakrishnan, 1974; Barrai, 1974; Chakraborty and Tateno, 1976; Gajdusek, Leyshon, Kirk, Blake, Keats, and McDermid, 1978; Ghosh, Kirk, Joshi, and Bhatia, 1977; Jacquard, 1974; Jorde, 1978; Kirk, 1976; Krzanowski, 1971; Lefevre-Witier and Vergnes, 1977; Rothhammer, Chakraborty, and Llop, 1977; Saha, Kirk, Shanbhag, Joshi, and Bhatia, 1976; Sanghvi and Balakrishnan, 1972; Wright, 1978).

In addition, Hedrick (1975) calculated correlations for several distance measures that were applied to theoretical gene frequency distributions (unimodal, bimodal, uniform, and U-shaped). All correlations were greater than 0.85.

2.2. Measures of Population Differentiation: F Statistics

In a panmictic population the fixation index, F, of Sewall Wright (1921, 1951) is defined as

$$F = 1 - \frac{H_o}{H_e} \tag{2.8}$$

where H_o is the observed number of heterozygotes, H_e is the expected number of heterozygotes for a panmictic population in Hardy–Weinberg equilibrium, or $2pq$. The genotype frequencies can then be expressed as

$$p^2 + pqF, \qquad 2pq(1-F), \qquad q^2 + pqF$$

F, then, can be used as a measure of deviation from panmixia.

Wahlund (1928), in a classic paper, demonstrated that subdivision of a population (into "isolates", a term he first coined) increases the frequency of homozygotes (and thus F) for a gene by the amount σ_p^2 (the variance of p across all subdivisions). This implies that greater homozygosis will result when the subdivisions display greater differences in gene frequency. Wahlund assumed no migration among subdivisions, no mutation, and no selection. Also, he assumed panmixia within each subdivision. Sinnock (1975) has extended the Wahlund effect to the two-locus case, showing that subdivision results in an increase of double homozygotes.

Because of the effect of subdivision on F, it is important to examine F in a more detailed fashion. Wright (1943, 1951, 1965, 1969, 1973) originated F statistics for this purpose. Three basic statistics can be defined:

1. F_{IS}: the correlation between uniting gametes relative to the gametes of the subdivision, averaged over all subdivisions — sometimes called "local inbreeding". Under *some* circumstances,

$$F_{IS} = \sum_i w_i \left(1 - \frac{H_i}{2p_i q_i} \right) \tag{2.9}$$

where w_i is the proportion of the total population living in subdivision i, H_i is the observed frequency of heterozygotes in subdivision i, and $q_i = 1 - p_i$.

2. F_{ST}: the correlation between random gametes within subdivisions, relative to those of the total population. For diallelic loci, this statistic is most often estimated as

$$F_{ST} = \frac{\sigma_p^2}{\bar{p}\bar{q}} \qquad (2.10)$$

where σ_p^2 is the variance of p across subdivisions, as in Wahlund's effect, and $\bar{p}$ is the weighted mean of p across subdivisions. In practice, F_{ST} is equivalent (or nearly so) to Harpending's R_{ST}, Morton's $\Phi(0)$, and Cavalli-Sforza's f_θ. Nei (1965) has shown how to estimate F_{ST} for multiallelic loci.

3. F_{IT}: the correlation between uniting gametes, relative to those of the entire population. This is most often estimated by

$$F_{IT} = \frac{H_T}{2\bar{p}\bar{q}} \qquad (2.11)$$

where H_T is the observed proportion of heterozygotes in the total population. When certain assumptions are met, the following relation holds:

$$F_{ST} = \frac{F_{IT} - F_{IS}}{1 - F_{IS}} \qquad (2.12)$$

Expressed in terms of the panmictic index, $P(= 1 - F)$, it is

$$P_{ST} = \frac{P_{IT}}{P_{IS}} \qquad (2.13)$$

Kirby (1975) has shown that F_{IS} can be averaged as in (2.9) only if $F_{NM} - F_{GM} = 0$ (F_{NM} is the covariance of F_{IS} with the square of the gene frequency; F_{GM} is the covariance of F_{IS} with gene frequency itself). The importance of these quantities was noted by Barrai (1971). When $p \neq 0.5$, F_{IS} should be computed as

$$F_{IS} = \sum_i \frac{w_i p_i q_i F_{IS_i}}{w_i p_i q_i} \qquad (2.14)$$

Wright (1951) pointed out that F_{IT} and F_{IS} can be negative (excess heterozygotes), while F_{ST} is "necessarily positive." This is always true when F_{ST} is computed from pedigrees (as was the case in Wright's early work). However, when F_{ST} is estimated from gene frequencies, a correction factor for sampling bias should be subtracted (see Harpending and Jenkins, 1974, or Workman et al., 1973, for discussion). When samples are small, subtraction of the bias factor can result in a negative F_{ST} value. These workers justify this theoretically by noting that F_{ST} was defined as a correlation between gametes and that any correlation can legitimately be negative (Workman, Lucarelli, Agostino, Scarabino, Scacchi, Carapella, Palmarino, and Bottini, 1975). Jacquard (1975) provides another discussion of the problem of sampling error and demonstrates how to separate variance due to sampling from that due to actual heterogeneity.

Negative values of F_{IS} are often attributed to selection in favor of heterozygotes. However, selection which acts to keep genes in linkage disequilibrium can also cause F_{IS} to be negative, even though the alleles themselves can be selectively neutral (Kirby, 1975). The avoidance of consanguineous mating can also lead to a negative F_{IS} (Wright, 1965; Cockerham, 1973). Cannings and Edwards (1969) treat the problem of excess heterozygosis due to small deme size and derive a correction factor for it. Robertson (1965) has demonstrated that a difference in gene frequencies between males and females can lead to excess heterozygotes, and Purser (1966) has shown that differential fertility between genotypes can lead to more heterozygotes than predicted by the Hardy–Weinberg relation. Finally, Harpending, Workman, and Grove (1973) show that simple exogamy can lead to a negative F_{IS} estimate. Since the effects of mating practice and subdivision are confounded, they place little confidence in estimates of F_{IS}. A good review of most of the factors involved in producing excess heterozygosis is given by Workman (1969).

Nei and Chakravarti (1977), noting that Wright assumed an infinite number of subpopulations in his model, show that, when the number of subdivisions is small, the variance of F_{ST} due to drift becomes quite large. To overcome this problem when doing genetic analysis, it is necessary to use a large number of loci so that the error variance is reduced. MacCluer (1974), using simulation, obtained a similar result.

Thus far, the discussion of F statistics has centered on the "traditional" approach developed by Wright. At least three other approaches, which differ somewhat in their theory and methodology (but *not* very much in their empirical results), will be discussed briefly.

Nei (1973b, 1977) has criticized traditional F statistics because of the assumptions of a diallelic locus and an infinite number of subdivisions. He cites evidence from molecular genetics which demonstrates the invalidity of the assumption that forward and backward mutation preserve a locus in only two allelic states. Since many mutations will create a completely new allele, a statistic appropriate for the multiallelic case is needed. Nei also criticizes the "equilibrium" approach of F statistics, which assumes that recurrent mutation and selection act to maintain equilibrium frequencies, which are estimated by the mean frequencies of the population (see Harpending, 1974, for a similar discussion). Since these forces are probably not as important as once thought, Nei prefers the gene identity approach, which does not directly use mean gene frequencies. Nei's G_{ST}, which is identical in interpretation to F_{ST}, is computed using the gene identity method. It can be used for multiallelic loci, and an infinite number of subpopulations is not assumed. Furthermore, Nei maintains it is independent of patterns of selection, migration, mutation, and method of reproduction. The drift variance (due to finite sample size) of G_{ST} has been calculated for some breeding systems (Nei and Chakravarti, 1977; Nei, Chakravarti, and Tateno, 1977).

It is interesting, given the criticism accorded by Nei to the F statistics approach, that G_{ST} is equal to a weighted mean of F_{ST} across alleles (Nei, 1973b). Thus, for practical empirical purposes, the two approaches are identical.

A lesser known approach is that of Cockerham (1969), who used a correlation method to derive his version of F statistics as intraclass correlations. He later extended the model for use on subdivisions of unequal size (Cockerham, 1973). Spielman, Neel, and Li (1977) point out that this approach lends a well-defined statistical interpretation to Wright's rather ambiguous phraseology (e.g., "relative to gametes of the total population"). A disadvantage of Cockerham's method is that it can be used only for codominant diallelic loci.

Finally, Rothman, Sing, and Templeton (1974) present a model in which a multinomial Dirichlet distribution is the likelihood function which is maximized in the estimation of F statistics. Empirically, they find that their technique gives results quite similar to those of Cockerham's least-squares approach. Spielman, Neel, and Li (1977) mention that this method suffers from considerable estimation bias. Nevertheless, as Spielman, Neel, and Li (1977) demonstrate empirically, all four of the approaches discussed give very similar results.

It is common to compare degrees of population differentiation, measured by F_{ST}, in various populations (e.g., Cavalli-Sforza, 1969b; Harpending and Jenkins, 1974). Caution must be exercised in interpreting differences in F_{ST}, however, for a number of reasons. First, the size of the subdivision chosen can greatly affect F_{ST}. Neel and Ward (1972), for example, have criticized Workman and Niswander (1970) for lumping Papago villages into districts in their analysis. They caution that this could mask a great deal of variability at the village level, lowering F_{ST} and possibly causing F_{IS} to become negative.[†] Nei and Imaizumi (1966a.b,c) examined F_{ST} in Japanese populations grouped into several administrative levels. They found higher values of F_{ST} when using smaller units as their total population. At first glance, this might seem counterintuitive, since one might expect small units (e.g., districts, rather than the entire country) to be more homogeneous. But, since the subdivisions of these smaller units are themselves quite small (e.g., villages rather than districts), a large amount of between-subdivision variability can arise from genetic drift and founder effect. When villages are lumped into districts, much of this genetic variability can be canceled out. Thus, one can vary F_{ST} values considerably by the choice of subdivision size.

A second related problem comes about when comparing large technologically advanced countries with small "primitive" groups like the Yanomama, the Bundi of New Guinea, or the Bougainville population. The advanced groups tend to be defined by political boundaries and often encompass a diversity of social, cultural, and economic subgroups. Unless the subdivisions in such populations

---

[†] However, Workman (personal communication) points out that the actual village sizes in the Papago population were usually too small (many less than 30) to enable reliable genetic analysis at this level.

are carefully defined, they too will each include a great deal of variability. The primitive or isolated groups on the other hand, tend to be defined by traditional cultural boundaries; thus a typical sample will cut across much less variability. As a result, the "differentiation" measured in the advanced countries might be much lower simply because each subdivision spans most of the existing variability.

A third difficulty is that of variability in genetic sample size. For obvious reasons, the sample sizes from European populations, for example, are much larger than those from South American Indians. Most writers who have computed F_{ST} have not subtracted the estimation bias factor (see Workman et al., 1973, for discussion). For the large samples, usually taken from advanced groups, bias will be negligible, but for primitive groups, with smaller samples, it can become quite considerable.

All these factors together can account for some of the differences in F_{ST} observed between populations at different levels of development. Of course, this variation will also be due in part to differences in the development of transportation and communication facilities, etc. Indeed, a temporal decline in F_{ST} for several populations is shown below: this is certainly due for the most part to increased migration levels brought on by technological advances.

Table 1 summarizes F_{ST} values for a number of populations. Where possible, census size, sample size, and number of subdivisions have been included. F_{ST} can be calculated on migration and isonymy data as well as genetics and pedigrees, and it is interesting to compare estimates of F_{ST} derived from different sources for the same population. When data are available for several time periods, a decrease in F_{ST} through time is usually observable.

Workman and Niswander (1970) show that F_{ST} is related to the heterogeneity chi-square statistic computed on intersubdivision gene frequency differences:

$$F_{ST} = \frac{\chi^2}{2N_T(k-1)} \tag{2.15}$$

where N_T is genetic sample size and k is the number of alleles at the locus. This equation assumes that σ_p^2 is equal across all alleles at the locus. When this is not the case, another, slightly more complex, equation is given by Workman and Niswander. When differentiation is random, the expected value of χ^2 is equal to its degrees of freedom: $(s-1)(k-1)$, where s is the number of subdivisions in the population. Thus, under random differentiation,

$$F_{ST} = \frac{(s-1)(k-1)}{2N_T(k-1)} = \frac{s-1}{2N_T} \tag{2.16}$$

When comparing a large number of populations, one might expect, on the basis of this relationship, that F_{ST} and s should be positively related, while F_{ST} and N_T should be negatively related. Indeed, Fig. 1 demonstrates a significant positive relationship between F_{ST} and s for 34 populations from Table 1 on

Table 1. F_{ST} Values

F_{ST}	Number of subdivisions	Sample size	Census size	Data type	Population	Reference
0.011[a]	6	490	—	genetics	North India (Delhi)	Roychoudhury, 1974
0.012[a]	4	1,218	—	genetics	West India (Bombay)	Imaizumi, 1974
0.000295[a]	5	53,294	5,199,000	genetics	Scotland	
0.000337[a]	13	381,096	46,253,830	genetics	England	
0.000913[a]	19	447,215	54,186,700	genetics	Great Britain	
0.001375[a]	20	508,475	55,710,700	genetics	United Kingdom	
0.00122[a]	21	48,609	103,540,000	genetics—MN	Japan	Nei and Imaizumi, 1966a
0.00069[a]	45	599,342	103,540,000	genetics—ABO	Japan	
0.0224[a]	12	24,880	289,015	genetics	Isolated Japanese populations	Nei and Imaizumi, 1966b
0.00192[a]	16	6,926	1,962,998	genetics	Kagoshima Prefecture, Japan	Nei and Imaizumi, 1966c
0.00475[a]	14	3,467	847,279	genetics	Tokushima Prefecture, Japan	
0.0067[a]	8[b]	2,623[b]	—	genetics	Mean for 6 Japanese districts	
0.0198	10	681	5,102	genetics	Papago	Workman and Niswander, 1970
0.0358	10	—	—	migration	Papago, 1900–1909	Workman et al., 1973
0.0297	10	—	—	migration	Papago, 1910–1919	
0.0128	10	—	—	migration	Papago, 1920–1929	
0.0077	10	—	—	migration	Papago, 1930–1939	
0.0056	10	—	—	migration	Papago, 1940–1949	
0.0027	10	—	—	migration	Papago, 1950–1959	
0.0077	10	—	—	migration	Papago, entire period	
0.0208	10	713	5,102	genetics	Papago (origin)	
0.0140[a]	10	713	5,102	genetics	Papago (residence)	
0.0108[a]	5	687	10,000	genetics	Tinos Island, Greece	Roberts, Luttrell, and Slater, 1965
0.0324	5	—	819	migration	Juang tribe ("advanced"), India	Ray, 1975
0.0131	5	—	819	pedigree	Juang tribe ("advanced"), India	
0.0045	16	—	1,570	migration	Juang tribe ("primitive")	
0.0016	16	—	1,570	pedigree	Juang tribe ("primitive")	
0.0438	21	—	3,000,000	genetics	Dhangar castes, India	Chakraborty, Chakravarti, and Malhotra, 1977
0.0053	—	—	—	genetics	Western Greenland	Persson, 1968
0.0031	14	1,404	—	genetics	N. Sweden, 1871–1890	Beckman, et al., 1972
0.0024	14	3,493	—	genetics	N. Sweden, 1891–1900	
0.0037	14	5,242	—	genetics	N. Sweden, 1900–1910	
0.0050	14	7,149	—	genetics	N. Sweden, 1911–1920	

Table 1. (continued)

F_{ST}	Number of subdivisions	Sample size	Census size	Data type	Population	Reference
0.0043	14	9,017	—	genetics	N. Sweden, 1921–1930	
0.0060	14	10,209	—	genetics	N. Sweden, 1931–1940	
0.0029	14	15,528	—	genetics	N. Sweden, 1941–1950	
0.0019	14	4,338	—	genetics	N. Sweden, 1951–1960	
0.0018	14	3,481	—	genetics	N. Sweden, 1961–	
0.0008[a]	14	59,862	—	genetics	N. Sweden, entire period	
0.00087[a]	13	35,442	50,775,000	genetics	France	Thoma, 1970
0.00031[a]	7	174,206	14,467,000	genetics	Czechoslovakia	Thoma, 1970
0.0382[a]	43	3,982	122,022	genetics	E. Highlands, N. Guinea	Wiesenfeld and Gajdusek, 1976
0.0201[a]	19	1,766	13,529	genetics	Fore, New Guinea	and Simmons, Graydon, Gajdusek, Alpers, and Hornabrook, 1972
0.094[a]	32	14,117	—	genetics	S. American Indian populations	Gershowitz and Neel, 1978
0.057[a]	29	10,166	—	genetics	S. American Indian populations	Salzano, 1975b
0.046	18	—	—	genetics	Uzbekistan	Ginter, Garkavtseva, and Revazov, 1980
0.060	—		—	genetics	S. African populations	
0.0067[a]	6	883	2,200	genetics	Pure !Kung populations	Harpending and Jenkins, 1973
0.0028[a]	9	1,523	5,700	genetics	Mixed !Kung populations	Harpending and Jenkins, 1974
0.0045	9	512	5,700	migration	Mixed !Kung populations	
0.0492	15	1,128	—	migration	Bougainville	
0.0477[a]	18	2,008	—	genetics	Bougainville	Friedlaender, 1975
0.0082[a]	14	1,240	50,309	genetics	Sardinia	Workman et al., 1975
0.0022[a]	8	5,536	4,682,000	genetics	Finland (counties)	Workman, Mielke, and Nevanlinna, 1976
0.0050[a]	27	5,536	4,682,000	genetics	Finland (districts)	
0.0633[a]	37	2,416	12,000	genetics	Yanomama	Neel and Ward, 1972
0.0358[a]	7	539	2,000	genetics	Makiritare	
0.0067[a]	3	455	1,500–2,000	genetics	Xavante	
0.0116	—			migration	Parma Valley	Cavalli-Sforza, 1958, 1963
0.0356[a]	75	≅3,000	300,000	genetics	Parma Valley	Cavalli-Sforza, et al., 1964
0.0132	33	—	—	genetics	Irish Counties	Tills, 1977
0.0109	15	7,603	11,405	migration	Åland Islands, 1750–1799	Mielke et al., 1976
0.0098	15		12,888	(matrimonial)	Åland Islands, 1800–1849	
0.0066	15	—	18,365		Åland Islands, 1850–1899	
0.0037	15	—	24,841		Åland Islands, 1900–1909	
0.0051	15	—	21,356		Åland Islands, 1910–1919	
0.0035	15	—	20,423		Åland Islands, 1920–1929	

F_{ST}					Population	Reference
0.0010	15	—	19,705	migration	Aland Islands, 1930–1939	Workman and Jorde, 1980
0.0008	15	—	21,196	(parent–offspring)	Aland Islands, 1940–1949	
0.0048	11	1,277	18,365	genetics	Aland Islands, pre-1900	
0.0029	12	2,904	20,285	genetics	Aland Islands, 1900–1929	
0.0009	12	1,871	20,245	genetics	Aland Islands, post-1929	
0.0106	11	279	18,365	genetics	Aland Islands, pre-1900	Jorde, 1978
0.0126	12	742	20,285	genetics	Aland Islands, 1900–1929	
0.0115	12	447	20,245	genetics	Aland Islands, post-1929	
0.0097[a]	12	1,459	19,362	genetics	Aland Islands, entire period	
0.015	—	—	—	migration	Pygmies	Cavalli-Sforza, 1969b
0.02	—	1,600	—	genetics	Pygmies	
0.040	—	—	500	genetics	Australian tribes	
0.042	—	—	30,000	genetics	African "main groups"	
0.38	—	—	—	genetics	Major human races	
0.00078[a]	11	9,965	131,659	genetics	Sweden	Beckman et al., 1972 and Beckman, 1959
0.00050	6	—	1,796	genetics	Skane county, Sweden	
0.0034	6	—	1,442	genetics	Gotland county, Sweden	
0.00184	17	—	5,013	genetics	Goteborg county, Sweden	
0.00464	20	—	8,311	genetics	Vasterbotten county, Sweden	
0.013	6	—	14,570	migration	Mayan villages, Guatemala	Cavalli-Sforza and Bodmer, 1971
0.014	6	—	14,570	genetics	Mayan villages, Guatemala	Cavalli-Sforza and Bodmer, 1971
0.00037	9	467	78,470	migration	Iceland (1900)	Jorde et al., n.d.
0.00123[a]	9	27,128	180,000	genetics	Iceland	Wright, 1978
0.1248	7	—	—	genetics	Major human races	
0.00036	12	—	—	migration	Connecticut R. valley, Massachusetts, 1790–1809	A. C. Swedlund and J. H. Mielke, personal communication
0.00029	12	—	—	migration	Connecticut R. valley, Massachusetts, 1810–1829	
0.00017	12	—	—	migration	Connecticut R. valley, Massachusetts, 1830–1849	

[a] Indicates F_{ST} values used in regression analysis.
[b] These were calculated as mean values over the six districts.

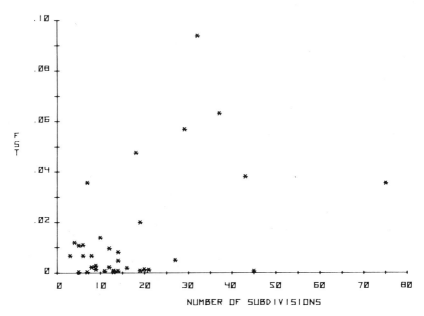

FIGURE 1. F_{ST} (y axis) and number of subdivisions (x axis). Pearson's $r = 0.471$ ($p < 0.003$).

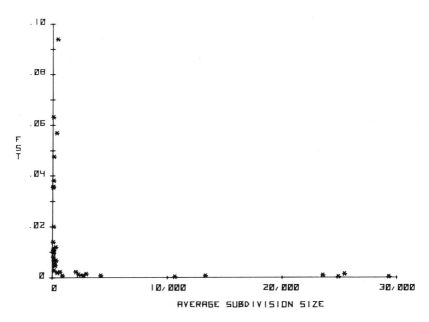

FIGURE 2. F_{ST} (y axis) and average genetic sample size per subdivision (x axis). Pearson's $r = 0.319$ ($p < 0.034$).

which genetics sample sizes were available. The relationship between the average sample size per subdivision and F_{ST} is shown in Fig. 2. Here, the expected negative relationship, while statistically significant, is less well defined than in Fig. 1, with a large number of populations clustering near the origin.

These results demonstrate that some of the observed variation in F_{ST} may well be due to extraneous factors such as sample size and number of subdivisions. Of course, sample size in these studies is often correlated with the level of technological advancement, which, as discussed above, can be legitimately expected to lower F_{ST} due to increased migration rates, etc. Nevertheless, comparisons of F_{ST} across populations would be much more useful if factors such as sample size and number of subdivisions were controlled for.

Lewontin and Krakauer (1973) have developed a controversial method to detect natural selection by examining heterogeneity in F_{ST} across loci. They attribute this idea to Cavalli-Sforza (1966), but Nei (1965) also mentioned it briefly. Basically, Lewontin and Krakauer posit that, since the action of "breeding structure" (i.e., migration, drift, and inbreeding) should affect all loci to the same degree, any significant heterogeneity by locus in F_{ST} can be attributed to the action of selection, which will of course act on different alleles to different degrees. By studying the distributional patterns of F_{ST}, they have developed tests to determine whether observed differences in F_{ST} are due to selection.

Two tests were formulated to test for selective neutrality. The first test develops a statistic defined, for the ith locus, as

$$\frac{(n-1)F_{ST_i}}{\bar{F}_{ST}}$$

where n is the number of subpopulations in the sample and $\bar{F}_{ST}$ is the mean of F_{ST}, calculated across all loci.

This statistic is then compared with a chi-square distribution with $(n-1)$ degrees of freedom, which is the theoretically expected distribution under neutrality. Lewontin and Krakauer use the chi-square goodness of fit test to determine whether the observed distribution differs significantly from the theoretical distribution.

The second test compares the theoretical variance of F_{ST} with the observed variance. The former is defined as

$$\sigma^2 = \frac{K\bar{F}_{ST}^2}{(n-1)} \tag{2.17}$$

where $K = 2$ for binomially distributed gene frequencies.

The ratio $S_{F_{ST}}^2/\sigma^2$ is calculated (the numerator is the observed variance of F_{ST}); the ratio is distributed as $\chi^2/(n-1)$. Significant departure from this distribution indicates that selection has acted on some loci.

Regarding the first test, Ewens and Feldman (1976) emphasize the assumption that all alleles used in calculating F_{ST} values are independent, identically distributed normal random variables. Certainly, this is an unreasonable assumption for most natural populations, including humans.

Nei and Maruyama (1975) point out that correlations in gene frequencies among subdivisions (which can result from high migration rates) will inflate the ratio used in performing the second test. Furthermore, Ewens and Feldman (1976) show that such correlations can lead to a violation of the assumption that the upper limit of K is 2, an important component of the second test.

Robertson (1975) demonstrates a number of ways in which hierarchical population structure can affect the Lewontin–Krakauer statistic. "Genetic sampling" due to historical events (founder effect, bottlenecks, etc.) will often have great effects on F_{ST} at different loci. Robertson maintains that these objections cannot be obviated by the random sampling techniques suggested by Lewontin and Krakauer. Furthermore, he demonstrates that a very large number of loci would be needed to get reasonably precise estimates of the variance components required for the test. Gillespie (1976) concludes that Wright's island model is probably the only breeding structure in which this test is applicable. Also, Nei and Chakravarti (1977) demonstrate that assumptions of this test are violated even under a pure genetic drift process.

Lewontin and Krakauer (1975) have responded to some of these criticisms by imposing a set of strict constraints on the use of their test. Unfortunately, these restrictions tend to make the test inapplicable in most situations.

A modification of the model has been offered by Tsakas and Krimbas (1976), who suggest that many of Robertson's objections can be overcome if only pairs of populations are compared. In addition to its inconvenience, this approach still requires that there be no gene flow between populations after they have split, a condition which, for human populations, is quite unlikely.

Before leaving this discussion, it should be mentioned that Wood (1978) has recently applied the Lewontin–Krakauer test to data from New Guinea, using the method proposed by Robertson (1975) to correct for the inflation of $\sigma^2_{F_{ST}}$ due to hierarchical structure. Interestingly, the difference between the corrected result and the original was slight.

Closely related to F_{ST} and also used to examine intersubdivision differentiation is the heterogeneity chi-square statistic. Workman and Niswander (1970) discuss it well, and they apply it to their Papago data. It has also been used by Imaizumi and Morton (1970) and by Cavalli-Sforza (1963).

Smouse and Kojima (1972) developed a maximum-likelihood criterion to test the hypothesis of equal gene frequencies across subdivisions. They show that their λ is asymptotically identical to χ^2; divergence occurs when samples become small, however. For an application of this method, see Kojima, Smouse, Yang, Nair, and Brncic (1972).

Smith (1969, 1977) has criticized the χ^2 approach to measuring population differentiation, noting that it tests the null hypothesis "that X and Y are randomly chosen samples from the same population" (1977:477), an assumption which, he says, is "usually nonsensical." While it is true that significance tests on χ^2 probably have little meaning, the statistic is nevertheless valuable as a comparative measure. Of course, the cautions noted above for F_{ST} apply equally to χ^2.

2.3. Clines

Often, subdivided populations exhibit systematic spatial gradients in gene frequency. "Clines" were first defined by Huxley (1938), and a number of models have been developed for their analysis. The first analytic treatment of them is Fisher's (1937) model of a dynamic cline (i.e., a gene "wave" spreading through a population). Fisher derived the diffusion rate for a selectively advantageous allele in a population uniformly distributed in a one-dimensional habitat. Kimura (1957) extended Fisher's work to two dimensions. Holgate (1964) has given a modification of this model, and a number of other extensions are reviewed in Felsenstein (1976). Cavalli-Sforza and Bodmer (1971) have applied Fisher's model to the distribution of eye and hair pigmentation in Europe. The result of their application — that the "gene" would move two kilometers per generation — is highly questionable since the selection coefficient for the trait is completely unknown and since the actual spread of the gene would be two dimensional, not one dimensional.

Another application of Fisher's model to human populations is given by Weiss and Maruyama (1976), who used it to compare the plausibility of the "phyletic" versus the "replacement" hypotheses of the evolution of human races. They demonstrate that a gene could diffuse within the time frame specified by the phyletic model. Their two-dimensional diffusion model (which had to be analyzed by simulation) gave the same result. These models are single-gene models, however, while most of the traits used to distinguish races are polygenic (e.g., skin color, anthropometric measures). Presumably, the rate of spread of polygenes would be different than that of single genes.

Other simulations of gene diffusion processes for human populations have been conducted by Livingstone (1969) and by Brues (1972).

Haldane (1948) was the first to develop a model of a stable cline. His model assumed a population uniformly distributed on an infinite plane. On one side of a boundary, AA and Aa would have a selective advantage; on the other side, aa would have the advantage. A similar model was derived by Fisher (1950), who assumed that there is no dominance and that the selection coefficient changes gradually near the boundary between the two populations. Fisher's paper, incidentally, demonstrates the first use of a computer in genetics (Felsenstein, 1976).

Cavalli-Sforza and Bodmer (1971) applied these models to the distribution of ABO frequencies in Japan. The two models gave remarkably similar results, both indicating that the cline in ABO frequencies would have required 20,000 generations for its formation presuming that present selection coefficients were responsible for the cline. Given the implausibility of this result, Cavalli-Sforza and Bodmer concluded that factors other than selection (such as migration) were responsible for the cline.

The most common method of analyzing clines is some form of multiple regression of gene frequencies on geographic coordinates. Examples of the use of this technique for single gene include Beckman, Cedergren, Collinter, and Rasmuson (1972) (N. Sweden), Imaizumi (1974) (United Kingdom), Imaizumi and Morton (1969) (Japan), Imaizumi and Morton (1970) (New Guinea), Morgan and Holmes (n.d.) (Yanomama), Morton (1964) (N.E. Brazil), Morton, Yasuda, Miki, and Yee (1968) (Switzerland), and Nei and Imaizumi (1966a) (Japan). This method has also been used for clines of genetically complex traits. Roberts (1973b) tested Bergmann's and Allen's rules for human populations, finding significant results in the expected direction for both rules.

A slight variation of the regression approach has been used by Ward and Neel (1976) on their Yanomama data. On the advice of Smouse (1974), they use a logit transformation of gene frequencies in their regression equation:

$$\ln \left[\frac{p_i}{1 - p_i} \right] = \beta_0 + \beta_1 (\text{latitude}) + \beta_2 (\text{longitude}) \qquad (2.18)$$

The advantage of this transformation is that it forces the predicted values, $\hat{p}_i$, to lie between zero and one.

Ward and Neel acknowledge that the regression model assumes that the set of gene frequencies derive from independent samples, within and between populations. Smith (1969) has pointed out that this assumption is violated in nearly all human genetics samples. Ward and Neel conclude that significance tests are probably meaningless here, but that, as in the case of the χ^2 statistic, the regression coefficients are of value for comparative purposes. Using the data of Ward and Neel, Morgan and Holmes (n.d.) found that a nonlinear ("second-order geographical surface") model got better results than a linear model in some cases.

Recently, Menozzi, Piazza, and Cavalli-Sforza (1978) introduced an application of principal components analysis to the mapping of clinal distributions. Essentially, the technique involves the computation of the loadings of each population on the eigenvectors derived in the reduction of the matrix of gene frequencies. The method provides a convenient graphic display of clinal variation (or of any type of spatial variation). These authors used this technique to investigate genetic evidence on the diffusion of agriculture in Europe.

A number of models have been developed which have not yet been applied to subdivided human populations. These are given in papers by Clarke (1966), Endler (1973), Felsenstein (1975b), Karlin and Richter-Dyn (1976), Slatkin (1973), and Slatkin and Maruyama (1975b). Much of this work is discussed nicely in May, Endler, and McMurtie (1975); this paper is particularly concerned with the application of these models to field data. An excellent and up-to-date review of nearly all the literature on clines is given in Endler's (1977) book.

3. Migration Models

When studying large populations over long periods of time, attention is usually focused on adaptation, and the action of natural selection is of great importance. In addition, large population sizes allow its detection. In most studies of human population structure, however, relatively small populations are examined over a rather short period of time. Here, the effects of genetic drift and migration become much more important objects of study. Indeed, micro-evolutionary processes are usually dominated by migration (Morton, 1975b; Morton, Klein, Hussels, Dodinval, Todorov, Lew, and Yee, 1973; Spieth, 1974; Smith, 1969) to such an extent that any effects of selection and mutation are "swamped." Therefore, the models discussed below, which tend to focus on the mutual influence of drift and migration, are particularly important in human population structure.

Before discussing the migration models themselves, it is important to elaborate on two of their most important parameters: effective population size and effective migration rate. Population size is important in these models because it is often used to estimate the effect of genetic drift. Wright (1931) introduced the concept of *effective* population size in order to deal with the fact that most populations are not ideal panmictic units; thus, the proportion of the population which effectively contributes to the gene pool at any given time is N_e rather than N. The factors influencing the value of N_e include differential fertility, the presence of more than one generation in a population, the fact that generations overlap, the presence of consanguineous mating, sex ratios not equal to unity, variation through time in population size, and migration (see Fierre-Maia, 1974; Morton *et al.*, 1971; and Weiss and Ballonoff, 1975, for further definition).

Kimura and Crow (1963) distinguish two types of effective size: *inbreeding* and *variance* effective size. The former relates to the increase in homozygosity due to the probability of identity by descent of two homologous genes in a finite population. The latter is due to the sampling variance in gene frequency (i.e., drift), which also leads to an increase in homozygosity. The two effects are often equal. Some errors have been pointed out in Kimura and Crow's equations (Felsenstein, 1971; Crow and Kimura, 1972).

Most of the factors listed above in the definition of N_e act to raise or lower the proportion of homozygotes (as pointed out in the discussion on F statistics). Those effects which increase homozygosis will tend to lower N_e; conversely, those which decrease homozygosis will raise N_e. For example, MacCluer and Schull (1970), in a computer simulation, demonstrate that avoidance of consanguineous mating causes excess heterozygosis,‡ which, in addition to giving negative F_{IS} values, raises effective size.

Variation in population size through time is usually controlled for by using a harmonic mean of population sizes to compute N_e, which tends to emphasize low values in population size. Thus, the effect of "bottlenecks" on genetic structure is accounted for. Cavalli-Sforza and Bodmer (1971) present a useful review of these effects and the formulas commonly used to measure them.

In some respects, formulations for effective size are quite robust. Felsenstein (1971) has shown that haploid models for the estimation of N_e are generally applicable to diploid populations. Also, Hill (1972) demonstrates that measures intended for populations with discrete generations are usually valid for those with overlapping generations.

In studies on human populations, data on fertility, sex ratio, etc., are not always readily available. Therefore, a large number of workers have estimated N_e between $N/4$ and $N/2$ (usually, as $N/3$) (Cavalli-Sforza and Bodmer, 1971; Crow and Morton, 1955; Eriksson, Fellman, Workman, and Lalonel, 1973a; Felsenstein, 1971; Harpending and Jenkins, 1974; Imaizumi, Morton, and Harris 1970; Morton, 1969; Morton, Smith, Hill, Frackiewicz, Lew, and Yee, 1976; Pollock, Lalouel, and Morton, 1972; Roberts, 1975; Salzano, 1971; Smith, 1969; Wagener, 1973). Justification for a N_e/N ratio of 1/3 is given by Bodmer and Cavalli-Sforza (1976). In most contemporary populations, there are three generations: a prereproductive, a reproductive, and a postreproductive age group, each comprising roughly one-third of the population. Since N_e is intended to deal with the reproductive portion of the population, its value will be about 1/3. Of course, age structure will greatly affect the validity of this approach, as Langaney, Gessain, and Robert (1974) demonstrate empirically. Further demonstration of this effect has been given by Cavalli-Sforza (1958), who calculated the proportion of the "genetically active" population of the Parma Valley to be 0.88. Estimates of N_e have in fact varied from 0.12 (Morton and Lalouel, 1973b) to 1.67 (Kimura and Crow, 1963). Nei (1970:695) comments that "the N_e/N ratio in human populations is never constant either spatially or temporally." Thus, estimation of N_e should be made with caution, since arbitrary designations may be seriously in error.

The concept of effective migration, also introduced by Wright (1967), has been discussed much less than that of effective size. The idea is similar, however: migrants into a population usually do not differ much in genetic composition from the resident population, since most immigrants come from neighboring gene pools, rather than from an equilibrium (mean) gene pool. Therefore, m_e is usually smaller than m, the actual migration rate. Wright (1969) gives the following equation for estimating m_e:

---

‡ This effect was demonstrated first by Robbins (1918), who showed analytically that avoidance of brother–sister mating increases heterozygosis in a stationary population.

$$m_e = m\left[\frac{q - Q_0}{q - Q}\right] \qquad (3.1)$$

where q is the frequency of an allele in the population which is receiving immigrants, Q_0 is the frequency of the allele in the immigrants, and Q is the frequency of the allele in the population as a whole. Morton et al. (1971) have contributed a good discussion of m_e and the procedure for estimating it from kinship coefficients in successive generations.

3.1. Discrete Models

The Island Models. Sewall Wright (1931, 1940, 1943) modeled a subdivided population in which each subdivision is panmictic, is of size N_e, and receives a random sample of immigrants from the other subdivisions. In his analysis, Wright considered the dynamics of a single subdivision (or "island"). Genetic drift in the island is inversely proportional to N_e. Drift is balanced by migration (m_e) from other subdivisons (sometimes considered to be a "continent"), and the island will approach the same gene frequencies as the continent when $4N_e m_e \gg 1$. At equilibrium [when $F(t) = F(t - 1)$], for small m_e,

$$F \cong \frac{1}{4N_e m_e + 1} \qquad (3.2)$$

The island model has been applied to human population data in a number of studies. Having determined F from genetic data, Tills (1977) used the equilibrium equation (3.2) to predict the amount of migration necessary to balance the effects of drift in Ireland. Nei and Imaizumi (1966b) have used the same approach to determine the expected value of m for a set of isolated Japanese populations. Roberts (1975) reviews several other studies in which the island model has been applied.

As with nearly all mathematically elegant models, the island model suffers from a number of unfulfilled assumptions. One of these was recognized by Wright himself: "In most cases, the actual immigrants to a population come from immediately surrounding localities in excess and thus are not a random sample of the species" (1943:116). This phenomenon — isolation by distance — was treated by Wright and others and will be discussed below. Also, the equilibrium assumption used in calculating F in (3.2) is usually not met.

Moran (1959) extended the island model to treat more than one island in his analysis of the decay of heterozygosity in a subdivided population. Maynard Smith (1970) studied a similar model in order to determine the effects of migration, population size, and mutation on population differentiation. He demonstrated that the genetic similarity between any pair of "islands" is due only to mutation and migration and that population size has no effect. Spieth

(1974) studied this model further and concluded that, as a rule of thumb, a migration rate on the order of one per generation would be sufficient to override the effects of drift. He then inferred that, since observed differences among subpopulations will seldom be due to drift, differential selection must be responsible.

In evaluating these results, some of which are rather questionable, the criticisms leveled at Wright's version of the island model still hold. In addition, the rate of migration *itself* will often depend on the relative sizes of the subdivisions, as predicted by the gravity model of migration.

Another classic extension of the island model is Levene's (1953) model of random migration into different niches. Here, selection intensity varies by niche. Some of the many modifications of this model are cited in Felsenstein (1976).

Gillespie (1976) has also studied an island model in which selection and migration are considered. In his model, a stochastic element is provided by random fluctuations in the environment, rather than by gametic sampling. The principal conclusion is what would be expected in an island model: when migration increases, gene frequency variance diminishes. A number of other models treat the interaction of migration and selection in subdivided populations. For a summary, consult Karlin (1976).

The Stepping Stone Model. A discrete model in which each subdivision exchanges migrants only with its nearest neighbor was studied by Malécot (1950) and by Kimura (1953). This stepping stone model was studied further and extended to two and three dimensions by Kimura and Weiss (1964) and Weiss and Kimura (1965). In two dimensions, an infinite number of subdivisions are located at the nodes of a rectangular lattice. Symmetric migration takes place once each generation, each subdivision exchanging with its four nearest neighbors (two neighbors in the linear case, six in three dimensions). Systematic pressure, in the form of mutation and migration from outside the population, is included in the model, as is random drift. Kimura and Weiss demonstrate that their model approximates Wright's island model when intercolony migration is zero. Also, the model can be converted to continuous form by simply allowing the intercolony distances to approach zero. Kimura and Weiss study the genetic correlation between subdivisions as well as gene frequency variance. They find that the correlation between colonies decreases as distance between them increases, and that the rate of decrease increases with higher-dimensional models. It is particularly interesting that they find the form of the function to be negative exponential, since this form of the isolation by distance function was derived independently by Malécot (1948, 1959).

In addition to studying genetic correlation, stepping stone models have been used to examine the rate of decay of heterozygosity in subdivided populations (Maruyama, 1970a) (see Maruyama, 1970e,f, 1971a,b,c, 1972a,b, 1973, 1974a,b for additional approaches to the study of heterozygosity decay). One of the most interesting results of Maruyama's work is that the rate of approach to homozygosity appears to be independent of population structure.

Fleming and Su (1974) studied a continuous approximation to a finite one-dimensional stepping stone model. They incorporated boundary effects and considered gene frequency covariance and the probability of identity of genes sampled from the one-dimensional habitat.

A stepping stone model was applied to study the rate of approach to linkage equilibrium in subdivided populations by Feldman and Christiansen (1975). Nei and Li (1973) also discuss the effects of subdivision on linkage disequilibrium. They show that, when there is genetic covariance between subdivisions, the total population may be in equilibrium even though the subdivisions are in disequilibrium.

One of the assumptions of the stepping stone model which is obviously invalid is that the number of subdivisions is infinite. Also, symmetric migration is often not found in natural populations. Maruyama (1969, 1970b,c,d, 1971b) has treated stepping stone models in which these two assumptions are removed. He has studied both rectangular and circular stepping stone models. One advantage of a circular (or a torus, in two dimensions) model is that each subdivision has an equal number of neighbors: "edge effects" are not a problem. Maruyama demonstrated that, for the rectangular model, marked local differentiation results when $N_e m < 1$, a result which would also be predicted by Wright's island model. When $N_e m \geqslant 4$, the population appears approximately panmictic. In his torus model, the criterion for local differentiation is

$$2mN_e < \frac{K}{\pi^2} \tag{3.3}$$

where K is the number of subdivisions. Much of this work is reviewed in Kimura and Maruyama (1971) and Maruyama (1977).

At least two further criticisms of the stepping stone model are worth mentioning (following Bodmer and Cavalli-Sforza, 1974, and Schull and Mac-Cluer 1968). First, the results are based on an equilibrium situation. Clearly, most human populations are not at equilibrium. Second, migration rates are assumed to be constant and isotropic (i.e., the migration rate of a subdivision is independent of its spatial location), a condition which rarely prevails.

Matrix Methods. Several related methods have been derived to deal directly with matrices of actual migration rates between subdivisions. These methods generally proceed from a model in which drift, intercolony migration, and systematic pressure (long-range migration, mutation, linear selection) are specified. Wright (1943) gives the original definition of systematic pressure, and Felsenstein (1976) points out that systematic pressure can be assumed to be linear (i.e., selection is linear) only when gene frequencies are at or near equilibrium.

The end result of the matrix approach is a matrix of kinship coefficients or a variance–covariance matrix, both of which predict the genetic relationships between all pairs of populations. These methods convey the advantage of dealing with the migration rates specific to each subdivision; thus, the unrealistic assumption of equal, isotropic migration contained in the island and stepping stone models is obviated. The principal disadvantage of the migration matrix approach is that it lacks the elegance and generality of the other models. Essentially, the matrix methods are computer simulations which predict population structure on the basis of input parameters.

The migration matrix, M, is a Markov transition matrix whose elements, m_{ij}, give the probability of moving from subdivision i to subdivision j (see Morton, 1973a, for elaboration). The probabilities are preferably based on the birthplaces of parents and their offspring. Matrimonial migration data can also be used to form M; however, to use this type of data one must assume no correlation between differential fertility and migration. Empirical evidence (e.g., Eriksson *et al.*, 1973a) indicates that this assumption is quite often met. Since the effects of mutation and linear selection are usually negligible, systematic pressure is measured as the proportion of long-range migration into the population (Morton, 1973a). Some workers (Harrison, Hiorns, and Küchemann, 1970; Langaney and Gomila, 1973; Morton, 1973a) prefer to make the migration matrix, M' (i.e., the matrix of raw counts – not the transition matrix) symmetric, since asymmetry implies changes in population size through time. This is done by simply averaging m'_{ij} and m'_{ji}. The disadvantage of this approach is that it distorts the actual migration patterns. While Morton (1973a) concludes that asymmetric matrices and their symmetric versions will usually yield similar results when migration matrix algorithms are applied, it is apparent that the results will differ more with matrices which deviate further from perfect symmetry.

The first matrix method to be discussed here is that of Bodmer and Cavalli-Sforza (1968, 1974). They use a backward stochastic migration matrix (i.e., the matrix is formed such that its elements specify the probability that a gene in i came from j) to derive a matrix of predicted genetic variances and covariances. The drift process is simulated by binomial sampling of gametes, and the angular transformation is used to make the gene frequency variance independent of the frequency itself. The expectation of gene frequency at generation n, $p_i^{(n)}$, is given by

$$p_i^{(n)} = \sum_{j=1}^{k} (1 - \alpha_i) m_{ij} p_j^{(n-1)} + \alpha_i x_i \tag{3.4}$$

where k is the number of subdivisions, α_i is the proportion of immigrants to subdivision i from outside the population (i.e., systematic pressure), x_i is the gene frequency (assumed constant) of the immigrants, and M is the stochastic migration matrix. The covariance of the transformed gene frequencies between subdivisions in the nth generation is given by

$$\text{cov}[\theta_i^{(n)}\theta_j^{(n)}] = \frac{1}{8} \sum_{l=i}^{k} \frac{1}{N(l)} \sum_{r=1}^{n-1} (m_{il}^{(r)} m_{jl}^{(r)}) \tag{3.5}$$

where $\theta_i^{(n)}$ and $\theta_j^{(n)}$ are transformed gene frequencies in subdivisions i and j in the nth generation, $N(l)$ is the population size of the lth generation, and $m_{il}^{(r)}$ is the ilth element of the rth power of $(1 - \alpha_i)M_{il}$. When M is a diagonal matrix, this model reduces to Wright's island model. The equation is iterated until the variance–covariance matrix converges.

Bodmer and Cavalli-Sforza point out that, without systematic pressure, which exerts a constant directional force, all alleles eventually will become lost or fixed. Generally, the principal effect of varying systematic pressure is to speed convergence of the process with higher systematic pressure. Often, this has little effect on the ultimate configuration of the relationship matrix (Harpending and Jenkins, 1974).

A number of criticisms of the Bodmer–Cavalli-Sforza model are given in Imaizumi, Morton, and Harris (1970).

Wagener (1973) changed the Bodmer–Cavalli-Sforza model slightly, allowing the vector α to become a matrix, A, where a_{ir} represents the contribution to the ith colony by the rth external source. This way, the effect of systematic pressure from more than one outside source can be accounted for. Applying her method to the Makiritare data of Ward and Neel (1970), Wagener found little difference between her equilibrium results and those obtained using Bodmer and Cavalli-Sforza's method.

A matrix model remarkably similar to that of Bodmer and Cavalli-Sforza was derived independently by C. A. B. Smith (1969). The principal difference incorporated in his model is that the angular transformation is not used.

Imaizumi, Morton, and Harris (1970), working from a recurrence relation given originally by Malécot (1950), demonstrate a matrix method by which a kinship matrix, Φ, is calculated. ϕ_{ii} gives the probability of identity by descent of two homologous genes drawn from population i, and ϕ_{ij} gives the probability of identity by descent of a gene drawn from population i and a homologous gene drawn from j. Their model works directly from a backward transition matrix to Φ, with no angular transformation or expectation of gene frequencies calculated. The recurrence equation for Φ at time t is expressed as three sums:

$$\phi_{ij}^{(t)} = (1 - m_i)(1 - m_j) \sum_{k=1}^{n} \frac{p_{ki}p_{kj}}{2N_k} + \sum_{k=1}^{n} p_{ki}p_{kj}\left(1 - \frac{1}{2N_k}\right)\phi_{kk}^{(t-1)}$$

$$+ \sum_{k \neq 1} p_{ki}p_{hj}\phi_{hk}^{(t-1)} \tag{3.6}$$

where m_i is a vector of systematic pressure values (one for each subdivision), P is the stochastic migration matrix, and N_k are the effective sizes of each subdivision. The term under the first summation is the probability that, for two genes drawn from populations i and j at generation t, both genes derived from the same gene in population k at generation $t-1$. The second term, $p_{ki}p_{kj}(1-1/2N_k)$, is the probability that the two genes are derived from two different genes in k at $t-1$. In the last sum, $p_{ki}p_{hj}$ is the probability that the two genes came from two different populations, h and k, at $t-1$.

Equation (3.6) can be condensed slightly, giving

$$\phi_{ij}^{(t)} = (1-m_i)(1-m_j) \sum_{h=1}^{n} \sum_{k=1}^{n} p_{ki}p_{hj}\phi_{hk}^{(t-1)} + \sum_{k=1}^{n} \frac{p_{ki}p_{kj}[1-\phi_{kk}^{(t-1)}]}{2N_k}$$

(3.7)

Morton (1973a) gives the first sum of this equation incorrectly [as $\sum_{k=1}^{n} \sum_{k=1}^{n} p_{ki}p_{kj}\phi_{kj}^{(t-1)}$]. This is worth pointing out, since the erroneous equation is being replicated in other papers (e.g., Mielke, Workman, Fellman, and Eriksson, 1976).

In Malécot's (1950) original version of this model, m (systematic pressure) represented the mutation rate and was therefore a scalar. Morton's group also used a single value for m (long-range migration) in their early papers (Morton, 1969; Imaizumi, Morton, and Harris, 1970). This allows one to give (3.7) in matrix notation as

$$\Phi(t) = \sum_{r=1}^{t} (1-m)^{2r}P'^r D^{(r-1)}P^r$$

(3.8)

where P is the stochastic migration matrix, P' is its transpose, and $D^{(r-1)}$ is a diagonal matrix which has $[1-\phi_{kk}^{(r-1)}]/2N_k$ in its diagonal. As Cannings and Cavalli-Sforza (1973) point out, it is more realistic to use a vector of long-range migration values rather than the average value, m. This has been done in some more recent publications (Workman et al., 1973; Mielke et al., 1976). However, in both of these papers, (3.8) is cited as the appropriate equation. The correct version of this equation when using a vector of systematic pressure would be

$$\Phi(t) = \sum_{r=1}^{t} M^r P'^r D^{(r-1)}P^r$$

(3.9)

where P and D are defined as in (3.8) and $M = (1-m_i) \otimes (1-m_j)$ [i.e., M is a matrix defined by the outer product of the vectors $(1-m_i)$ and $(1-m_j)$]. Again, this recurrence equation is iterated until Φ converges.

Harpending and Jenkins (1974) show that the "a priori" kinship matrix, Φ, is best transformed to a "conditional" kinship matrix R as follows:

$$r_{ij} = \frac{\phi_{ij} + \bar{\phi}.. - \bar{\phi}_i. - \bar{\phi}._j}{1 - \bar{\phi}..}$$

(3.10)

where $\bar{\phi}_i. = \Sigma_k w_k \phi_{ik}$ (due to symmetry, $\bar{\phi}_i. = \bar{\phi}._j$), w is defined as in (2.9), and $\bar{\phi}.. = \Sigma_{i,k} w_i w_k \phi_{ik}$. This R matrix specifies kinship relative to a *contemporary* array of gene frequencies, rather than to the ancestral array. Note that the quantity $R_{ST} = \Sigma_i w_i r_{ii}$ is a direct estimate of Wright's F_{ST}.

Another matrix approach is that of Hiorns, Harrison, Boyce, and Küchemann (1969). Their method differs considerably from the others in that they begin with a hypothetical population whose subdivisions are unrelated. Their recurrence model is then iterated until a prescribed level of homogeneity is obtained. Application of their model to Oxfordshire migration data yields the prediction of very rapid convergence to 95% common ancestry. They remark on the rapidity of the convergence; however, this should not be surprising, since their model ignores the effect of genetic drift, which would certainly slow the convergence process considerably (for small populations). One of the more interesting features of their approach is Hiorns' (1971) addition of a linear function that models a decrease in endogamy through time.

This group has also applied their migration model to data on migration between social classes in England (Harrison, Hiorns, and Küchemann 1970; Harrison, Küchemann, Hiorns, and Carrivick, 1974a; Hiorns, Harrison, and Gibson, 1977; Hiorns, Harrison, and Küchemann, 1973). In spite of rather strong assortative mating by class, their model predicts homogeneity (assessed by their 95% criterion) in only nine generations, when exchange matrices from marriage and parent–offspring mobility are combined.

Recently, Carmelli and Cavalli-Sforza (1976) have formulated a "star model" of migration. Basically, the model consists of "strings" of colonies between which migration can occur; all are connected to a central population, and each string has a unique external source of gene flow. At equilibrium, clines are formed along the strings. This model would be particularly applicable for centripetal or centrifugal migration processes (e.g., urbanization).

As Carmelli and Cavalli-Sforza, among others, have pointed out, a drawback of all matrix methods is that they assume a matrix of migration probabilities that remain constant through time. Since many human populations have recently undergone drastic changes in both the magnitude and direction of their migration, a model which projects current migration rates to an equilibrium solution must be regarded with caution. Wood (1977) has dealt with this problem and concludes that "the observed migration rates must have been constant for at least as many generations as the number of powerings it takes for M to converge" (p.311). Wood's position is a bit too conservative, however, since the number of iterations required for convergence of the migration model is subject to a number of purely artificial constraints. The most salient of these is the convergence criterion itself, which can be varied arbitrarily in the computer program and has no real biological relevance. A more stringent convergence criterion will of course lead to a larger number of required iterations.

One way to test the plausibility of equilibrium results is to examine the first eigenvector of the transition matrix, which gives the equilibrium distribution of population sizes (Bodmer and Cavalli-Sfora, 1968, 1974). This can then be compared to the actual proportions of population sizes $(w_1, w_2, \ldots, w_k)$ to determine whether the present migration pattern would maintain w approximately in its present form. Cavalli-Sforza and Zei (1967) found a fairly good agreement between observed and equilibrium values for the Parma Valley migration data, as did Malcolm, Booth, and Cavalli-Sforza (1971) for Bundi clans in New Guinea. For populations which have been undergoing substantial changes in their migration pattern, one would not expect good agreement between the two vectors, and this has been found in at least one case: the Åland Islands, Finland (Jorde, 1978).

Wood (1977) has suggested another method for evaluating the stability of migration patterns. He examines the eigenvalues of a matrix of partial derivatives which describe changes in population sizes due to growth (exponential growth is assumed) and migration. If all eigenvalues are less than zero, the system is stable. The most obvious difficulty with this technique is the assumption of exponential growth of the populations. Certainly, this growth pattern in any human population is not conducive to long-term stability! The method would be much more useful if a more realistic growth pattern could be used (an oscillatory pattern, perhaps, or even logistic growth).

Another often-violated assumption of the matrix method is that migrants are a random sample of the population from which they came. Kempton (1971) has demonstrated that "selective" migration can easily lead to genetic divergence between two populations. Harrison et al. (1974b) discuss this problem and give some empirical evidence for differential migration by I.Q. score. Also, Shapiro and Hulse (1939) showed that Japanese immigrants to the United States were not physically representative of the population of Japan. There are cases, however, in which immigrants do appear to represent a random sample of the parent population (e.g., Susanne, 1979).

Fix (1978) has also treated this problem in his study of kin-structured migration (also termed the "lineal effect"). He demonstrates empirically, with data from the Semai Senoi of Malaysia, that this type of migration is generally less effective in reducing heterogeneity than would be the migration of random samples. Using simulation, he shows the same effect; in fact, under some circumstances, kin-structured migration can increase heterogeneity.

The Gravity Model. A fundamentally different way to treat migration is to assume that the probability of migrating to another subdivision is directly proportional to the subdivision's size and inversely proportional to the distance traveled to the subdivision. Appropriately, this has been called a gravity model; the number of exchanges between i and j, n_{ij}, can be given by

$$n_{ij} = \frac{CN_iN_j}{d_{ij}^r} \qquad (3.11)$$

where N_i and N_j are the population sizes of i and j, d is the distance between i and j, and C and r are fitted by a least-squares method. The gravity model shown here follows a Pareto distribution. Courgeau (1974) summarizes several interesting applications of this model to data from human populations. Also, Cavalli-Sforza (1958) applied this model to migration data from the Parma Valley and got a good fit for short distances (95% of his sample). He also applied it to a Swedish parish and the city of Philadelphia with good results. Lalouel and Langaney (1976) have also applied the model in several forms, with moderate success, to migration data from Senegal. The model has additionally been used sometimes to predict migration rates when they are not known (e.g., Morton *et al.*, 1971b; Pollock, Lalouel, and Morton, 1972).

Graph Theoretic Approaches. A migration matrix is a directed graph. At least two graph theoretic approaches have been applied to migration matrices. Lalouel and Langaney (1976) show how to calculate the mean first passage time for a migration matrix. This specifies the average number of generations it would take a gene to get from i to j under a given migration pattern. Workman and Jorde (1979) have introduced the use of a connectivity measure for migration matrices. Connectivity, as they apply it, specifies the percentage of pairwise combinations of subdivisions that will be "connected" by migration in a given number of generations.

3.2. Continuous Models

Wright's Neighborhood Model. As noted above, Wright recognized that the lack of isolation by distance in his island model was a severe liability. His "neighborhood" model (Wright, 1943, 1951, 1969), which assumes a uniformly distributed population, does incorporate the isolation by distance property. This is accomplished by restricting the distribution of the parent–offspring migration distance. The neighborhood size has been defined as "the effective population number in an area from which the parents may be assumed to be drawn at random" (Wright, 1951:332). Mathematically, this is given by $2\pi\sigma^2$, where σ is the standard deviation of the parent–offspring migration distances. Wright assumed that the parent–offspring migration distribution was normal; however, he was aware that it was usually quite leptokurtic. In his 1951 paper he commented that neighborhood size seemed to be largely independent of the form of this distribution, and in his 1969 text he provides evidence for this. Another assumption is that σ^2 for grandparent–grandchild migration distances is twice that of parent–offspring distances, and so on for each preceding ancestral generation.

Wright demonstrated the relation between F and neighborhood size in one- and two-dimensional models. He also gave an approximate relation for the decline of gametic correlation with distance. Applications of this model to human data are cited in Harrison and Boyce (1972) and in Roberts (1975), and Wright (1978) lists a number of applications to other organisms.

Many of the assumptions of this model are open to question. Human populations are seldom distributed continuously, and panmixia within neighborhoods rarely obtains. Normality of the parent—offspring distances, while perhaps not too important, is certainly questionable. Roberts (1975) has summarized several other criticisms of the model.

Rohlf and Schnell (1971) used computer simulation to investigate this model. They were particularly interested in measuring genetic differentiation over many generations. They found that, after a large number of generations, the amount of differentiation given by one-, two-, or three-dimensional models differed very little. This is of course different from the results of most other investigators (Kimura and Weiss, 1964; Malécot, 1948; Wright, 1951). Also, the predicted rate at which the inbreeding coefficient increased through time differed considerably from that predicted analytically by Wright.

The question of the actual distribution of parent—offspring and matrimonial migration distances has stimulated a number of curve-fitting attempts. Generally, observed distributions are leptokurtic and skewed to the left. Brownlee (1911), who was studying the spread of epidemics, was apparently the first to notice this. Sutter and Tran-Ngoc-Toan (1957) fitted a negative exponential distribution to their French data and obtained a reasonably good fit. Cavalli-Sforza (1958) used the same distribution on his Parma Valley data, with good results except in the zero distance class. This distribution has been used more recently by Boyce, Küchemann, and Harrison (1967) (Oxfordshire), Fix (1974) (Malaysia), and Swedlund (1972) (historic Deerfield, Massachusetts), all of whom were interested in the effect of "neighborhood knowledge" on migration distance. Cavalli-Sforza (1962) suggested forms of the gamma distribution (including a truncated gamma to eliminate the zero distance problem), and Gedde-Dahl (1973) has applied an augmented gamma distribution to matrimonial migration distances in Norway, with fairly good results. Imaizumi (1977, 1978) applied gamma and negative exponential distributions to matrimonial migration distances from Japanese cities and districts, failing to get good fits. The gamma distribution was also applied to matrimonial migration data from Ann Arbor, Michigan, by Spuhler and Clark (1961). Here the distribution provided a good approximation to the data. Yasuda and Kimura (1973) obtained a surprisingly good fit to a parent—offspring distribution from Japan using a normal distribution (the zero class was again a problem, however). For matrimonial migration data, the normal distribution did not fit well, and an exponential and a "K" distribution was used. The K distribution, derived by Malécot, is a combination of Bessel and gamma functions. Yasuda (1975), using a random walk model, also applied the K distribution, obtaining a good fit to data from Japan and the Parma Valley.

This diversity of models and results is due in part to the effects of many different factors on the distribution of migration distances. A number of these, including population density, marital age, occupation, and social class, have been discussed by Coleman (1973) and by Küchemann, Harrison, Hiorns, and Carrivick (1974).

Malécot's Isolation by Distance Model. During the past ten years, the approach to isolation by distance of Malécot (1948, 1950, 1959, 1973) has largely supplanted the use of Wright's neighborhood model. Morton and colleagues (Imaizumi, Morton, and Harris, 1970; Morton, 1969; Yasuda and Morton, 1967), have been responsible for popularizing the use of Malécot's model in the evaluation of kinship coefficients estimated from genetic or anthropometric data, or predicted from migration data.

The model assumes a population distributed uniformly along an infinite line; the probability of migration depends only upon distance. Also, it is assumed that no clines in gene frequency exist. The mean kinship coefficient, $\phi(d)$, for individuals who are a distance d apart can be expressed as

$$\phi(d) = ae^{-bd} \tag{3.12}$$

where a is a measure of local kinship and can be estimated by

$$a \cong \frac{1}{1 + 4N_e \sigma m^{1/2}} \tag{3.13}$$

where N_e is effective population size, σ is the standard deviation of the distribution of marital migration distances, and m is systematic pressure. b specifies the rate of exponential decline of $\phi(d)$ and can be estimated by

$$b = \frac{(8m)^{1/2}}{\sigma} \tag{3.14}$$

In practice, a and b are usually estimated by a nonlinear regression technique.

Malécot (1959), recognizing that local kinship would be affected by the dimensionality of the migration process, reformulated (3.12) as

$$\phi(d) = ae^{-bd}d^{-c} \tag{3.15}$$

where $c = 0$ for a linear model, $1/2$ for a two-dimensional model, and, as Kimura and Weiss (1964) showed, 1 for a three-dimensional model.

It has since been demonstrated that, for the rather short distances commonly encountered in human population structure studies, c is effectively zero for all forms of migration (Imaizumi, Morton, and Harris, 1970; Morton, 1972).

Because $\phi(d)$ is estimated from sample mean gene frequencies, it occasionally becomes negative at large distances. Since it is a probability measure, it has little meaning when negative. Accordingly, Morton, Miki, and Yee (1968) modified the equation:

$$\phi(d) = (1 - L)ae^{-bd} + L \tag{3.16}$$

where L is interpreted theoretically as a correction factor to account for the deviation of the contemporary population from the ancestral founding population, or, more simply, as "kinship at large distances" (Morton and Lalouel, 1973b). Harpending (1971, 1973a, 1974; see also Morton, 1971) has criticized the use of this scalar as an *ad hoc* procedure which has no theoretical justification.

Since the existence of areas of high population density can significantly alter estimates of a, Morton *et al.* (1968) offer a transformation which gives constant density.

The Malécot approach has been evaluated critically in review papers by Cannings and Cavalli-Sforza (1973) and Cavalli-Sforza (1973). They feel that the definitions of a and b are rather vague and that short-range migration (on which a depends) and long-range migration (on which b depends) are difficult to distinguish realistically. They note also that the equilibrium assumption of the model is difficult to fulfill and that most areas are sufficiently heterogeneous to make the assumption of a uniform distribution questionable. Harrison and Boyce (1972) have called into question the assumption that systematic pressure operates uniformly on all populations. And Workman and his colleagues (Mielke *et al.*, 1976; Workman, Mielke, and Nevanlinna, 1976) have demonstrated that treating subdivisions separately often reveals interesting patterns of isolation by distance which would be masked using the conventional Malécot approach.

Felsenstein (1975a) maintains that the assumptions of Malécot's model are internally inconsistent and that, since the evolution of lines of descent is a branching process, most lines will go extinct in time and eventually clumps of populations will form along the linear dimension in Malécot's model. Only as the line goes to infinity will a uniform distribution occur. Therefore, Felsenstein dismisses Malécot's model as "biologically irrelevant" and concludes that stepping stone models are much more useful and realistic.

Lalouel (1977) has answered these objections in detail, demonstrating some misinterpretation of Malécot's assumptions as well as a mathematical error in Felsenstein's analysis.*

One of the advantages of the Malécot approach is that it allows the study of huge numbers of subdivisions. For example, Morton *et al.* (1968) studied over 3000 Swiss communes; certainly, a migration matrix approach would not have been feasible here. Another advantage is that the structures of various populations can be compared by examining their a and b values (Morton 1974a, 1977). Morton, Dick, Allan, Izatt, Hill, and Yee (1971) have generalized that large values of a (> 0.03) tend to be found in island and primitive populations, and large b values are found in continental isolates (e.g., Swiss Alpine isolates), but not in hunter–gatherer or oceanic island populations. This type of generalization has been criticized by Workman, *et al.* (1973), who point out that population size is an important factor influencing a and b. Mielke *et al.*. (1976), who found a large b value (about 0.5) for an island population, question Morton's

---

* For the most recent discussion of this issue, see Felsenstein, J. (1979), Isolation by distance: reply to Lalouel and Morton, *Ann. Hum. Genet.*, **42**:523–527; Lalouel, J. M. (1979), Comment on Felsenstein's reply to Lalouel and Morton, *Ann. Hum. Genet.*, **42**:529.

Table 2. Malécot's a and b Values[a]

Morton's classif.	a	b	System	Population	Reference
Hunter–gather and horticulturalist populations					
2	0.057	0.002[b]	genetics	Australian aborigines	Keats, 1977
2	0.040	0.046[b]	genetics	New Guinea aborigines	Friedlaender, 1971a, b
2	0.051	0.105[b]	genetics	Bougainville Islanders	
2	0.059	0.095[b]	migration	Bougainville Islanders	
2	0.054	0.232[b]	anthropometrics	Bougainville Islanders	
2	0.053	0.040[b]	genetics	Makiritare	Lalouel and Morton 1973
2	0.038	0.003[b]	genetics	South and Central American Indians	Roisenberg and Morton, 1970, Lalouel and Morton, 1973
2	0.030	0.052[b]	genetics	New Guinea	Imaizumi and Morton, 1970
1	0.033	0.001[b]	genetics	Micronesia	
3	0.014	0.001[b]	isonymy	N.E. Brazil	Azevedo, Morton, Miki, and Yee, 1969
3	0.083	0.006[b]	race + height		
3	0.026	0.014[b]	blood pressure		
3	0.003	0.002[b]	genetics		
3	0.017	0.0002[b]	pedigree		
3	0.055	0.002[b]	genetics	E. Caroline Islands	Morton and Lalouel, 1973
1	0.057	0.002[b]	anthropometrics		
1	0.043	0.005[b]	migration	Marshall Island atolls	Pollock, Lalouel, and Morton, 1972
2	0.045	0.009[b]	migration	Western New Guinea aborigines	Gajdusek et al., 1978
2	0.044	0.013[b]	migration	Bedik, E. Senegal	Langaney and Gomila, 1973
2	0.010	0.069[b]	migration	Niokholonko, E. Senegal	
2	0.018	0.046[b]	genetics	Bedik	Langaney, Gomila, Bouloux, 1972
2	0.018	0.066[b]	genetics	Papago (residence)	Workman et al., 1973
2	0.047	0.013	genetics	Papago (origin)	
2	0.013	0.005[b]	migration	Papago	
	$\bar{a} = 0.038$	$\bar{b} = 0.035$			

Table 2. (continued)

Morton's classif.	a	b	System	Population	Reference
Modern continental populations					
2	0.005	0.862 [b]	migration	Oxfordshire	Imaizumi, Morton, and Harris, 1970
2	0.003	0.011 [b]	genetics	Swiss Alpine towns	Morton et al., 1973
2	0.007	0.064 [b]	genetics	Swiss Alpine isolates	
2	0.002	0.083 [b]	isonymy	Swiss Alpine towns	
2	0.004	0.126 [b]	isonymy	Swiss Alpine isolates	
3	0.006	0.026 [b]	genetics	Ferrera Province, Italy	Zanardi, Dell'Acqua, Menini, Barrai, 1977
3	0.001	0.025 [b]	genetics	Belgian recruits	Dodinval, 1970
3	0.001	0.008 [b]	genetics	Japan	Imaizumi and Morton, 1969
3	0.002	0.005 [b]	genetics	Sweden	
3	0.002	0.096 [b]	pedigree	Norway	Gedde-Dahl, 1973
3	0.003	0.002 [b]	pedigree	Gyoda City, Japan	Imaizumi, 1977
3	0.004	0.023 [b]	pedigree	Hasuda City, Japan	
3	0.003	0.048 [b]	pedigree	Minami-cho District (rural), Japan	Imaizumi, 1978
3	0.007	0.212 [b]	pedigree	Shinsie-cho District, Japan	
3	0.009	0.007 [b]	migration	Kumamoto Prefecture, Japan	Imaizumi, 1971
3	0.018	0.941 [b]	migration	Uto City, Japan	
3	0.014	0.214 [b]	migration	Shimomashiki *gun*, Japan	
3	0.015	1.724 [b]	migration	Tomiai village, Japan	
3	0.004	0.004 [b]	pedigree	Japan (entire)	
3	0.001	0.002 [b]	migration	Yokohama City, Japan	
3	0.0021	0.023 [b]	genetics	Switzerland	Morton et al., 1968
	$\bar{a} = 0.005$	$\bar{b} = 0.215$			

Modern island populations

1	0.005	1.242[b]	isonymy	Barra Island, Scotland	Morton et al., 1968
	0.004	0.031	isonymy	Barra, with other areas in Scotland	
1	0.010	0.006[b]	genetics	Barra Island	
1	0.010	0.100[b]	genetics	Sardinia	Workman et al., 1975
1	0.006	0.006[b]	genetics	Lewis Island, Scotland	Morton et al., 1977
1	0.013	0.008[b]	genetics	Orkney Island, Scotland	
	0.0091	0.0360	migration	Åland Islands, Finland, 1750–1799	Mielke et al., 1976
	0.0086	0.0412	(matrimonial)	1800–1849	
	0.0050	0.0400		1850–1899	
	0.0026	0.0376		1900–1909	
	0.0018	0.0364		1910–1919	
	0.0014	0.0368		1920–1929	
	0.0003	0.0217		1930–1939	
1	0.0002	0.0214[b]		1940–1949	
	0.0156	0.539	genetics	Åland Islands, Finland	
	0.0099	0.0361	migration	Åland Islands, Finland, pre–1900	Workman and Jorde, 1980
1	0.0069	0.0332[b]	(parent–	1900–1929	
	0.0034	0.0375	offspring)	post–1929	
	0.0151	0.1999	genetics	Åland Islands, Finland, pre–1900	
1	0.0168	0.5000	genetics	1900–1929	
	0.0149	0.5000	genetics	post–1929	
1	0.0135	0.5000[b]	genetics	all periods	

$\bar{a} = 0.008$ $\bar{b} = 0.181$

[a] When several values are given for different time periods, only the most recent time period (or the entire period value) was used in making Figs. 3 and 4. Also, values of b above 0.4 were plotted as 0.4 in the figures.
[b] Values used in plotting Figs. 3 and 4.

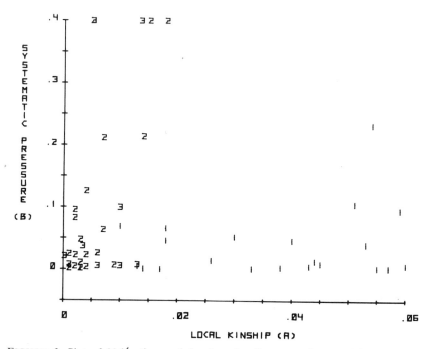

FIGURE 3. Plot of Malécot's *a* and *b* values. 1 – Hunger–gatherer and horticulturalist populations; 2 – modern continental populations; 3 – modern island populations.

generalization, as do Spielman, Neel, and Li (1977), who note the importance of size of the study area, heterogeneity of subdivisions, assortative mating, and social and ethnic stratification.

To examine empirically the generalizations that can be made about *a* and *b*, a fairly complete summary of computed *a* and *b* values has been compiled in Table 2. It is interesting to note, as in Table 1, the decline in kinship values through time in those studies in which temporal stratification was possible.

The populations are divided here into three groups, based on cultural and ecological characteristics: hunter–gatherers and horticulturalists, modern island populations, and modern continental populations. Patterns of variation of *a* and *b* in these groups are summarized in Fig. 3, where values of *a* and *b* for each group are plotted against each other (only the values in Table 2 which are accompanied by a "*b*" are used). From the figure, it is apparent that group 1 (hunter-gatherers and horticulturalists) has higher *a* values than the other two groups. This was confirmed by a *t* test of mean *a* values (see Table 3).[§] There is, however, no significant difference between groups 2 and 3 (islands and continental populations) in terms of local inbreeding. This indicates that, for most

---

§ Since some of the assumptions of this test are violated by these data, the significance values must not be taken too literally. They are, however, useful for comparison.

Table 3. T values from t Tests on Mean Values of Malécot's Parameters

	Author's classification		Morton's classification	
Groups	a	b	a	b
1–2	$7.40(p = 0.001)$	$-1.88(p = 0.0370)$	$-1.06(p = 0.150)$	$0.52(p = 0.307)$
1–3	$6.58(p = 0.001)$	$-1.32(p = 0.115)$	$1.37(p = 0.093)$	$0.00(p = 0.500)$
2–3	$-1.29(p = 0.115)$	$-0.14(p = 0.445)$	$2.86(p = 0.004)$	$-0.59(p = 0.279)$

technologically advanced populations, transportation facilities have virtually erased differences in inbreeding between these two types of populations. A one-way analysis of variance of the *a* values yielded a significant F value ($F = 35.52$, $p < 0.001$).

An examination of *b* values indicates less variation between populations with respect to this parameter. The only significant difference is between populations 1 and 2: island populations show a more rapid decline of kinship with distance than do hunter–gatherer/horticulturalist populations. As expected, analysis of variance of the *b* values yields a nonsignificant ($p = 0.13$) F value.

Since Morton (1973d) has also used a three-group classification of *a* and *b*, it is of interest to summarize his categories as well. He grouped the populations according to "ecological" considerations: oceanic islands, isolates, and conti-nental regions. Figure 4 is a plot of *a* against *b*, using this classification (see

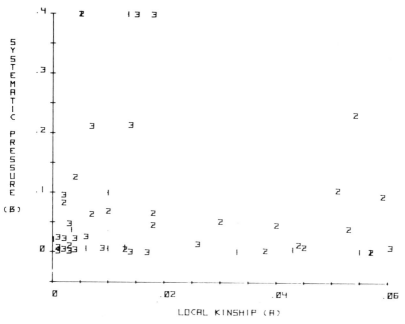

FIGURE 4. Plot of Malécot's *a* and *b* values, using Morton's classification system. 1 – Oceanic islands; 2 – isolates; 3 – continental populations.

Table 2 for a designation of which populations were grouped into each of Morton's categories). There appears to be somewhat less "clustering" of Morton's three groups than of the groups presented in Fig. 3. This is borne out by the analysis of variance, which gives considerably lower F values for a ($F = 4.094$, $p = 0.023$) and b ($F = 0.188$, $p = 0.830$). Similarly, Table 3 shows only one significant t value using these categories: the a value, for isolates vs. continental populations.

These comparisons indicate that a classification which takes culture type into consideration results in better differentiation of a and b values than one which considers only the ecological setting of the populations. However, Table 2 and Figs. 3 and 4 show that both classifications result in a great deal of within-groups variation. Thus, generalizations regarding "categories" of a and b values must be viewed with caution.

4. Display Methods

Similarity and distance matrices computed from genetics, migration or other data can be difficult to interpret when the number of subdivisions exceeds five or so. Two approaches to the convenient graphic display of these matrices are commonly used: the topology, or "map," approach, and the "tree" approach. These will be discussed briefly, and a comparison will be made of their relative advantages and disadvantages.

4.1. Topology

This approach is based on principal components analysis and its variations. The eigenvectors of a variance—covariance matrix provide a dimensional reduction of the matrix; often, the first two or three eigenvectors account for enough of the total variance to allow a good representation of the matrix. Apparently, the first application of this technique to data on human population structure was that of Rao (1952), who applied it to a matrix of Mahalanobis' D^2 values compiled from anthropometric measures. Cavalli-Sforza (1963, 1966) was the first to use principal components analysis on human genetics data in an analysis of worldwide gene frequencies. Harpending and Jenkins (1973) provide an excellent discussion of the details of principal components analysis and an application to human genetics data (for further discussion of this and related techniques, see Lalouel, this volume).

Gower (1966) has outlined a method quite similar to principal components analysis, called principal coordinates analysis. This method is a "Q-technique" (while principal components analysis is an "R-technique") and extracts eigenvalues and eigenvectors from a genetic distance matrix. If principal components and principal coordinates analysis are applied to the same standardized data set, their results will be identical (Sneath and Sokal, 1973).

Gower (1971a,b), Lalouel (1973), and Schönemann and Carroll (1970) have developed useful modifications and extensions of these techniques. Numerous examples of their application are given in the population structure analyses of Morton and his colleagues.

A method whose end result is very similar to that of principal coordinates analysis is nonmetric multidimensional scaling (MDS). However, the method itself is quite different (see Kruskal, 1964a,b, for discussion of one type of MDS). Since MDS is a nonmetric technique which analyzes the rank orders of distances, it can occasionally overcome problems to which distribution-sensitive metric techniques are prone (Lalouel, 1973). However, the configurations computed by MDS are generally very much like those of principal coordinates analysis (Gower, 1972; Harpending, 1974). A few examples of the use of MDS in population structure are given in Fix and Lie-Injo (1975), Kendall (1971), Morton *et al.* (1977), and Neel, Rothhammer, and Lingoes (1974).

Sometimes a two-dimensional reduction does not account for a sufficient amount of the variance of the original data set. Harpending (1973b) has applied a method suggested by Andrews (1972) for plotting multidimensional data structures. Basically, each population is expressed as a trigonometric series and the line for its equation is plotted. Any number of dimensions can be plotted this way. However, when the number of populations exceeds ten or so, the plot becomes rather cluttered. Gnanadesikan (1977) has suggested a modification of the method which largely overcomes this problem.

4.2. Trees

The theory and methodology of estimating evolutionary trees has been the subject of much more analysis, discussion, and controversy than has the use of the topology approach. In part, this is due to the fact that the goals of the tree approach are much more ambitious. In addition to providing a graphic display, trees are usually intended to give information about the *evolutionary* relationships of populations, particularly with regard to the length of time that has elapsed since any pair or group of populations split apart. Much of the controversy surrounding the use of trees centers on whether this goal is achievable.

Evolutionary tree models were first applied to human populations by Cavalli-Sforza and Edwards (1963) (see Cavalli-Sforza, Barrai, and Edwards, 1964, Cavalli-Sforza, 1966, Cavalli-Sforza and Edwards, 1967, and Edwards, 1971b, for elaboration). In essence, their model envisions the pattern of evolution as a random drift process which can be transformed into a Brownian motion process in a Euclidean space. The drift process is a branching process in which gene frequencies undergo a random walk after each node in the tree. Populations split according to a simple birth process (a Yule process). Genetic variance is proportional to elapsed time, since $\sigma_p^2 = \bar{p}(1 - \bar{p})(1 - e^{-t/2N})$. By using the angular transform of gene frequencies, gene frequency variance is independent of $\bar{p}$.

The preferred approach to estimating the configuration and time scale of such a tree would be maximum-likelihood estimation. Since they encountered singularities in the likelihood surface, Cavalli-Sforza and Edwards resorted to a rather *ad hoc* approach to approximate a maximum-likelihood solution: the "minimum evolution" method. Viewing the tree as an undirected graph, this technique searches for the tree which minimizes the total length of all edges connecting the populations. In the parlance of graph theory, this is the minimal Steiner tree. The only way to determine which unrooted tree (of all possible configurations) best satisfies this criterion is to test directly each configuration. Since the number of possible trees for N populations is given by

$$\prod_{i=3}^{N} (2i - 5)$$

the task of finding the "best" tree can soon become quite arduous.

There is little theoretical basis for the minimum evolution approach. Indeed, Cavalli-Sforza and colleagues admit that "it is not easy to justify minimum length evolutionary trees in other ways than through the generally accepted principle of parsimony" (Cavalli-Sforza and Piazza, 1975:321). Nevertheless, this is the method which has thus far been applied most often in deriving evolutionary trees.

A second technique is a least-squares approach called the "additive-tree" method (Cavalli-Sforza and Edwards, 1963, 1967). Again, a random evolutionary process is assumed, and, to quote Cavalli-Sforza and Edwards (1963:925):

> the total difference existing between two populations is the sum of the differences accumulated in evolving from a common ancestral population. The pathway connecting two points in the net is then equated to the actual difference between them. A system of a large number of equations (as many as the number of pairs of populations being examined) is then created, where the unknowns are the edges of the net.

Obviously, a drawback here is the number of equations which must be solved for a set of populations (e.g., 105 equations for 15 populations). The theoretical justification for this method is the same as that for the minimum evolution method.

A third method, proposed by Edwards and Cavalli-Sforza (1965) is a divisive cluster analysis technique in which the ratio of between- to within-groups variance is maximized. To do this, all possible combinations of groups must be tested. Again, this is extremely time consuming, even with very fast computers. Cavalli-Sforza and Piazza (1975) provide a complex extension of this method.

The properties of these three methods have been compared by Kidd and Cavalli-Sforza (1971) and by Kidd, Astolfi, and Cavalli-Sforza (1974).

Felsenstein (1973) has pursued the likelihood approach to tree estimation. He points out that one of the reasons for the singularities encountered by Cavalli-Sforza and Edwards was that they tried to estimate too many parameters. He estimates the topology and branching time of the tree, ignoring the estimation of phenotypes at the nodes of the tree. Felsenstein's method is essentially one of trial and error, however, since parameter values are guessed; then the likelihood is evaluated. As Thompson (1975) points out, this procedure is not very informative of the shape of the likelihood surface. In her book, which provides the best and most complete treatment of evolutionary trees currently available, Thompson has gone a step beyond Felsenstein's work by developing an iterative technique to derive the maximum-likelihood estimate of a tree. She also demonstrates that her technique is superior to previous approaches in terms of both reliability and economy of computer time. Felsenstein (1977), however, does not feel that Thompson's method is "entirely correct," due to the existence of "nuisance parameters" in the model.

One of the objections frequently voiced to these techniques is the huge amount of computer time required to use them (Blackith and Reyment, 1971; Gower, 1967). A number of agglomerative clustering techniques have been used in population structure, all of which are much more efficient in terms of computer time than the above models (e.g., Fitch and Margoliash, 1967; Harpending and Jenkins, 1973; Malyutov, Passekov, and Rychkov, 1972; Morton and Lalouel, 1973a; Spuhler, Gluckman, and Pori, (1976).

A more important theoretical objection is to the assumption that an accurate estimate of divergence time can be made by considering a pure drift process. The criticisms here are the same as noted above for Nei's attempts to estimate the number of codon substitutions: the magnitude of past migration, selection, mutation, and random historical effects simply is not known for human populations. Thus, while trees can give a good two-dimensional description of the relations among populations, one must view estimates for divergence times with skepticism.

It should be noted that Piazza, Sgaramella-Zonta, Gluckman, and Cavalli-Sforza (1975) discuss a method by which the "treeness" (i.e., the plausibility of evolution by random drift) of a structure can be tested. Those populations which do not conform to the assumption are discarded from the analysis.

A number of investigators have used the tree approach in portraying their data. Some examples are the papers by Blanco and Chakraborty (1975), Chakraborty, Blanco, Rothhammer, and Llop (1976), Gajdusek *et al.* (1978), Harpending and Jenkins (1973), Kirk (1976), Morton *et al.* (1976), Saha *et al.* (1976), Spuhler (1979), and Szathmary and Ossenberg (1978).

In comparing map and tree methods, it can be concluded first that the eigenvector approach is more efficient, with regard to computer time, than most or all of the tree methods. Second, at this time, the divergence times estimated in the tree approach are probably not reliable. As a means of simply displaying population structure, a tree often defines relations between closely related populations more exactly than does a map, while maps tend to give more accurate descriptions of the relations among larger groups of subdivisions (i.e., the nodes near the base of the tree) (Sneath and Sokal, 1973). Both techniques suffer from the distortion inherent in projecting a k-dimensional distance/similarity matrix on a two-dimensional space. A number of workers have reported good congruence between the two approaches when both were applied to their data (Cavalli-Sforza and Edwards, 1963; Harpending and Jenkins, 1973; Undevia, Balakrishnan, Kirk, Blake, Saha, and McDermid, 1978). Generally, then, either approach will give a sufficient reduction of a matrix, and the choice depends largely on whether the investigator prefers to look at trees or maps. A more polemical discussion of the trees vs. maps issue can be found in the papers by Cavalli-Sforza (1973, 1974), Lalouel (1974), and Morton (1974b).

5. Other Types of Subdivision

5.1. Hierarchical Subdivision

Wright (1943) pointed out that his F statistics could be extended to populations in which there exists a hierarchy of subdivisions (i.e., the subdivisions are themselves subdivided). Nei (1973) demonstrated that his G_{ST} could be extended the same way. While these measures apparently have not been used directly in studying hierarchical subdivision, this type of structure has been studied in other ways. The most commonly studied form of hierarchical subdivision is the division of the human species into races, which are in turn subdivided into local populations. Lewontin (1972) studied the between- and within-groups diversity of human races and found that most variation (about 85%) occurs within races. Nei and Roychoudhury (1974b), using Nei's heterozygosity measure, arrived at the same conclusion. Mitton (1977), however, used a "multilocus" generalization of Hedrick's (1971) gene identity measure and found a great deal more between-race variation. This conclusion has sparked considerable critical comment (Chakraborty, 1978; Lewontin, 1978; Mitton, 1978; Powell and Taylor, 1978).

Spuhler (1972) examined mean genetic distance between and within linguistic groups of American Indians. More recently (Spuhler 1979), he has applied discriminant analysis to 53 American Indian populations grouped into ten language phyla. The analysis used three loci and classified 64.7% of the populations into the correct language grouping. When the populations were grouped into "culture areas" 58.5% were classified correctly by the discriminant functions. Zegura (1975) has used discriminant analysis on anthropometric data for linguistic groupings of Eskimo populations. And Carmelli and Cavalli-Sforza (1979) have recently used this approach in a study of genetic affinities and origins of four major groups of Jewish populations.

Multivariate analysis of variance was applied by Rhoads and Friedlaender (1975) to examine hierarchical subdivision in the Bougainville data. Here, villages were grouped into linguistically similar divisions. Their analysis demonstrated most variation to be at the within-village level.

Imaizumi (1971) examined the values of the inbreeding coefficient and Malécot's a and b values at four different levels of subdivision in Japan. She found that all three parameters increased as smaller subdivisions were studied.

In studying hierarchical subdivision, one encounters a problem already discussed in regard to evaluating F statistics: the definition of subdivision size and boundaries can be of critical importance. Also, the size and definition of the populations composing each subdivision must be considered carefully. This must be given special attention when making sweeping generalizations about similarities and differences among human races.

5.2. Temporal Subdivision

While it is common to consider subdivision in terms of spatial, linguistic, or cultural groupings, subdivision models have seldom been applied to populations which are subdivided temporally.

Morton et al. (1976) have applied Malécot's isolation by distance model to isonymy data to study the decrease in kinship over several generations. Most studies treating temporal change, however, simply document a change in the inbreeding coefficient, endogamy rate, or rate of consanguineous marriage. Usually, the pattern is one of decrease of inbreeding (or of endogamy) through time. Examples of this are numerous: Beckman et al. (1972) (Sweden), Blanco and Chakraborty (1975b) (Chile), Crawford (1980) (Acceglio, Italy), Ellis and Starmer (1978) (Törbel, Switzerland), Gedde-Dahl (1973) (Norway), Imaizumi (1977, 1978) (Japan), Kirkland and Jantz (1977) (Appalachia), Küchemann, Lasker, and Smith (1979) (Otmoor villages), Lasker, Chiarelli, Mosali, Fedele, and Kaplan (1972) (Italian Alpine villages), Mielke et al. (1976) (Åland Islands —matrimonial migration), Morton et al. (1971b) (Pingelap Atoll), Saugstad (1977b) (Norway), Sutter and Tran-Ngoc-Toan (1957) (France), Tanaka (1963) (Japan), Workman and Jorde (1980) (Åland Islands — parent—offspring migration), Workman et al. (1973) (Papago).

Generally, this pattern of decreasing isolation is attributed to advances in transportation, communication, etc. Schull (1972), summarizing the trends in Italy, Belgium, and France, maintains that the proportion of consanguineous marriages probably increased until about 1850, after which it declined. He attributes this to population growth, which, he says, would increase the probability that one of one's relatives would be of marriageable age and sex. A related consideration is the fact that, with increased village sizes, fewer persons would find it necessary to look outside their own community for a mate, thereby increasing endogamy and the possibility of consanguineous marriage. Beckman (1961) has suggested that this may have occurred in northern Sweden.

A phenomenon related to decreasing endogamy and consanguinity is the temporal increase of migration distances noted in some populations [Küchemann, Boyce, and Harrison, 1967 (Oxfordshire); Spuhler and Clark, 1961 (Ann Arbor,

Michigan)]. Beckman and Cedergren (1971) note a temporal decrease in short-range Swedish migration, while long-range migration has increased.

A few studies have demonstrated little temporal change in inbreeding or endogamy (Roberts, Lutrell, and Slater, 1965 in Tinos Island, Greece, and Lasker, 1968, in San Jose, Peru); several others have shown a temporal *increase* [Morton *et al.*, 1971b (Mokil Atoll); LaJeunesse, 1979 (Cape Barren Island); Roberts, 1975, 1979 (Tristan da Cunha); Spuhler and Kluckhohn, 1953 (Ramah Navajo)]. It is not surprising that the populations in which F increased temporally are small, highly isolated populations founded (partially, in the case of Mokil) within the past 200 years.

Roberts and Rawling (1974), in an analysis of isonymy based on 17th and 18th century Anglican parish records, provide a very nice demonstration of the effects of historical and demographic events on fluctuations in F through time. A similar type of study has been done for Italy by Moroni (1969, cited in Roberts, 1975). Here it was demonstrated that consanguineous marriage (first-cousin) increased prior to World War I. Interestingly, these marriages took place in order to avoid the breakup of family farming lands.

6. Discussion

6.1. Concordance of Data Types

Inference on human population structure can be based on several different data sources, including genetics, migration, anthropometrics, isonymy, and pedigrees. The use of each of these sources entails certain assumptions, which will be discussed in this section. Often the degree of concordance between the different data sources is an indication of how closely these assumptions are met. Table 4 lists a number of empirical correlations reported between various types of data.

Migration. Migration data are often used to assess human population structure, and, as seen above, a sophisticated methodology has evolved to deal with them. There is great variation in the literature on the degree of concordance between genetics and migration. For example, Cavalli-Sforza and Bodmer (1971) have reported good agreement for F_{ST} values computed from genetics and migration data for Guatemalan Indians, Babinga Pygmies, and Bundi clans in New Guinea. Skolnick, Cavalli-Sforza, Moroni, and Siri (1976) demonstrate congruity of F_{ST} values from the Parma Valley data. And Hiorns, Harrison, and Gibson (1977) obtained good agreement for the Oxfordshire–Otmoor data. On the other hand, a definite lack of agreement between genetics and migration relationship matrices has been found for the Papago (Workman *et al.* 1973) and the Åland Islands (Jorde, 1978; Workman and Jorde, 1980).

There are several reasons for these differences. Workman and Jorde (1979) point out that, while the migration matrix method of Imaizumi, Morton, and

Table 4. Correlations of Different Data Types[a]

Systems	Population	Correlation	Reference
Genetics–linguistics	9 S. American Indian groups	$r = 0.000$	Murillo, Rothhammer, and Llop, 1977
Genetics–linguistics	North American Indians	$r = -0.33$	Spuhler, 1972
Genetics–linguistics	Ge-speaking Indians, Brazil	$r = -0.27$	Salzano et al., 1977
Genetics–anthropometrics	Yanomama	$\tau = 0.30$	Neel, Rothhammer, and Lingoes, 1974
Genetics–dermatoglyphics		$\tau = 0.34$	
Anthropometrics–dermatoglyphics		$\tau = 0.08$	
Genetics–linguistics	New Guinea Highland villages	$r = 0.0132$	Livingstone, 1963
Genetics–cultural dissimilarity	Chilean Indians	$r = 0.775$	Chakraborty et al., 1976
Linguistics–cultural dissimilarity	Chilean Indians	$r = 0.032$	
Migration (matrix)–genetics (distance)	Semai Senoi, Malaysia	$\rho = -0.543$	Fix and Lie-Injo, 1975
Genetics–migration	Bougainville	$\tau = 0.34$	Sanghvi, 1953
Genetics–anthropometrics	5 endogamous groups in India	$\tau = 0.545$	Morgan and Holmes, n.d.
Genetics–anthropometrics	Yanomama	$\tau = 0.13$	da Rocha, Spielman, and Neel, 1974
Genetics–anthropometrics	7 S. American Indian populations	$\tau = 0.315$	Szathmary and Ossenberg, 1978
Genetics–osteometrics	American Indian and Eskimo populations	$\tau = 0.19$	Chakraborty and Yee, 1973a,b
Genetics–anthropometrics	5 tribes from Orissa, India	$\tau = 0.287$	White and Parsons, 1973
Genetics–linguistics	Australian aborigines	$r = 0.44$	Sofaer et al., 1972
Genetics–odontometrics	Pima, Papago, Zuni	$\tau = 0.333$	Rothhammer and Spielman, 1971
Genetics–anthropometrics	Aymará Indians, N. Chile	$\rho = 0.333$	Spielman, 1973
Genetics–anthropometrics	19 Yanomama villages	$\rho = 0.19$	
Anthropometrics–geography		$\rho = 0.80$	Jorde, 1978
Genetics–migration	Åland Islands, pre–1900	$\tau = -0.03$	
Genetics–migration	1900–1929	$\tau = 0.01$	
Genetics–migration	post–1929	$\tau = 0.07$	
Genetics–migration	entire sample	$\tau = 0.09$	
Anthropometrics–linguistics	Bougainville	$r = 0.42$	Howells, 1966

[a] Many of the correlations given in this table were computed by the author.

Harris (1970) projects populations to an equilibrium state, a genetic distance matrix represents the sum of past processes which are generally not measurable and do not necessarily reflect equilibrium conditions. Due to the equilibrium assumption of the migration models, one might expect closer congruence between migration and genetics in populations whose migration pattern is near equilibrium. Indeed, this appears to be the pattern in the studies mentioned here: the Bundi, Parma Valley, and Pygmy groups have all been shown to have a relatively stable migration pattern, while the Åland Islands have migration patterns which are not at equilibrium.

Harpending (1974) notes that migration matrix approaches assume that migration is a Markovian process, when in fact it may often be non-Markovian, (e.g., when individuals migrate back to the residence of their grandparents).

Finally, Cavalli-Sforza (1969b) has pointed out that, while stabilizing and differential selection can greatly vary the F_{ST} values measured by genetics data, they will have no effect on the F_{ST} values predicted from a migration matrix.

Anthropometrics. A number of problems present themselves when using anthropometric data in studying human population structure. Most important among these is the fact that many anthropometric traits are quite sensitive to environmental variation (e.g., altitude, temperature) (Boas, 1911; Cavalli-Sforza, 1969b; Cavalli-Sforza and Piazza, 1975; Kaplan, 1954; Morton and Greene, 1972; Spielman, 1973). This apparent increase in sensitivity to environmental variation may contribute to the lack of agreement between trees computed for the major races based on anthropometrics and gene frequencies. Guglielmino-Matessi, Gluckman, and Cavalli-Sforza (1979) recently attempted to correct for this discrepancy by eliminating the effect of climate on anthropometric variation using linear regression. The fact that the two trees remained discordant after the regression procedure led them to conclude that factors other than climate are responsible for the observed lack of fit.

Workman and Niswander (1970) suggested that, since polygenic anthropometric traits are generally subjected to greater selection than genetic markers, one should expect less intersubdivision differentiation when using anthropometric data (assuming, of course, that selection does not differ by subdivision, in which case the opposite effect would be expected).

A final problem with anthropometric measures is observer error, which has been shown to be quite high in some cases (Sofaer, Niswander, MacLean, and Workman, 1972; Spielman, da Rocha, Weitkamp, Ward, Neel, and Chagnon, 1972).

Isonymy. Crow and Mange (1965), following an approach suggested by G. H. Darwin in 1875, first demonstrated that F statistics could be estimated from the frequency of isonymous ("same name") marriages in a population. Lasker (1968, 1969) applied their technique to human populations (see Lasker, 1977, for a good review of other isonymy studies). Isonymy data can also be used to estimate between-population relationships, as demonstrated by Lasker

(1977). However, it has been shown that this approach tends to overestimate kinship between populations (Lasker, 1978).

Undoubtedly the most serious problem encountered in using isonymy data is "polyphyletism": surnames often have multiple ancestral origins, which means that many isonymous marriage partners can be unrelated. Failure to meet the assumption of monophyletism has been cited for the lack of agreement between isonymy and pedigree results in the Swiss isolates of Saas (Hussels, 1969; Morton and Hussels, 1970) and Kippel (Friedl and Ellis, 1974). Because polyphyletism so often causes F to be overestimated, isonymy results should perhaps be regarded only as estimates of the upper limit of F.

Another important assumption, noted by Lasker (1977), is that "surname flow" is an accurate reflection of actual gene flow. This assumption is not met, for example, when names are inherited patrilaterally while most migrating individuals are females.

Sometimes, customs of designating surnames can make isonymy data useless, as in Scandinavia, where patronyms are often taken as surnames.

Ellis and Starmer (1978) provide a nice demonstration of the pitfalls of isonymy in their comparative study of isonymy and pedigree data in Törbel, Switzerland. Because they have pedigree information, they are able to correct the isonymy estimates, which are inflated by polyphyletism and/or outmarriage. After these corrections are made, fairly good agreement is obtained between isonymy and pedigree results.

Pedigrees. The most accurate assessment of population structure can be made when a full pedigree of a population is available, extending back to the founding population (as in Tristan da Cunha or the Ramah Navajo). Commonly, available pedigrees extend back only a few generations, leading to the conclusion that "the fraction of kinship actually ascertained through pedigrees is discouragingly small" (Lalouel and Morton, 1973). Because of this problem, pedigree results usually should be considered estimates of the lower limit of F.

6.2. Determinants of Population Structure

Geographic Distance. The average genetic map, tree, or F statistic is eminently uninteresting unless accompanied by an attempt to elucidate some of the underlying processes. Perhaps the most commonly studied causative factor in genetic structure is the effect of geographic distance on migration and genetic relationship. (Many of the theoretical effects of geographic distance as an isolating factor are discussed above.) Cavalli-Sforza (1962) advocates the use of road distances (or travel time) rather than straight-line distances, while Morton *et al.* (1973) point out that straight-line distances have Euclidean properties and offer a "standard" means of comparison.

Table 5 lists a number of correlations between geography and genetic distance, and Table 6 gives correlations between relationship matrices derived from

Table 5. Correlations between Genetic and Geographic Distance Matrices[a]

Correlation	Population	Reference
$r = 0.494$	Papago	Workman and Niswander, 1970
$r = 0.10-0.28$	Hutterites	Martin, 1973
$r = 0.007$	9 South American Indian populations	Murillo, Rothhammer, and Llop, 1977
$r = 0.26$	Ferrera Province, Italy	Zanardi *et al.*, 1977
$\tau = 0.134$	Bedik, Senegal	Langaney, Gomila, and Bouloux, 1972
$r = 0.503$	New Guinea	Wyber, 1970
$r = 0.468$	22 South American Indian populations	Blanco and Chakraborty, 1975
$\tau = 0.51$	Yanomama	Neel, Rothhammer, and Lingoes, 1974
$r = 0.156$	New Guinea highland villages	Livingstone, 1963
$r = 0.716$	Chilean Indians	Chakraborty *et al.*, 1976
$r = 0.85$	4 S.W. Indian populations	Workman *et al.*, 1974
$r = 0.51$	Sardinia	Workman *et al.*, 1975
$\tau = 0.54$	Bougainville	Friedlaender, 1975
$\tau = 0.28$	Yanomama	Morgan and Holmes, n.d.
$r = 0.43$	Australian aborigines	White and Parsons, 1973
$\tau = 0.099$	United Kingdom	Imaizumi, 1974
$\rho = 0.018$	Aymará Indians, Northern Chile	Rothhammer and Spielman, 1971
$\rho = 0.39$	19 Yanomama villages	Spielman, 1973
$\tau = 0.20$	Åland Islands, Finland, pre-1900	Jorde, 1978
$\tau = 0.28$	1900-1929	
$\tau = 0.30$	post-1929	
$\tau = 0.32$	all periods	
$r = 0.81$	Australian aborigines	Sanghvi, Kirk, and Balakrishnan, 1971

[a] Many of the correlations given in this table were computed by the author.

Table 6. Correlations between Migration and Geographic Distance Matrices

Correlation	Population	Reference
$r = 0.301$	Papago	Workman *et al.*, 1973
$r = 0.502$	Papago, using ln transformation of Φ	
$R_c{}^a = 0.811$	Bedik and Niokholonko, Senegal	Lalouel and Langaney, 1976
$r = 0.94, 0.60$	Barra Island, Scotland — correlations of first two eigenvectors with geography	Morton *et al.*, 1976
$\tau = 0.36$	Bougainville	Friedlaender, 1975
$\tau = -0.36$	Åland Islands, Finland, pre-1900 (kinship with geographic distance)	Jorde, 1978
$\tau = -0.17$	1900-1929	
$\tau = -0.04$	post-1929	
$\tau = -0.10$	all periods	

[a] R_c is the correlation between eigenvectors calculated by the MATFIT program of Lalouel (1973).

migration and geographic distance. Most correlations are moderate, ranging between 0.2 and 0.6.

Significance levels are not given for these correlations, since the degrees of freedom for pairwise comparisons of two matrices of intercorrelated populations cannot be specified (Gower, 1971b; Lalouel, 1973). Some work has been done on this problem, using simulation (Spielman, 1973), but no general means of determining degrees of freedom has yet been derived. Due to the nonlinearity and nonnormality of these distances, it is preferable to use nonparametric correlations in comparing them.

In addition to those reported in Table 5, a number of other studies have reported the degree of congruence between genetic and geographic distance, without specifying statistical correlations. Those reporting "good" agreement include Cavalli-Sforza and Edwards (1963), Crawford, Leyshon, Brown, Lees, and Taylor (1974), Malyutov, Passekov, and Rychkov (1972), Roychoudhury (1975), and Wiesenfeld and Gajdusek (1976). Several others have reported a "poor" fit: Bjarnason, Bjarnason, Edwards, Fridriksson, Magnusson, Mourant, and Tills (1973), Giles Walsh, and Bradley (1966a,b), Kirk, Keats, Blake, McDermid, Ala, Karimi, Nickbin, Shabazi, and Kmet (1977), Livingstone (1973), Rightmire (1976), and Salzano, Pages, Neel, Gershowitz, Tanis, Moreno, and Franco (1978).

The effect of geographic distance is, of course, to limit migration. At very low levels of migration, one might expect geographic distance to have little correlation with genetic distance, since drift would be a more important factor in determining gene frequencies. At very high levels of migration, the effects of geographic isolation would be swamped, again resulting in a low correlation. It is at some intermediate level of migration that one would expect the highest correlation between geographic and genetic distance. Certainly subdivision sizes must also be considered, since this affects the magnitude of random drift.

Population History. Genetically inferred relationship has been compared to the known history of some groups; Boyd (1963) reviews several classic studies. Good concordance between history and genetic relationships has also been demonstrated for the Yanomama (Ward, 1972, 1973; Ward and Neel, 1976) and for Finland (Workman, Mielke, and Nevanlinna, 1976). In addition, several studies have compared genetic structure to oral tradition and have found close agreement (Ghosh *et al.*, 1977; Kirk, 1976; Sinnett, Blake, Kirk, Lai, and Walsh, 1970).

Linguistics. Linguistic differences often provide significant barriers to mating and can influence population structure considerably. Correlations between linguistic similarity (e.g., percent of shared cognates) or distance and genetic distance are given in Table 4. Several workers have studied the effects of linguistic grouping on genetic structure, including Brown, Hanna, Dahlberg, and Strandskov (1958), Crawford, Mielke, Dykes, and Polesky (1979), Friedlaender (1975), Gajdusek *et al.* (1978), Giles *et al.* (1966b), Imaizumi and Morton (1970),

Kumer and Mukherjee (1975), Livingstone (1973), Rightmire (1976), Salzano, Neel, Gershowitz, and Migliazza (1977), Spielman, Migliazza, and Neel (1974), and Spuhler (1972, 1979).

Cultural Factors. A number of other cultural variables can affect population structure. Chakraborty (1976; Chakraborty *et al.* 1976) compiled a cultural dissimilarity index for seven Chilean Indian populations, entering the index in a multiple regression equation with geographic distance as another independent variable and genetic distance as the dependent variable. He showed geographic distance to be a more important determinant of genetic distance than was cultural dissimilarity. His procedure has been criticized by Greene (1977).

Langaney, Gomila, and Bouloux (1972; see also Lalouel and Langaney, 1976) found a significant "ethnic barrier" reflected in the genetic structure of the Bedik and Niokholonko of Senegal. Morton, Imaizumi, and Harris (1971) considered the effect of clan divisions on genetic structure by using simulation; they found surprisingly little effect.

Several studies have examined the relationship between culture level and heterozygosity. Ray (1975) has compared "primitive" and "advanced" Indian populations, finding a much lower kinship coefficient in the former group. This is due perhaps to the more nomadic lifestyle of the "primitive" population. Harpending and Chasko (1976) found that Southern African hunter–gatherers had higher levels of heterozygosity than did settled Bantu agriculturalists, again due probably to higher mobility in the former. Salzano (1975a) found little association between heterozygosity and the level of acculturation of five South American Indian groups. Beals and Kelso (1975), in a more comprehensive study, found a general increase in heterozygosity in going from band to tribe to chiefdom to state. Here again, the effect of subdivision size could be quite important.

Differences in population structure often exist between rural and urban populations in the same region. Saugstad (1977b) found a lower F in rural Norwegian populations than in urban ones. The reverse case is more common, however (e.g., Imaizumi, 1977; Schull, Komatsu, Nagano, and Yamamoto, 1968).

Demographic Effects. A number of demographic variables have already been shown to affect genetic structure (e.g., sex ratio, age structure). Population density also exerts important influences on structure. The levels of inbreeding and consanguineous marriage, for example, are usually correlated negatively with population density [Cavalli-Sforza, 1958 (Parma Valley); Nevanlinna, 1972 (Finland); Saugstad, 1977a (Norway)].

Another important consideration is the effect of population size on mate availability. For instance, Workman and Jorde (1979) tested the relationship between genetic distance and the quantity $1/N_{e_i} + 1/N_{e_j}$ for each pair of subdivisions, i and j, in the Åland Islands. The latter quantity was used as an indicator of the potential for genetic drift between each pair of populations. The expected positive relationship was shown to exist for all populations except one.

This population had the lowest census size (about 300), but exhibited low, rather, than high, genetic distances from all other populations. Examination of migration data showed that about one-fourth of the women in the population had immigrated from Sweden, since, due to small population size, there were not enough unrelated marriageable women available. Since the Swedish gene frequencies are nearly identical to the mean Åland gene frequencies, this population was genetically "close" to the other populations in Åland because of its female immigrants. This result leads to the prediction that the relationship between population size and genetic distance will often tend to be quadratic in form, since very small populations will be forced to increase their migration rates to provide mates.

Random Events. Random historical events can also influence population structure, particularly in small populations. Roberts (1967, 1968, 1971, 1975, 1980) provides the best documented example of such effects in his studies of the isolated island of Tristan da Cunha. A seafaring accident, for example, killed most of the male population of the island, and Roberts was able to show with pedigree analysis that this event significantly altered the proportionate contribution of previous generations to the gene pool.

In any small population, a "bottleneck" due to population reduction will tend to raise the inbreeding coefficient. Chance migrations of individuals with differing gene frequencies will lower it. In large populations, these effects tend to be attenuated.

7. Conclusions

As this review has shown, there are a large number of theoretical approaches to the study of population structure. Similarly, there is no lack of methodology, and a large amount of data has been collected. There is, however, a substantial divergence between the scope and orientation of most of the theoretical studies and those which address empirical questions. Workman and Jorde (1979) have discussed this problem, and Lewontin (1974) has noted that much of the theory of population genetics is based on parameters which are not measurable. The result of this "empirical insufficiency" is that many theoretical models, while mathematically interesting, tell us little about the real world.

As mentioned earlier in this paper, natural selection, which is responsible for most of the interesting aspects of macroevolution, is difficult to measure in most human populations. Thus, gene flow and genetic drift have been emphasized in empirical studies of human population structure, while selection has been more the province of theoretical studies. This has led Harpending (1974) to suggest that the empirical analysis of human population genetics can yield information on the history of a specific population but can contribute little to our understanding of human evolution.

This apparent dichotomy between data-oriented microevolutionary studies and theory-oriented macroevolutionary studies is a major shortcoming in human population genetics. Lewontin's (1974) suggestion that theory should be formulated so that it can be tested is certainly worth heeding. In addition, more attention should be paid to ways in which the masses of data already collected can be used to gain inference on processes of macroevolution and to test predictions deduced from theoretical models. Some areas appear particularly fruitful for such endeavors. These include the effects of genetic structure on the evolution and distribution of disease and the effects of patterns of population movement and variation in demographic parameters on genetic evolution.

Clearly, data on genetics alone are insufficient to achieve these goals. Only by considering genetic data in conjunction with data on migration patterns, ethnohistory, economic history, ecology, and demography can we hope to broaden our understanding of the role of genetic structure in human evolution.

ACKNOWLEDGMENTS

I am grateful for suggestions and comments from Dorit Carmelli, Henry Harpending, Alan Rogers, and James Spuhler. I am especially indebted to Peter Workman, who spent many hours discussing this chapter and related issues with me. Partial financial support for this work was provided by National Science Foundation Grant No. SM176-22857.

References

Andrews, D. F. (1972), Plots of high dimensional data, *Biometrics* **28**:125–136.

Antonelli, P. L., and Strobeck, C. (1977), The geometry of random drift. I. Stochastic distance and diffusion. *Adv. Appl. Probab.* **9**:238–249.

Antonelli, P. L., Chapin, J., Lathrop, G. M., and Morgan, K. (1977), The geometry of random drift. II. The symmetry of random genetic drift, *Adv. Appl. Probab.* **9**: 250–259.

Azevedo, E., Morton, N. E., Miki, C., and Yee, S. (1969), Distance and kinship in northeastern Brazil, *Am. J. Hum. Genet.* **21**:1–22.

Balakrishnan, V. (1974), Comparison of some commonly-used genetic distance measures, in *Human Population Genetics in India* (L. D. Sanghvi, V. Balakrishnan, H. M. Bhatia, P. K. Sukumaran, and J. V. Undevia, eds.), pp. 173–186, Orient Longman, New York.

Balakrishnan, V., and Sanghvi, L. D. (1968), Distance between populations on the basis of attribute data, *Biometrics* **24**:859–865.

Balakrishnan, V., Sanghvi, L. D., and Kirk, R. L. (1975), *Genetic Diversity among Australian Aborigines*, Australian Institute of Aboriginal Studies, Canberra.

Barrai, I. (1971), Subdivision and inbreeding, *Am. J. Hum. Genet.* **23**:95–96.

Barrai, I. (1974), Indicators of genetic distance, in *Genetic Distance* (J. F. Crow and C. Denniston, eds.), pp. 1–4, Plenum Press, New York.

Beals, K. L., and Kelso, A. J. (1975), Genetic variation and cultural evolution, *Am. Anthropol.* 77:566–579.

Beckman, L. (1959), A contribution to the physical anthropology and genetics of Sweden. Variation of the ABO, Rh, MN, and P blood groups, *Hereditas* 45:1–189.

Beckman, L. (1961), Breeding patterns of a North Swedish parish, *Hereditas* 47:72–80.

Beckman, L., and Cedergren, B. (1971), Population studies in Northern Sweden. I. Variation of matrimonial migration distances in time and space, *Hereditas* 68:137–142.

Beckman, L., Cedergren, B., Collinter, E., and Rasmuson, M. (1972), Population studies in northern Sweden. III. Variations of ABO and Rh blood group gene frequencies in time and space, *Hereditas* 72:183–200.

Bhattacharyya, A. (1946), On a measure of divergence between two multinomial populations, *Sankhya* 7:401–406.

Bjarnason, O., Bjarnason, V., Edwards, J. H., Fridriksson, S., Magnusson, M., Mourant, A. E., and Tills, D. (1973), The blood groups of Icelanders, *Ann. Hum. Genet.* 36:425–458.

Blackith, R. E., and Reyment, R. A. (1971), *Multivariate Morphometrics*, Academic Press, London.

Blanco, R., and Chakraborty, R. (1975a), Genetic distance analysis of twenty-two South American Indian populations, *Hum. Hered.* 25:177–193.

Blanco, R., and Chakraborty, R. (1975b), Consanguinity and demography in some Chilean populations, *Hum. Hered.* 25:477–487.

Boas, F. (1911), Changes in bodily form in the descendants of immigrants, from *Abstract of the Report on Changes in Bodily Form of Descendants of Immigrants*, U.S. Government Printing Office, Washington, D.C. [reprinted in *Source Book for Anthropology* (A. L. Kroeber and T. T. Waterman, eds.), pp. 141–154, Harcourt, Brace, and Co., New York].

Bodmer, W. F., and Cavalli-Sforza, L. L. (1968), A migration matrix model for the study of random genetic drift, *Genetics* 59:565–592.

Bodmer, W. F., and Cavalli-Sforza, L. L. (1974), The analysis of genetic variation using migration distances, in *Genetic Distance* (J. F. Crow and C. Denniston, eds.), pp. 45–61, Plenum Press, New York.

Bodmer, W. F., and Cavalli-Sforza, L. L. (1976), *Genetics, Evolution, and Man*, W. H. Freeman, San Francisco.

Boyce, A. J., Küchemann, C. F., and Harrison, B. A. (1967), Neighborhood knowledge and the distribution of marriage distances, *Ann. Hum. Genet.* 30:335–338.

Boyd, W. C. (1963), Four achievements of the genetical method in physical anthropology, *Am. Anthropol.* 65:243–252.

Brown, K. S., Hanna, B. C., Dahlberg, A. A., and Standskov, H. H. (1958), The distribution of blood group alleles among Indians of Southwest North America, *Am. J. Hum. Genet.* 10:175–195.

Brownlee, J. (1911), The mathematical theory of random migration and epidemic distribution, *Proc. R. Soc. Edinburgh* 31:262–289.

Brues, A. M. (1972), Models of race and cline, *Am. J. Phys. Anthropol.* 37:389–399.

Cannings, C., and Cavalli-Sforza, L. L. (1973), Human population structure, in *Advances in Human Genetics*, Vol. 4 (H. Harris and K. Hirschhorn, eds.), pp. 105–171, Plenum Press, New York.

Cannings, C., and Edwards, A. W. F. (1969), Expected genotypic frequencies in a small sample: deviations from Hardy–Weinberg equilibrium, *Am. J. Hum. Genet.* 21:245–247.

Carlson, R., and Welch, Q. B. (1977), A new model for measuring breeding genetic distance, *Ann. Hum. Genet.* 40:455–461.

Carmelli, D., and Cavalli-Sforza, L. L. (1976), Some models of population structure and evolution, *Theor. Popul. Biol.* 9:329–359.

Carmelli, D., and Cavalli-Sforza, L. L. (1979), The genetic origin of the Jews: a multivariate approach, *Hum. Biol.* **51**:41–61.

Cavalli-Sforza, L. L. (1958), Some data on the genetic structure of human populations, in *Proceedings of the 10th International Congress on Genetics*, Vol. 1; pp. 389–407, University of Toronto Press, Toronto.

Cavalli-Sforza, L. L. (1962), The distribution of migration distances: models and applications to genetics, in *Les Déplacements Humains* (J. Sutter, ed.), pp. 139–166, Hachette, Paris.

Cavalli-Sforza, L. L. (1963), Genetic drift for blood groups, in *The Genetics of Migrant and Isolate Populations* (E. Goldschmidt, ed.), pp. 34–39, Williams and Wilkins, New York.

Cavalli-Sforza, L. L. (1966), Population structure and human evolution, *Proc. R. Soc. London Ser. B.* **164**:362–379.

Cavalli-Sforza, L. L. (1969), Human diversity, *Proc. XII Int. Congr. Genet.* **31**:405–416.

Cavalli-Sforza, L. L. (1973), Analytic review: some current problems of human population genetics, *Am. J. Hum. Genet.* **25**:82–104.

Cavalli-Sforza, L. L. (1974), Controversial issues in human population genetics, *Am. J. Hum. Genet.* **26**:266–271.

Cavalli-Sforza, L. L., and Bodmer, W. F. (1971), *The Genetics of Human Populations*, Freeman, San Francisco.

Cavalli-Sforza, L. L., and Edwards, A. W. F. (1963), Analysis of human evolution, *Proc. XI Int. Congr. Genet.* **3**:923–933.

Cavalli-Sforza, L. L., and Edwards A. W. F. (1967), Phylogenetic analysis: models and estimation procedures, *Evolution* **21**:550–570; *Am. J. Hum. Genet.* **23**:235–252.

Cavalli-Sforza, L. L., and Piazza, A. (1975), Analaysis of evolution: evolutionary rates, independence and treeness, *Theor. Popul. Biol.* **8**:127–165.

Cavalli-Sforza, L. L., and Zei, G. (1967), Experiments with an artificial population, in *Proceedings of the Third International Congress of Human Genetics* (J. F. Crow and J. V. Neel, eds.), pp. 473–478. Johns Hopkins University Press, Baltimore.

Cavalli-Sforza, L. L., Barrai, I., and Edwards, A. W. F. (1964), Analysis of human evolution under random genetic drift, *Cold Spring Harbor Symp. Quant. Biol.* **29**:9–20.

Cavalli-Sforza, L. L., Zonta, L. A., Nuzzo, F., Bernini, L., DeJong, W. W. W., Meera Khan, P., Ray, A. K., Went, L. N., Siniscalco, M., Nijenhuis, L. E., Vanloghen, E., and Modiano, G. (1969), Studies on African Pygmies. I. A pilot investigation of Babinga Pygmies in the Central African Republic (with an analysis of genetic distances), *Am. J. Hum. Genet.* **21**:252–274.

Chakraborty, R. (1974), A note on Nei's measure of gene diversity in a substructured population, *Humangenetik* **21**:85–88.

Chakraborty, R. (1975), Estimation of race admixture – a new method, *Am. J. Phys. Anthropol.* **42**:507–511.

Chakraborty, R. (1976), Cultural, language and geographic correlates of genetic variability in Andean highland Indians, *Nature* **264**:350–352.

Chakraborty, R. (1978), Single-locus and multilocus analysis of genetic differentiation of the races of man: a critique, *Am. Nat.* **112**:1134–1138.

Chakraborty, R., and Nei, M. (1974), Dynamics of gene differentiation between incompletely isolated populations of unequal sizes, *Theor. Popul. Biol.* **5**:460–469.

Chakraborty, R., and Tateno, Y. (1976), Correlations between some measures of genetic distance, *Evolution* **30**:851–853.

Chakraborty, R., and Yee. S. (1973a), Phenotypic bioassay of five tribes of Orissa, India, *Hum. Hered.* **23**:270–279.

Chakraborty, R., and Yee, S. (1973b), Five tribes of Orissa, India: Anthropometry and kinship, *Hum. Hered.* **23**:301–307.

Chakraborty, R., Blanco, R., Rothhammer, F., and Llop, E. (1976), Genetic variability in Chilean Indian populations and its association with geography, language, and culture, *Soc. Biol.* **23**:73–81.

Chakraborty, R., Chakravarti, A., and Malhotra, K. C. (1977), Variation in allele frequencies among caste groups of the Danghars of Maharashtra, India: an analysis with Wright's F_{ST} statistic, *Ann. Hum. Biol.* **4**:275–280.

Clarke, B. (1966), The evolution of morph-ratio clines, *Am. Nat.* **100**:389–402.

Cockerham, C. C. (1969), Variance of gene frequencies, *Evolution* **23**:72–84.

Cockerham, C. C. (1973), Analysis of gene frequencies, *Genetics* **74**:679–700.

Coleman, D. A. (1973), Marriage movement in British cities, in *Genetic Variation in Britain* (D. F. Roberts and E. Sunderland, eds.), pp. 35–57, Taylor and Francis, London.

Courgeau, D. (1974), Migration, in *Genetic Structure of Populations* (A. Jacquard, ed.), pp. 351–387. Springer-Verlag, New York.

Crawford, M. H. (1980), The breakdown of reproductive isolation in an Alpine genetic isolate: Acceglio, Italy, in *Population Structure and Genetic Disease* (A. W. Eriksson, H. Forsius, H. R. Nevanlinna, and P. L. Workman, eds.), Academic Press, New York.

Crawford, M. H., and Workman, P. L. (eds.) (1973), *Methods and Theories of Anthropological Genetics*, University of New Mexico Press, Albuquerque.

Crawford, M. H., Leyshon, W. C., Brown, K., Lees, F., and Taylor, L. (1974), Human biology in Mexico: II. A comparison of blood group, serum and red cell enzyme frequencies, and genetic distances of the Indian populations of Mexico, *Am. J. Phys. Anthropol.* **41**:251–268.

Crawford, M. H., Mielke, J. H., Dykes, D. D., and Polesky, H. F. (1979), Population structure of Alaskan and Siberian indigenous communities, paper delivered at the 48th annual meeting of the American Association of Physical Anthropologists, San Francisco.

Crow, J. F., and Kimura, M. (1970) *An Introduction to Population Genetics Theory*, Harper and Row, New York.

Crow, J. F., and Kimura, M. (1972), The effective number of a population with overlapping generations: a correction and further discussion, *Am. J. Hum. Genet.* **24**:1–10.

Crow, J. F., and Mange, A. P. (1965), Measurement of inbreeding from the frequency of marriages between persons of the same surname, *Eugen. Q.* **12**:199–203.

Crow, J. F., and Morton, N. E. (1955), Measurement of gene frequency drift in small populations, *Evolution* **9**:202–214.

Dodinval, P. A. (1970), Population structure of A, B, O and AB blood groups in Belgium, *Hum. Hered.* **20**:169–177.

Edwards, A. W. F. (1971a), Distance between populations on the basis of gene frequencies, *Biometrics* **27**:873–881.

Edwards, A. W. F. (1971b), Mathematical approaches to the study of human evolution, in *Mathematics in the Archeological and Historical Sciences* (F. R. Hodson, D. G. Kendall, and P. Tautu, eds.), pp. 347–353, Aldine-Atherton, Chicago.

Edwards, A. W. F., and Cavalli-Sforza, L. L. (1964), Reconstruction of evolutionary trees, in *Phenetics and Phylogenetic Classification* (V. E. Heywood and J. McNeill, eds.), pp. 67–76, The Systematics Association, London.

Edwards, A. W. F., and Cavalli-Sforza, L. L. (1965), A method for cluster analysis, *Biometrics* **21**:362–375.

Edwards, A. W. F., and Cavalli-Sforza, L. L. (1972), Affinity as revealed by differences in gene frequencies, in *The Assessment of Population Affinities in Man* (J. S. Weiner, and J. Huizinga, eds.), pp. 37–47, Clarendon Press, Oxford.

Ellis, W. S., and Starmer, W. T. (1978), Inbreeding as measured by isonymy, pedigrees and population size in Törbel, Switzerland, *Am. J. Hum. Genet.* **30**:366–376.

Endler, J. A. (1973), Gene flow and population differentiation, *Science,* **179**:243–250.

Endler, J. A. (1977), *Geographic Variation, Speciation, and Clines*, Princeton University Press, Princeton.

Eriksson, A. W., Fellman, J. O., Workman, P. L., and Lalouel, J. M. (1973a), Population studies on the Åland Islands. I. Prediction of kinship from migration and isolation by distance, *Hum. Hered.* **23**:422–433.

Eriksson, A. W., Eskola, M.-R., Workman, P. L., and Morton, N. E. (1973b), Population studies on the Åland Islands. II. Historical population structure: inference from bioassay of kinship and migration, *Hum. Hered.* **23**:511–534.

Eriksson, A. W., Forsius, H., Nevanlinna, H. R., and Workman, P. L. (eds.), (1980), *Population Structure and Genetic Disease*, Academic Press, New York.

Ewens, W. J., and Feldman, M. W. (1976), The theoretical assessment of selective neutrality, in *Population Genetics and Ecology* (S. Karlin and E. Nevo, eds.), pp. 303–337, Academic Press, New York.

Feldman, M. W., and Christiansen, F. B. (1975), The effect of population subdivision on two loci without selection, *Genet. Res.* **24**:151–162.

Felsenstein, J. (1971), Inbreeding and variance effective numbers in populations with overlapping generations, *Genetics* **68**:581–597.

Felsenstein, J. (1973), Maximum-likelihood estimation of evolutionary trees from continuous characters, *Am. J. Hum. Genet.* **25**:471–492.

Felsenstein, J. (1975a), A pain in the torus: some difficulties with models of isolation by distance, *Am. Nat.* **109**:359–368.

Felsenstein, J. (1975b), Genetic drift in clines which are maintained by migration and natural selection, *Genetics* **81**:191–207.

Felsenstein, J. (1976), The theoretical population genetics of variable selection and migration, *Ann. Rev. Genet.* **10**:253–280.

Felsenstein, J. (1977), Review of *Human Evolutionary Trees*, *Q. Rev. Biol.* **52**:231.

Fisher, R. A. (1930), The distribution of gene ratios for rare mutants, *Proc. R. Soc. Edinburgh* **50**:204–219.

Fisher, R. A. (1937), The wave of advance of advantageous genes, *Ann. Eugen.* **7**:355–360.

Fisher, R. A. (1950), Gene frequencies in a cline determined by selection and diffusion, *Biometrics* **6**:353–361.

Fitch, W. M., and Margoliash, E. (1967), Construction of phylogenetic trees, *Science*, **155**:279–284.

Fix, A. G. (1974), Neighborhood knowledge and marriage distance: the Semai case, *Ann. Hum. Genet.* **37**:327–332.

Fix, A. G. (1978), The role of kin-structured migration in genetic microdifferentiation, *Ann. Hum. Genet.* **41**:329–339.

Fix, A. G., and Lie-Injo, L. E. (1975), Genetic microdifferentiation in the Semai Senoi of Malaysia, *Am. J. Phys. Anthropol.* **43**:47–56.

Fleming, W. H., and Su, C.-H. (1974), Some one-dimensional migration models in population genetics theory, *Theor. Popul. Biol.* **5**:431–449.

Freire-Maia, N. (1957), Inbreeding levels in different countries, *Eugen. Q.* **4**:127–138.

Freire-Maia, N. (1974), Population genetics and demography, *Hum. Hered.* **24**:105–113.

Friedl, J., and Ellis, W. E. (1974), Inbreeding, isonymy and isolation in a Swiss community, *Hum. Biol.* **46**:699–712.

Friedlaender, J. S. (1971a), The population structure of South-Central Bougainville, *Am. J. Phys. Anthropol.* **35**:13–26.

Friedlaender, J. S. (1971b), Isolation by distance in Bougainville, *Proc. Natl. Acad. Sci. U.S.A.* **68**:704–707.

Friedlaender, J. S. (1975), *Patterns of Human Variation: The Demography, Genetics, and Phenetics of Bougainville Islanders*, Harvard University Press, Cambridge.

Gajdusek, D. C., Leyshon, W. C., Kirk, R. L., Blake, N. M., Keats, B., and McDermid, E. M.

(1978), Genetic differentiation among populations in Western New Guinea, *Am. J. Phys. Anthropol.* **48**:47–64.

Gedde-Dahl, T. (1973), Population structure in Norway, *Hereditas* **73**:209–231.

Geoge, S. L., and Siciliano, M. J. (1973), Comparisons of methods of measuring genetic distances among several populations, *Genetics* **74**:592.

Gershowitz, H., and Neel, J. V. (1978), The immunoglobulin allotypes (Gm and Km) of twelve Indian tribes of Central and South America, *Am. J. Phys. Anthropol.* **49**: 289–302.

Ghosh, A. K., Kirk, R. L., Joshi, S. R., and Bhatia, H. M. (1977), A population genetic study of the Kota in the Nilgiri Hills, South India, *Hum. Hered.* **27**:225–241.

Giles, E., Walsh, R. J., and Bradley, M. A. (1966a), Microevolution in New Guinea: the role of genetic drift, *Ann. N. Y. Acad. Sci.* **134**:655–665.

Giles, E., Walsh, R. J., and Bradley, M. A. (1966b), Blood group genetics of natives of the Morobe District and Bougainville, Territory of New Guinea, *Arch. Phys. Anthropol. Oceania* **1**:135–154.

Gillespie, J. H. (1976), The role of migration in the genetic structure of populations in temporally and spatially varying environments. II. Island models, *Theor. Popul. Biol.* **10**:227–238.

Ginter, E. K., Garkavtseva, R. F., and Revazov, A. A. (1980), Population structure and hereditary disease in Uzbekistan, in *Population Structure and Genetic Disease* (A. W. Eriksson, H. Forsius, H. R. Nevanlinna, and P. L. Workman, eds.), Academic Press, New York, in press.

Gnanadesikan, R. (1977), *Methods for Statistical Analysis of Multivariate Observations*, Wiley, New York.

Goodman, M. M. (1972), Distance analysis in biology, *Syst. Zool.* **21**:174–186.

Goodman, M. M. (1974), Genetic distances: measuring dissimilarity among populations, *Yearb. Phys. Anthropol.* **17**:1–38.

Goodman, M., Barnabas, J., and Moore, G. W. (1974), Man, the conservative and revolutionary mammal: molecular findings, *Yearb. Phys. Anthropol.* **17**:71–97.

Gower, J. C. (1966), Some distance properties of latent root and vector methods used in multivariate analysis, *Biometrika* **53**:325–338.

Gower, J. C. (1967), A comparison of some methods of cluster analysis, *Biometrics* **23**: 623–637.

Gower, J. C. (1971a), An illustration of a new technique for comparing different distance analyses (abstract), *Am. J. Phys. Anthropol.* **35**:280.

Gower, J. C. (1971b), Statistical methods of comparing different multivariate analyses of the same data, in *Mathematics in the Archaeological and Historical Sciences* (F. R. Hodson, D. G. Kendall, and P. Tautu, eds.), pp. 138–149. Edinburgh University Press, Edinburgh.

Gower, J. C. (1972), Measures of taxonomic distance and their analysis, in *The Assessment of Population Affinities in Man* (J. S. Weiner and J. Huizinga, eds.), pp. 1–24, Clarendon Press, Oxford.

Greene, P. J. (1977), Culture and genetic variability, *Nature* **267**:375.

Guglielmino-Matessi, C. R., Gluckman, P., and Cavalli-Sforza, L. L. (1979), Climate and the evolution of skull metrics in man, *Am. J. Phys. Anthropol.* **50**:549–564.

Haldane, J. B. S. (1948), The theory of a cline, *J. Genet.* **48**:277–284.

Harpending, H. C. (1971), Inference on population structure studies, *Am. J. Hum. Genet.* **23**:536–538.

Harpending, H. C. (1973a), Discussion, in *Genetic Structure of Populations* (N. E. Morton, ed.), pp, 78–79, University of Hawaii Press, Honolulu.

Harpending, H. C. (1973b), Discussion, in *Genetic Structure of Populations* (N. E. Morton, ed.), pp. 150–152, University of Hawaii Press, Honolulu.

Harpending, H. C. (1974), Genetic structure of small populations, *Ann. Rev. Anthropol.* **3**:229–243.

Harpending, H. C., and Chasko, W. J. (1976), Heterozygosity and population structure in Southern Africa, in *The Measures of Man: Methodologies in Biological Anthropology* (E. Giles and J. S. Friedlaender, eds.), pp. 214–229, Peabody Museum Press, Cambridge.

Harpending, H. C., and Jenkins, T. (1973), Genetic distances among Southern African populations in *Methods and Theories of Anthropological Genetics* (M. H. Crawford and P. L. Workman, eds.), pp. 177–199, University of New Mexico Press, Albuquerque.

Harpending, H. C., and Jenkins, T. (1974), !Kung population structure, in *Genetic Distance* (J. F. Crow and C. F. Denniston, eds.), pp. 137–161, Plenum Press, New York.

Harpending, H. C., Workman, P. L., and Grove, J. (1973), Local genotypic disequilibrium in a generalized island model, *Hum. Biol.* **45**:359–362.

Harrison, G. A. (ed.) (1977), *Population Structure and Human Variation*, Cambridge University Press, Cambridge.

Harrison, G. A., and Boyce, A. J. (1972a), Migration, exchange, and the genetic structure of populations, in *The Structure of Human Populations* (G. A. Harrison and A. J. Boyce, eds.), pp. 128–145, Clarendon Press, Oxford.

Harrison, G. A., and Boyce, A. J. (eds.) (1972b), *The Structure of Human Populations*, Clarendon Press, Oxford.

Harrison, G. A., Hiorns, R. W., and Küchemann, C. F. (1970), Social class relatedness in some Oxfordshire parishes, *J. Biosoc. Sci.* **2**:71–80.

Harrison, G. A., Küchemann, C. F., Hiorns, R. W., and Carrivick, P. J. (1974a), Social mobility, assortative marriage and their interrelationships with marital distance and age in Oxford City, *Ann. Hum. Biol.* **1**:211–233.

Harrison, G. A., Gibson, J. B., Hiorns, R. W., Wigley, M., Hancock, C., Freeman, C. A., Küchemann, C. F., Macbeth, H. M., Saatcioglu, A., and Carrivick, P. J. (1974b), Psychometric, personality and anthropometric variation in a group of Oxfordshire villages, *Ann. Hum. Biol.* **1**:365–381.

Hedrick, P. W. (1971), A new approach to measuring genetic similarity, *Evolution* **25**: 276–280.

Hedrick, P. W. (1975), Genetic similarity and distance: comments and comparisons, *Evolution* **29**:362–366.

Hill, W. G. (1972), Effective size of populations with overlapping generations, *Theor. Popul. Biol.* **3**:278–289.

Hiorns, R. W. (1971), Statistical studies in migration, in *Mathematics in the Archaeological and Historical Sciences* (F. R. Hodson, D. G. Kendall, and P. Tautu, eds.), pp. 291–302, Aldine-Atherton, Chicago.

Hiorns, R. W., Harrison, G. A., Boyce, A. J., and Küchemann, C. F. (1969), A mathematical analysis of the effects of movement on the relatedness between populations, *Ann. Hum. Genet.* **32**:237–250.

Hiorns, R. W., Harrison, G. A., and Küchemann, C. F. (1973), Factors affecting the genetic structure of populations: an urban–rural contrast in Britain, in *Genetic Variation in Britain* (D. F. Roberts and E. Sunderland, eds.), pp. 17–32, Taylor and Francis, London.

Hiorns, R. W., Harrison, G. A., and Gibson, J. B. (1977), Genetic variation in some Oxfordshire villages, *Ann. Hum. Biol.* **4**:197–210.

Holgate, P. (1964), Genotype frequencies in a section of a cline, *Heredity* **19**:507–509.

Howells, W. W. (1966), Population distances: biological, linguistic, geographical, and environmental, *Curr. Anthropol.* **7**:531–540.

Hussels, I. (1969), Genetic structure of Saas, a Swiss isolate, *Hum. Biol.* **41**:469–479.

Huxley, J. S. (1938), Clines: an auxiliary taxonomic principle, *Nature* **142**:219–220.

Imaizumi, Y. (1971), Variation of inbreeding coefficient in Japan, *Hum. Hered.* **21**:216–230.

Imaizumi, Y. (1974), Genetic structure in the United Kingdom, *Hum. Hered.* **24**:151–159.

Imaizumi, Y. (1977), A demographic approach to population structure in Gyoda and Hasuda, Japan, *Hum. Hered.* **27**:318–327.

Imaizumi, Y. (1978), Population structure in Kanoya population, Japan, *Hum. Hered.* **28**:7–18.

Imaizumi, Y., and Morton, N. E. (1969), Isolation by distance in Japan and Sweden compared with other countries, *Hum. Hered.* **19**:433–443.

Imaizumi, Y., and Morton, N. E. (1970), Isolation by distance in New Guinea and Micronesia, *Arch. Phys. Anthropol. Oceania* **5**:218–235.

Imaizumi, Y., Morton, N. E., and Harris, D. E., (1970), Isolation by distance in artificial populations, *Genetics* **66**:569–582.

Jacquard, A. (ed.) (1974), *The Genetic Structure of Populations*, Springer-Verlag, New York.

Jacquard, A. (1975), Inbreeding: one word, several meanings, *Theor. Popul. Biol.* **7**:338–363.

Jorde, L. B. (1978), Patterns of genetics and migration in the Åland Islands, paper presented at the 47th annual meeting of the American Association of Physical Anthropologists, Toronto.

Jorde, L. B., Eriksson, A. W., Morgan, K., and Workman, P. L. (1980), The population structure of Iceland, in preparation.

Kaplan, B. A. (1954), Environment and human plasticity, *Am. Anthropol.* **56**:780–800.

Karlin, S. (1976), Population subdivision and selection migration interaction, in *Population Genetics and Ecology* (S. Karlin and E. Nevo, eds.), pp. 617–657, Academic Press, New York.

Karlin, S., and Richter-Dyn, N. (1976), Some theoretical analyses of migration selection interaction in a cline: a generalized two range environment, in *Population Genetics and Ecology* (S. Karlin and E. Nevo, eds.), pp. 659–706, Academic Press, New York.

Karlin, S., Kenett, R., and Bonné-Tamir, B. (1979), Analysis of biochemical genetic data on Jewish populations. II. Results and interpretation of heterogeneity indices and distance measures with respect to standards, *Am. J. Hum. Genet.* **31**:341–365.

Keats, B. (1977), Genetic structure of the indigenous populations in Australia and New Guinea, *J. Hum. Evol.* **6**:319–339.

Kempton, G. A. (1971), Difference in genetic composition between populations experiencing selective migration, *Ann. Hum. Genet.* **35**:25–34.

Kendall, D. G. (1971), Maps from marriages: an application of non-metric multidimensional scaling to parish register data, in *Mathematics in the Archaeological and Historical Sciences* (F. R. Hodson, D. G. Kendall, and P. Tautu, eds.), pp. 303–318, Aldine-Atherton, Chicago.

Kidd, K. K., Astolfi, P., and Cavalli-Sforza, L. L. (1974), Error in the reconstruction of evolutionary trees, in *Genetic Distance* (J. F. Crow and C. Denniston, eds.), pp. 121–136, Plenum Press, New York.

Kidd, K. K., and Cavalli-Sforza, L. L. (1971), Number of characters examined and error in reconstruction of evolutionary trees, in *Mathematics in the Archaeological and Historical Sciences* (F. R. Hodson, D. G. Kendall, and P. Tautu, eds.), pp. 335–346, Aldine-Atherton, Chicago.

Kidd, K. K., and Sgaramella-Zonta, L. A. (1971), Phylogenetic analysis: concepts and methods, *Am. J. Hum. Genet.* **23**:235–252.

Kimura, M. (1953), Stepping stone model of population, *Ann. Rep. Nat. Inst. Genet. (Japan)* **3**:62–63.

Kimura, M. (1957), Some problems of stochastic processes in genetics, *Ann. Math. Stat.* **28**:882–901.

Kimura, M. (1968), Evolutionary rate at the molecular level, *Nature* **217**:624–626.

Kimura, M. (1969), The rate of molecular evolution considered from the standpoint of population genetics, *Proc. Natl. Acad. Sci. U.S.A.* **63**:1181–1188.

Kimura, M., and Crow, J. F. (1963), The measurement of effective population number, *Evolution* **17**:279–288.

Kimura, M., and Maruyama. T. (1971), Pattern of neutral polymorphism in a geographically structured population, *Genet. Res.* **18**:125–131.

Kimura, M., and Weiss. G. H. (1964), The stepping-stone model of population structure and the decrease of genetic correlation with distance, *Genetics* **49**:561–576.

King, J. L., and Jukes, T. H. (1969), Non-Darwinian evolution, *Science* **164**:788–798.

Kirby, G. C. (1975), Heterozygote frequencies in small populations, *Theor. Popul. Biol.* **8**: 31–48.

Kirk, R. L. (1976), The legend of Prince Vijaya – a study of Sinhalese origins, *Am. J. Phys. Anthropol.* **45**:91–100.

Kirk, R. L., Keats, B., Blake, N. M., McDermid, E. M., Ala, F., Karimi, M., Nickbin, B., Shabazi, H., and Kmet, J. (1977), Genes and people in the Caspian littoral: a population genetic study in northern Iran, *Am. J. Phys. Anthropol.* **46**:377–390.

Kirkland, J. R., and Jantz, R. L. (1977), Inbreeding, marital movement and genetic isolation of a rural Appalachian population, *Ann. Hum. Biol.* **4**:211–218.

Kojima, K., Smouse, P., Yang, S., Nair, P. S., and Brncic, D. (1972), Isozyme frequency patterns in *Drosophila pavani* associated with geographical and seasonal variables, *Genetics* **72**:721–731.

Korey, K. A. (1978), A critical appraisal of methods for measuring admixture, *Hum. Biol.* **50**:343–360.

Korey, K. A. (1979), Cherokee admixture and its estimation by the gene identity method: a critique, *Am. J. Phys. Anthropol.* **50**:51–56.

Kruskal, J. B. (1964a), Multidimensional scaling by optimizing goodness of fit to a nonmetric hypothesis, *Psychometrika* **29**:1–27.

Kruskal, J. B. (1964b), Nonmetric multidimensional scaling: a numerical method, *Psychometrika* **29**:115–129.

Krzanowski, W. J. (1971), A comparison of some distance measures applicable to multinomial data, using a rotational fit technique, *Biometrics* **27**:1062–1068.

Küchemann, C. F., Boyce, A. J., and Harrison, G. A. (1967), A demographic and genetic study of a group of Oxfordshire villages, *Hum Biol.* **39**:251–276.

Küchemann, C. F., Harrison, G. A., Hiorns, R. W., and Carrivick, P. J. (1974), Social class and marital distance in Oxford City, *Ann. Hum. Biol.* **1**:13–27.

Küchemann, C. F., Lasker, G. W., and Smith, D. I. (1979), Historical changes in the coefficient of relationship by isonymy among the populations of the Otmoor villages, *Hum. Biol.* **51**:63–77.

Kumer, H., and Mukherjee, D. P. (1975), Genetic distances among the Ho tribe and other groups of Central Indians, *Am. J. Phys. Anthropol.* **42**:489–494.

Kurczynski, T. W. (1970), Generalized distance and discrete variables, *Biometrics* **36**: 525–534.

LaJeunesse, R. A., and Littlewood, R. A. (1979), Founder's effect and inbreeding in the Cape Barren Island isolate, 1815–1974, paper delivered at the 48th annual meeting of the American Association of Physical Anthropologists, San Francisco.

Lalouel, J. M. (1973), Topology of population structure, in *Genetic Structure of Populations* (N. E. Morton, ed.), pp. 139–149, University of Hawaii Press, Honolulu.

Lalouel, J. M. (1974), Controversial issues in human population genetics, *Am. J. Hum. Genet.* **26**:262–265.

Lalouel, J. M. (1977), The conceptual framework of Malécot's model of isolation by distance, *Ann. Hum. Genet.* **40**:355–360.

Lalouel, J. M., and Langaney, A. (1976), Bedik and Niokholonko of Senegal: inter-village relationship inferred from migration data, *Am. J. Phys. Anthropol.* **45**:453–466.

Lalouel, J. M., and Morton, N. E. (1973), Bioassay of kinship in a South American Indian population, *Am. J. Hum. Genet.* **25**:62–73.

Langaney, A., and Gomila, J. (1973), Bedik and Niokholonko intra and inter-ethnic migration, *Hum. Biol.* **45**:137–150.

Langaney, A., Gomila, J., and Bouloux, C. (1972), Bedik: bioassay of kinship, *Hum. Biol.* **44**:475–488.

Langaney, A., Gessain, R., and Robert, J. (1974), Migration and genetic kinship in Eastern Greenland, *Soc. Biol.* **21**:272–278.

Langley, C. H., and Fitch, W. M. (1973), The constancy of evolution: a statistical analysis of the α and β hemoglobins, cytochrome c, and fibrinopeptide A, in *Genetic Structure of Populations* (N. E. Morton, ed.), pp. 246–262, University of Hawaii Press, Honolulu.

Lasker, G. W. (1968), The occurrence of identical (isonymous) surnames in various relationships in pedigrees: a preliminary analysis of the relation of surname combinations to inbreeding, *Am. J. Hum. Genet.* **20**:250–257.

Lasker, G. W. (1969), Isonymy (recurrence of the same surname in affinal relatives): a comparison of rates calculated from pedigrees, grave markers, and death and birth registers, *Hum. Biol.* **41**:309–321.

Lasker, G. W. (1977), A coefficient of relationship by isonymy: a method for estimating the genetic relationship between populations, *Hum. Biol.* **49**:489–493.

Lasker, G. W. (1978), Increments through migration to the coefficient of relationship between communities estimated by isonymy, *Hum. Biol.* **50**:235–240.

Lasker, G. W., Chiarelli, B., Mosali, M., Fedele, F., and Kaplan, B. A. (1972), Degree of human genetic isolation measured by isonymy and marital distances in two communities in an Italian Alpine valley, *Hum. Biol.* **44**:351–360.

Latter, B. D. H. (1972), Selection in finite populations with multiple alleles. III. Genetic divergence with centripetal selection and mutation, *Genetics* **70**:465–490.

Latter, B. D. H. (1973a), Measures of genetic distance between individuals and populations, in *Genetic Structure of Populations* (N. E. Morton, ed.), pp. 27–37, University of Hawaii Press, Honolulu.

Latter, B. D. H (1973b), The estimation of genetic divergence between populations based on gene frequency data, *Am. J. Hum. Genet.* **25**:247–261.

Lefevre-Witier, P., and Vergnes, H. (1977), Genetic structure of Ideles Ahaggar agricultural center – Algerian Sahara, *Yearb. Phys. Anthropol.* **20**:164–180.

Leven, H. (1953), Genetic equilibrium when more than one ecological niche is available, *Am. Nat.* **87**:331–333.

Lewontin, R. C. (1972), The apportionment of human diversity, *Evol. Biol.* **6**:381–398.

Lewontin, R. C. (1974), *The Genetic Basis of Evolutionary Change*, Columbia University Press, New York.

Lewontin, R. C. (1978), Single- and multiple-locus measures of genetic distance between groups, *Am. Nat.* **112**:1138–1139.

Lewontin, R. C., and Krakauer, J. (1973), Distribution of gene frequency as a test of the theory of the selective neutrality of polymorphism, *Genetics* **74**:175–195.

Lewontin, R. C., and Krakauer, J. (1975), Testing the heterogeneity of F values, *Genetics* **80**:397–398.

Li, C. C. (1978), On measuring genetic distance by selection intensity, *Ann. Hum. Genet.* **41**:501–504.

Li, W.-H. (1976), Effect of migration on genetic distance, *Am. Nat.* **110**:841–847.

Li, W.-H., and Nei, M. (1975), Drift variances of heterozygosity and genetic distance in transient states, *Genet. Res.* **25**:229–248.

Livingstone, F. B. (1963), Blood groups and ancestry: a test case from the New Guinea highlands, *Curr. Anthropol.* **4**:541–542.

Livingstone, F. B. (1969), Gene frequency clines of the beta hemoglobin locus in various human populations and their simulation by models involving differential selection, *Hum. Biol.* **41**:223–236.

Livingstone, F. B. (1973), Gene frequency differences in human populations: some problems of analysis and interpretation, in *Methods and Theories of Anthropological Genetics* (M. H. Crawford and P. L. Workman, eds.), pp. 39–66, University of New Mexico Press, Albuquerque.

MacCluer, J. W. (1974), Monte Carlo simulation: the effects of migration on some measures of genetic distance, in *Genetic Distance* (J. F. Crow and C. Denniston, eds.), pp. 77–95, Plenum Press, New York.

MacCluer, J. W., and Schull, W. J. (1970), Estimating the effective size of human populations, *Am. J. Hum. Genet.* **22**:176–183.

Mahalanobis, P. C. (1936), On the generalized distance in statistics, *Proc. Natl. Inst. Sci. India* **2**:49–55.

Malcolm, L. A., Booth, P. B., and Cavalli-Sforza, L. L. (1971), Intermarriage patterns and blood group gene frequencies of the Bundi people of the New Guinea highlands, *Hum. Biol.* **43**:187–199.

Malécot, G. (1948), *Les Mathématiques de l'Hérédité*, Masson, Paris (translated as *The Mathematics of Heredity* (1969), Freeman, San Francisco).

Malécot, G. (1950), Quelques schémas probabilistes sur la variabilité des populations naturelles, *Ann. Univ. Lyon Sci. Sect. A* **13**:37–60.

Malécot, G. (1959), Les modeles stochastiques en génétique de population, *Publ. Inst. Statist. Univ. Paris* **8**:173–210.

Malécot, G. (1973), Isolation by distance, in *Genetic Structure of Populations* (N. E. Morton, ed.), pp. 72–75, University of Hawaii Press, Honolulu.

Malyutov, M. B., Passekov, V. P., and Rychkov, Y. G. (1972), On the reconstruction of evolutionary trees of human populations resulting from random genetic drift, in *The Assessment of Population Affinities in Man* (J. S. Weiner and J. Huizinga, eds.), pp. 48–71. Clarendon Press, Oxford.

Martin, A. O. (1973), An empirical comparison of some descriptions of population structure in a human isolate, in *Genetic Structure of Populations* (N. E. Morton, ed.), pp. 195–202, University of Hawaii Press, Honolulu.

Maruyama, T. (1969), Genetic correlation in the stepping stone model with nonsymmetrical migration rates, *J. Appl. Probab.* **6**:463–477.

Maruyama, T. (1970a), On the fixation probability of mutant genes in a subdivided population, *Genet. Res.* **15**:221–225.

Maruyama, T. (1970b), Effective number of alleles in a subdivided population, *Theor. Popul. Biol.* **1**:273–306.

Maruyama, T. (1970c), Stepping stone models of finite length, *Adv. Appl. Probab.* **2**:229–258.

Maruyama, T. (1970d), Analysis of population structure. I. One-dimensional stepping stone models of finite length, *Ann. Hum. Genet.* **34**:210–219.

Maruyama, T. (1970e), On the rate of decrease of heterozygosity in circular stepping-stone models, *Theor. Popul. Biol.* **1**:101–119.

Maruyama, T. (1970f), Rate of decrease of genetic variability in a subdivided population, *Biometrika* **57**:299–311.

Maruyama, T. (1971a), The rate of decrease of heterozygosity in a population occupying a circular or a linear habitat, *Genetics* **67**:437–454.

Maruyama, T. (1971b), Analysis of population structure. II. Two-dimensional stepping stone models of finite length and other geographicallay structured populations, *Ann. Hum. Genet.* **35**:179–196.

Maruyama, T. (1971c), Speed of gene substitution in a geographically structured population, *Am. Nat.* **105**:253–265.

Maruyama, T. (1972a), Rate of decrease of genetic variability in a two-dimensional continuous population of finite size, *Genetics* **70**:639–651.

Maruyama, T. (1972b), The rate of decay of genetic variability in a geographically structured finite population, *Math. Biosci.* **14**:325–335.

Maruyama, T. (1973), Isolation by distance, genetic variability, the time required for a gene substitution. and local differentiation in a finite, geographically structured population, in *Genetic Structure of Populations* (N. E. Morton, ed.), pp. 80–81, University of Hawaii Press, Honolulu.

Maruyama, T. (1974a), A Markov process of gene frequency change in a geographically structured population, *Genetics* **76**:367–377.

Maruyama, T. (1974b), A simple proof that certain quantities are independent of the geographic structure of a population, *Theor. Popul. Biol.* **5**:148–154.

Maruyama, T. (1977), *Stochastic Problems in Population Genetics*, Springer-Verlag, Berlin.

May, R. M., Endler, J. A., and McMurtie, R. E. (1975), Gene frequency clines in the presence of selection opposed by gene flow, *Am. Nat.* **109**:659–676.

Maynard Smith, J. (1970), Population size, polymorphism, and the rate of non-Darwinian evolution, *Am. Nat.* **104**:231–237.

Menozzi, P., Piazza, A., and Cavalli-Sforza, L. L. (1978), Synthetic maps of human gene frequencies in Europeans, *Science* **201**:786–792.

Mielke, J. H., Workman, P. L., Fellman, J., and Eriksson, A. W. (1976), Population structure of the Åland Islands, Finland, in *Advances in Human Genetics*, Vol. 6 (H. Harris and K. Hirschhorn, eds.), pp. 241–321, Plenum Press, New York.

Mitra, S. (1975), On Nei and Roychoudhury's sampling variances of heterozygosity and genetic distance, *Genetics* **80**:223–226.

Mitra, S. (1976), More on Nei and Roychoudhury's sampling variances of heterozygosity and genetic distance, *Genetics* **82**:543–545.

Mitton, J. B. (1977), Genetic differentiation of races of man as judged by single locus and multilocus analyses, *Am. Nat.* **111**:203–212.

Mitton, J. B. (1978), Measurement of differentiation: a reply to Lewontin, Powell, and Taylor, *Am. Nat.* **112**:1142–1144.

Moran, P. A. P. (1959), The theory of some genetical effects of population subdivision, *Austral. J. Biol. Sci.* **12**:109–127.

Moran, P. A. P. (1962), *The Statistical Processes of Evolutionary Theory*, Clarendon Press, Oxford.

Morgan, K., and Holmes, T. M. (n.d.), On an attempt to estimate heritability of quantitiative characters from intervillage distances among the Yanomama Indians, unpublished manuscript.

Morton, N. E. (1964), Genetic studies of Northeastern Brazil, *Cold Spring Harbor Symp. Quant. Biol.* **29**:69–79.

Morton, N. E. (1969), Human population structure, *Ann. Rev. Genet.* **3**:53–73.

Morton, N. E. (1971a), Inference in population structure studies, *Am. J. Hum. Genet.* **23**: 538–539.

Morton, N. E. (1971b), Genetic structure of Northeastern Brazilian populations, in *The Ongoing Evolution of Latin American Populations* (F. M. Salzano, ed.), pp. 251–276, Thomas, Springfield, Illinois.

Morton, N. E. (1972), The future of human population genetics, in *Progress in Medical Genetics*, Vol. 8 (A. G. Steinberg and A. G. Bearn, eds.), pp. 103–124, Grane and Stratton, New York.

Morton, N. E. (ed.) (1973), *Genetic Structure of Populations*, University of Hawaii Press, Honolulu.

Morton, N. E. (1973a), Prediction of kinship from a migration matrix, in *Genetic Structure of Populations* (N. E. Morton, ed.), pp. 119–123, University of Hawaii Press, Honolulu.

Morton, N. E. (1973b), Kinship and population structure, in *Genetic Structure of Populations* (N. E. Morton, ed.), pp. 66–70, University of Hawaii Press, Honolulu.

Morton, N. E. (1973d), Population structure of Micronesia, in *Methods and Theories of Anthropological Genetics* (M. H. Crawford and P. L. Workman, eds.), pp. 333–366, University of New Mexico Press, Albuquerque.

Morton, N. E. (1974a), Controversial issues in human population genetics, *Am. J. Hum. Genet.* **26**:259–262.

Morton, N. E. (1974b), Kinship bioassay, in *Genetic Distance* (J. F. Crow and C. Denniston, eds.), pp. 97–104, Plenum Press, New York.

Morton, N. E. (1975a), Kinship, information and biological distance, *Theor. Popul. Biol.* **7**:246–255.

Morton, N. E. (1975b), Kinship, fitness, and evolution, in *The Role of Natural Selection in Human Evolution* (F. M. Salzano, ed.), pp. 133–154, American Elsevier, New York.

Morton, N. E. (1977), Isolation by distance in human populations, *Ann. Hum. Genet.* **40**: 361–365.

Morton, N. E., and Hussels, I. (1970), Demography of inbreeding in Switzerland, *Hum. Biol.* **42**:65–78.

Morton, N. E., Imaizumi, Y., and Harris, D. E. (1971), Clans as genetic barriers, *Am. Anthropol.* **73**:1005–1010.

Morton, N. E., and Lalouel, J. M. (1973a), Topology of kinship in Micronesia, *Am. J. Hum. Genet.* **25**:422–432.

Morton, N. E., and Lalouel, J. M. (1973b), Bioassay of kinship in Micronesia, *Am. J. Phys. Anthropol.* **38**:709–720.

Morton, N. E., Miki, C., and Yee, S. (1968), Bioassay of population structure under isolation by distance, *Am. J. Hum. Genet.* **20**:411–419.

Morton, N. E., Yasuda, N., Miki, C., and Yee, S. (1968), Population structure of the ABO blood groups in Switzerland, *Am. J. Hum. Genet.* **20**:420–429.

Morton, N. E., Yee, S., Harris, D. E., and Lew, R. (1971a), Bioassay of kinship, *Theor. Popul. Biol.* **2**:507–524.

Morton, N. E., Harris, D. E., Yee, S., and Lew, R. (1971b), Pingelap and Mokil Atolls: migration, *Am. J. Hum. Genet.* **23**:339–349.

Morton, N. E., Roisenberg, I., Lew, R., and Yee, S. (1971c), Pingelap and Mokil Atolls: genealogy, *Am. J. Hum. Genet.* **23**:350–360.

Morton, N. E., and Green, D. L. (1972), Pingelap and Mokil Atolls: Anthropometrics, *Am. J. Hum. Genet.* **24**:299–303.

Morton, N. E., Klein, D., Hussels, I. E., Dodinval, P., Todorov, A., Lew, R., and Yee, S. (1973), Genetic structure of Switzerland, *Am. J. Hum. Genet.* **25**:347–361.

Morton, N. E., Smith, C., Hill, R., Frackiewicz, A., Law, P., and Yee, S. (1976), Population structure of Barra, *Ann. Hum. Genet.* **39**:339–352.

Morton, N. E., Dick, H. M., Allan, N. C., Izatt, M. M., Hill, R., and Yee, S (1977), Bioassay of kinship in northwestern Europe, *Ann. Hum. Genet.* **41**:249–255.

Murillo, F., Rothhammer, F., and Llop, E. (1977), The Chipaya of Bolivia: dermatoglyphics and ethnic relationships, *Am. J. Phys. Anthropol.* **46**:45–50.

Neel, J. V., and Ward, R. H. (1972), Genetic structure of a tribal population, the Yanomama Indians. VI. Analysis by F-statistics, including a comparison with the Makiritare and Xavante, *Genetics* **72**:639–666.

Neel, J. V., Rothhammer, F., and Lingoes, J. C. (1974), The genetic structure of a tribal population, the Yanomama Indians. X. Agreement between representations of village distances based on different sets of characteristics, *Am. J. Hum. Genet.* **26**:281–303.

Nei, M. (1965), Variation and covariation of gene frequencies in subdivided populations, *Evolution* 19:256–258.

Nei, M. (1970), Effective size of human populations, *Am. J. Hum. Genet.* 22:694–696.

Nei, M. (1972), Genetic distance between populations, *Am. Nat.* 106:283–292.

Nei, M. (1973a), The theory and estimation of genetic distance, in *Genetic Structure of Populations* (N. E. Morton, ed.), pp. 45–51, University of Hawaii Press, Honolulu.

Nei, M. (1973b), Analysis of gene diversity in subdivided populations, *Proc. Natl. Acad. Sci. U.S.A.* 70:3321–3323.

Nei, M. (1975), *Molecular Population Genetics and Evolution*, North-Holland, Amsterdam.

Nei, M. (1976), Mathematical models of speciation and genetic distance, in *Population Genetics and Ecology* (S. Karlin and E. Nevo, eds.), pp. 723–765, Academic Press, New York.

Nei, M. (1977), F-statistics and analysis of gene diversity in subdivided populations, *Ann. Hum. Genet.* 41:225–233.

Nei, M., and Chakravarti, A. (1977), Drift variances of F_{ST} and G_{ST} statistics obtained from a finite number of isolated populations, *Theor. Popul. Biol.* 11:307–325.

Nei, M., and Feldman, M. W. (1972), Identity of genes by descent within and between populations under mutation and migration pressures, *Theor. Popul. Biol.* 3:460–465.

Nei, M., and Imaizumi, Y. (1966a), Genetic structure of human populations. I. Local differentiation of blood group gene frequencies in Japan, *Heredity* 21:9–36.

Nei, M., and Imaizumi, Y. (1966b), Genetic structure of human populations. II. Local differentiation of blood group gene frequencies among isolated populations, *Heredity* 21:183–190.

Nei, M., and Imaizumi, Y. (1966c), Genetic structure of human populations. III. Differentiation of ABO blood group gene frequencies in small areas of Japan, *Heredity* 21:461–472.

Nei, M., and Li, W.-H. (1973), Linkage disequilibrium in subdivided populations, *Genetics* 75:213–219.

Nei, M., and Maruyama, T. (1975), Lewontin-Krakauer test for neutral genes, *Genetics* 80:395.

Nei, M., and Roychoudhury, A. K. (1974a), Sampling variance of heterozygosity and genetic distance, *Genetics* 76:379–390.

Nei, M., and Roychoudhury, A. K. (1974b), Genic variation within and between the three major races of man, Caucasoids, Negroids, and Mongoloids, *Am. J. Hum. Genet.* 26:421–443.

Nei, M., Chakravarti, A., and Tateno, Y. (1977), Mean and variance of F_{ST} in a finite number of incompletely isolated populations, *Theor. Popul. Biol.* 11:291–306.

Nevanlinna, H. R. (1972), The Finnish population structure: a genetic and genealogical study, *Hereditas* 71:195–236.

Pearson, K. (1926), On the coefficient of racial likeness, *Biometrika* 18:105–117.

Persson, I. (1968), The distribution of serum types in West Greenland Eskimos, *Acta Genet. Statist. Med. (Basel)* 18:261–270.

Piazza, A., Sgaramella-Zonta, L., Gluckman, P., and Cavalli-Sforza, L. L. (1975), The fifth histocompatibility workshop gene frequency data: a phylogenetic analysis, *Tissue Antigens* 5:445–463.

Pollock, N., Lalouel, J. M., and Morton, N. E. (1972), Kinship and inbreeding on Namu Atoll, *Hum. Biol.* 44:459–474.

Powell, J. R., and Taylor, C. E. (1978), Are human races "substantially" different genetically? *Am. Nat.* 112:1139–1142.

Purser, A. F. (1966), Increase in heterozygote frequency with differential fertility, *Heredity* 21:322–327.

Rao, C. R. (1952), *Advanced Statistical Methods in Biometric Research*, Wiley, New York.

Ray, A. K. (1975), Population structure of the Juang tribe in Orissa, India, *Ann. Hum. Biol.* **2**:179–189.

Rhoads, J. G., and Friedlaender, J. S. (1975), Language boundaries and biological differentiation on Bougainville: multivariate analysis of variance, *Proc. Nat. Acad. Sci.* **72**:2247–2250.

Rightmire, G. P. (1976), Multidimensional scaling and the analysis of human diversity in Subsharan Africa, *Am. J. Phys. Anthropol.* **44**:445–452.

Robbins, B. B. (1918), Random mating with the exception of sister by brother mating, *Genetics* **3**:390–396.

Roberts, D. F. (1967), The development of inbreeding in an island population, *Cienc. Cult.* **19**:78–84.

Roberts, D. F. (1968), Genetic effects of population size reduction, *Nature* **220**:1084–1088.

Roberts, D. F. (1971), The demography of Tristan da Cunha, *Popul. Stud.* **25**:465–479.

Roberts, D. F. (1973a), Anthropological genetics: problems and pitfalls, in *Methods and Theories of Anthropological Genetics* (M. H. Crawford and P. L. Workman, eds.), pp. 1–17, University of New Mexico Press, Albuquerque.

Roberts, D. F. (1973b), *Climate and Human Variability*, Addison-Wesley, Menlo Park, California.

Roberts, D. F. (1975), Genetic studies of isolates, in *Modern Trends in Human Genetics*, Vol. 2 (A. E. H. Emery, ed.), pp. 221–269, Butterworths, London.

Roberts, D. F. (1980), Development of the genetic structure of an isolated population, in *Population Structure and Genetic Disease* (A. W. Eriksson, H. Forsius, H. R. Nevanlinna, and P. L. Workman, eds.), Academic Press, New York, in press.

Roberts, D. F., and Rawling, C. P. (1974), Secular trends in genetic structure: an isonymic analysis of Northumberland parish records, *Ann. Hum. Biol.* **1**:393–410.

Roberts, D. F., Luttrell, V., and Slater, C. P. (1965), Genetics and geography in Tinos, *Eugen. Rev.* **56**:185–193.

Robertson, A. (1965), The interpretation of genotypic ratios in domestic animal populations, *Anim. Prod.* **7**:319–324.

Robertson, A. (1975), Gene frequency distributions as a test of selective neutrality, *Genetics* **81**:775–785.

da Rocha, F. J., Spielman, R. S., and Neel, J. V. (1974), A comparison of gene frequency and anthropometric distance matrices in seven villages of four Indian tribes, *Hum. Biol.* **46**:295–310.

Rohlf, F. J., and Schnell, G. D. (1971), An investigation of the isolation-by-distance model, *Am. Nat.* **105**:295–324.

Roisenberg, I., and Morton, N. E. (1970), Population structure of blood groups in Central and South American Indians, *Am. J. Phys. Anthropol.* **32**:373–376.

Rothhammer, F., and Spielman, R. S. (1971), Anthropometric variation in the Aymara: genetic, geographic, and topographic contributions, *Am. J. Hum. Genet.* **24**:371–380.

Rothhammer, F., Chakraborty, R., and Llop, E. (1977), A collection of marker gene and dermatoglyphic diversity at various levels of population differentiation, *Am. J. Phys. Anthropol.* **46**:51–60.

Rothman, E. D., Sing, C. F., and Templeton, A. R. (1974), A model for analysis of population structure, *Genetics* **78**:943–960.

Roychoudhury, A. K. (1974), Gene differentiation among caste and linguistic populations of India, *Hum. Hered.* **24**:317–322.

Roychoudhury, A. K. (1975), Genetic distance and gene diversity among linguistically different tribes of Mexican Indians, *Am. J. Phys. Anthropol.* **42**:449–454.

Saha, N., Kirk, R. L., Shanbhag, S., Joshi, S. R., and Bhatia, H. M. (1976), Population genetic studies of the Kerala and the Nilgiris (Southwest India), *Hum. Hered.* **26**:175–197.

Salzano, F. M. (1971), Demographic and genetic interrelationships among the Cayapo Indians of Brazil, *Soc. Biol.* **18**:148–157.

Salzano, F. M. (ed.) (1975), *The Role of Natural Selection in Human Evolution*, American Elsevier, New York.

Salzano, F. M. (1975a), Degree of heterozygosity and population structure of South American Indians, in *Biosocial Interrelations in Population Adaptation* (E. S. Watts, F. E. Johnston, and G. W. Lasker, eds.), pp. 139–145, Mouton, The Hague.

Salzano, F. M. (1975b), Interpopulation variability in polymorphic systems, in *The Role of Natural Selection in Human Evolution* (F. M. Salzano, ed.), pp. 217–229, American Elsevier, New York.

Salzano, F. M., Neel, J. V., Gershowitz, H., and Migliazza, E. C. (1977), Intra and intertribal genetic variation within a linguistic group: the Ge-speaking Indians of Brazil, *Am. J. Phys. Anthropol.* **47**:337–348.

Salzano, F. M., Pages, F., Neel, J. V., Gershowitz, H., Tanis, R. J., Moreno, R., and Franco, M. H. L. P. (1978), Unusual blood genetic characteristics among the Ayoreo Indians of Bolivia and Paraguay, *Hum. Biol.* **50**:121–136.

Sanghvi, L. D. (1953), Comparison of genetical and morphological methods for a study of biological differences, *Am. J. Phys. Anthropol.* **11**:385–404.

Sanghvi, L. D., and Balakrishnan, V. (1972), Comparison of different measures of genetic distance between human populations, in *The Assessment of Population Affinities in Man* (J. S. Weiner and J. Huizinga, eds.), pp. 25–36, Clarendon Press, Oxford.

Sanghvi, L. D., Kirk, R. L., and Balakrishnan, V. (1971), A study of genetic distance among some populations of Australian aborigines, *Hum. Biol.* **43**:445–458.

Saugstad, L. F. (1977a), The relationship between inbreeding, migration, and population density in Norway, *Ann. Hum. Genet.* **40**:331–341.

Saugstad, L. F. (1977b), Inbreeding in Norway, *Ann. Hum. Genet.* **40**:481–491.

Schönemann, P. H., and Carroll, R. M. (1970), Fitting one matrix to another under choice of a central dilation and a rigid motion, *Psychometrika* **35**:245–255.

Schull, W. J. (1972), Genetic implications of population breeding structure, in *The Structure of Human Populations* (G. A. Harrison and A. J. Boyce, eds.), pp. 146–164, Clarendon Press, Oxford.

Schull, W. J., and MacCluer, J. W. (1968), Human genetics: structure of population, *Ann. Rev. Genet.* **2**:279–304.

Schull, W. J., Komatsu, I., Nagano, H., and Yamamoto, M. (1968), Hirado: temporal trends in inbreeding and fertility, *Proc. Natl. Acad. Sci.* **36**:671–679.

Shapiro, H. L., and Hulse, F. S. (1939), *Migration and Environment*, Oxford University Press, London.

Simmons, R. T., Graydon, J. J., Gajdusek, D. C., Alpers, M., and Hornabrook, R. W. (1972), Genetic studies in relation to Kuru. II. Blood group genetic patterns in Kuru patients and populations of the Eastern Highlands of New Guinea, *Am. J. Hum. Genet.* **24**: S39–S71.

Sinnett, P., Blake, N. M., Kirk, R. L., Lai, L. Y. C., and Walsh, R. J. (1970), Blood, serum protein and enzyme groups among Enga-speaking people of the Western Highlands, New Guinea, with an estimate of genetic distances between clans, *Arch. Phys. Anthropol. Oceania* **5**:236–252.

Sinnock, P. (1975), The Wahlund effect for the two locus model, *Am. Nat.* **109**:565–570.

Skolnick, M., Cavalli-Sforza, L. L., Moroni, A., and Siri, E. (1976), A preliminary analysis of the genealogy of Parma Valley, Italy, in *The Demographic Evolution of Human Populations* (R. H. Ward and K. M. Weiss, eds.), pp. 95–115, Academic Press, London.

Slatkin, M. (1973), Gene flow and selection in a cline, *Genetics* **75**:733–756.

Slatkin, M., and Maruyama, T. (1975a), The influence of gene flow on genetic distance, *Am. Nat.* **109**:597–601.

Slatkin, M., and Maruyama, T. (1975b), Genetic drift in a cline, *Genetics* **81**:209–222.

Smith, C. A. B. (1969), Local fluctuations in gene frequencies, *Ann. Hum. Genet.* **32**: 251–260.

Smith, C. A. B. (1977), A note on genetic distance, *Ann. Hum. Genet.* **40**:463–479.

Smith, C. A. B. (1978), Comments on C. C. Li's paper on measuring genetic distance, *Ann. Hum. Genet.* **41**:505.

Smouse, P. E. (1974), Likelihood analysis of geographic variation in allelic frequencies. II. The logit model and an extension to multiple loci, *Theor. Appl. Genet.* **45**:52–58.

Smouse, P. E., and Kojima, K. (1972), Maximum likelihood analysis of population differences in allelic frequencies, *Genetics* **72**:709–719.

Smouse, P. E., and Neel, J. V. (1977), Multivariate analysis of gametic disequilibrium in the Yanomama, *Genetics* **85**:733–752.

Sneath, P. H. A., and Sokal, R. R. (1973), *Numerical Taxonomy and the Principles and Practice of Numerical Classification*, W. H. Freeman, San Francisco.

Sofaer, J. A., Niswander, J. D., MacLean, C. J., and Workman, P. L. (1972), Population studies on Southwestern Indian tribes. V. Tooth morphology as an indicator of biological distance, *Am. J. Phys. Anthropol.* **37**:357–366.

Spielman, R. S. (1973), Differences among Yanomama Indian villages: do the patterns of allele frequencies, anthropometrics and map locations correspond?, *Am. J. Phys. Anthropol.* **39**:461–480.

Spielman, R. S., da Rocha, F. J., Weitkamp, L. R., Ward, R. H., Neel, J. V., and Chagnon, N. A. (1972), The genetic structure of a tribal population, the Yanomama Indians. VII. Anthropometric differences among Yanomama villages, *Am. J. Phys. Anthropol.* **37**:345–356.

Spielman, R. S., Migliazza, E. C., and Neel, J. V. (1974), Regional linguistic and genetic differences among Yanomama Indians, *Science* **184**:637–644.

Spielman, R. S., Neel, J. V., and Li, F. H. F. (1977), Inbreeding estimation from population data: models, procedures and implications, *Genetics* **85**:355–371.

Spieth, P. T. (1974), Gene flow and genetic differentiation, *Genetics* **78**:961–965.

Spuhler, J. N. (1972), Genetic, linguistic, and geographical distances in native North America, in *The Assessment of Population Affinities in Man* (J. S. Weiner and J. Huizinga, eds.), pp. 72–95, Clarendon Press, Oxford.

Spuhler, J. N. (1979), Genetic distances, trees, and maps of North American Indians, in *The First Americans: Origins, Affinities, and Adaptations* (W. S. Laughlin and A. B. Harper, eds.), pp. 135–183, Gustav Fisher, New York.

Spuhler, J. N., and Clark, P. J. (1961), Migration into the human breeding population of Ann Arbor, Michigan, 1900–1950, *Hum. Biol.* **33**:233–236.

Spuhler, J. N., and Kluckhohn, C. (1953), Inbreeding coefficients of the Ramah Navaho population, *Hum. Biol.* **25**:295–317.

Spuhler, J. N., Gluckman, P., and Pori, M. (1976), A method for grouping a phylogenetic tree based on gene frequencies, unpublished manuscript.

Steinberg, A. G., Bleibtreu, H. K., Kurczynski, T. W., Martin, A. O., and Kurczynski, E. M. (1967), Genetic studies of an inbred human isolate, in *Proceedings of the Third International Congress of Human Genetics* (J. F. Crow and J. V. Neel, eds.), pp. 267–289, Johns Hopkins University Press, Baltimore.

Susanne, C. (1979), Comparative biometrical study of stature and weight of Italian migrants in Belgium, *Am. J. Phys. Anthropol.* **50**:349–355.

Sutter, J., and Tran-Ngoc-Toan (1957), The problem of the structure of isolates and of their evolution among human populations, *Cold Spring Harbor Symp. Quant. Biol.* **22**: 379–383.

Swedlund, A. C. (1972), Observations on the concept of neighbourhood knowledge and the distribution of marriage distances, *Ann. Hum. Genet.* **35**:327–330.

Szathmary, E. J. E., and Ossenberg, N. S. (1978), Eskimo relationships: dogma disputed, paper presented at the 47th annual meeting of the American Association of Physical Anthropologists, Toronto.

Tanaka, K. (1963), Consanguinity study on Japanese populations, in *Genetics of Migrant and Isolate Populations* (E. Goldschmidt, ed.), pp. 169–176, Williams and Wilkins, New York.

Thoma, A. (1970), Selective differentiation of the ABO blood group gene frequencies in Europe, *Hum. Biol.* 42:450–468.

Thompson, E. A. (1975), *Human Evolutionary Trees*, Cambridge University Press, Cambridge.

Thompson, E. A. (1976), Population correlation and population kinship, *Theor. Popul. Biol.* 10:205–226.

Tills, D. (1977), The use of the F_{ST} statistic of Wright for estimating the effects of genetic drift, selection and migration in populations, with special reference to Ireland, *Hum. Hered.* 27:153–159.

Tsakas, S., and Krimbas, C. B. (1976), Testing the heterogeneity of F values: a suggestion and a correction, *Genetics* 84:399–401.

Undevia, J. V., Balakrishnan, V., Kirk, R. L., Blake, N. M., Saha, N., and McDermid, E. M. (1978), A population genetic study of the Vania Soni in Western India, *Hum. Hered.* 28:104–121.

Wagener, D. K. (1973), An extension of migration analysis to account for differential immigration from the outside world, *Am. J. Hum. Genet.* 25:47–56.

Wahlund, S. (1928), Zusammensetzung von populationen und korrelationsersheinungen vom standpunkt den vererbungslehre aus betrachtet, *Hereditas* 11:65–106 [English translation in *Demographic Genetics* (K. M. Weiss and P. A. Ballonoff, eds.), pp. 224–263, Dowden, Hutchinson and Ross, Stroudsburg].

Ward, R. H. (1972), The genetic structure of a tribal population, the Yanomama Indians. V. Comparison of a series of networks, *Ann. Hum. Genet.* 36:21–44.

Ward, R. H. (1973), Some aspects of genetic structure in the Yanomama and Makiritare: two tribes of southern Venezuela, in *Methods and Theories of Anthropological Genetics* (M. H. Crawford and P. L. Workman, eds.), pp. 367–388, University of New Mexico Press, Albuquerque.

Ward, R. H., and Neel, J. V. (1970), Gene frequencies and microdifferentiation among the Makiritare Indians: IV. A comparison of a genetic network with ethnohistory and migration matrices; a new index of genetic isolation, *Am. J. Hum. Genet.* 22:538–561.

Ward, R. H., and Neel, J. V. (1976), The genetic structure of a tribal population, the Yanomama Indians. XIV. Clines and their interpretation, *Genetics* 82:103–121.

Weiner, J. S., and Huizinga (eds.) (1972), *The Assessment of Population Affinities in Man*, Clarendon Press, Oxford.

Weiss, G. H., and Kimura, M. (1965), A mathematical analysis of the stepping stone model of genetic correlation, *J. Appl. Probab.* 2:129–149.

Weiss, K. M., and Ballonoff, P. A. (eds.) (1975), *Demographic Genetics*, Dowden, Hutchinson and Ross, Stroudsburg.

Weiss, K. M., and Maruyama, T. (1976), Archeology, population genetics and studies of racial ancestry, *Am. J. Phys. Anthropol.* 44:31–50.

White, N. G., and Parsons, P. A. (1973), Genetic and socio-cultural differentiation in the aborigines of Arnhem Land, Australia, *Am. J. Phys. Anthropol.* 38:5–14.

Wiesenfeld, S. L., and Gajdusek, D. C. (1976), Genetic structure and heterozygosity in the Kuru region, eastern highlands of New Guinea, *Am. J. Phys. Anthropol.* 45:177–190.

Wood, J. W. (1977), A stability test for migration matrix models of genetic differentiation, *Hum. Biol.* 49:309–320.

Wood, J. W. (1978), Population structure and genetic heterogeneity in the Upper Markham Valley of New Guinea, *Am. J. Phys. Anthropol.* 48:463–470.

Workman, P. L. (1969), The analysis of simple genetic polymorphisms, *Hum. Biol.* **41**:97–114.

Workman, P. L., and Jorde, L. B. (1980), The genetic structure of the Åland Islands, in *Population Structure and Genetic Disease* (A. W. Eriksson, H. Forsius, H. R. Nevanlinna, and P. L. Workman, eds.), Academic Press, New York, in press.

Workman, P. L. and Niswander, J. D. (1970), Population studies on Southwestern Indian tribes. II. Local genetic differentiation in the Papago, *Am. J. Hum. Genet.* **22**:24–49.

Workman, P. L., Harpending, H. C., Lalouel, J. M., Lynch, C., Niswander, J. D., and Singleton, R. (1973), Population studies on Southwestern Indian tribes. VI. Papago population structure: a comparison of genetic and migration analyses, in *Genetic Structure of Populations* (N. E. Morton, ed.), pp. 166–194, University of Hawaii Press, Honolulu.

Workman, P. L., Niswander, J. D., Brown, K. S., and Leyshon, W. C. (1974), Population studies on Southwestern Indian tribes. IV. The Zuni. *Am. J. Phys. Anthropol.* **41**:119–132.

Workman, P. L., Lucarelli, P., Agostino, R., Scarabino, R., Scacchi, R., Carapella, E., Palmarino, R., and Bottini, E. (1975), Genetic differentiation among Sardinian villages, *Am. J. Phys. Anthropol.* **43**:165–176.

Workman, P. L., Mielke, J. H., and Nevanlinna, H. R. (1976), The genetic structure of Finland, *Am. J. Phys. Anthropol.* **44**:341–368.

Wright, S. (1921), Systems of mating, *Genetics,* **6**:111–178.

Wright, S. (1931), Evolution in Mendelian populations, *Genetics* **16**:97–159.

Wright, S. (1940), Breeding structure of populations in relation to speciation, *Am. Nat.* **74**:232–248.

Wright, S. (1943), Isolation by distance, *Genetics* **28**:114–138.

Wright, S. (1951), The genetical structure of populations, *Ann. Eugen.* **15**:323–354.

Wright, S. (1965), The interpretation of population structure by F-statistics with special regard to systems of mating, *Evolution* **19**:395–420.

Wright, S. (1967), Stochastic processes in evolution, in *Proceedings of a Symposium on Stochastic Models in Medicine and Biology* (J. Gurland, ed.), pp. 199–244, University of Wisconsin Press, Madison.

Wright, S. (1969), *Evolution and the Genetics of Populations, Vol. 2 The Theory of Gene Frequencies,* University of Chicago Press, Chicago.

Wright, S. (1973), The origin of the F-statistics for describing the genetic aspects of population structure, in *Genetic Structure of Populations* (N. E. Morton, Ed.), pp. 3–26, University of Hawaii Press, Honolulu.

Wright, S. (1978), *Evolution and the Genetics of Populations, Vol. 4. Variability within and among Natural Populations,* University of Chicago Press, Chicago.

Wyber, S. (1970), Population structure in New Guinea (abstract), *Am. J. Hum. Genet.* **22**:29a–30a.

Yasuda, N. (1975), A random walk model of human migration, *Theor. Popul. Biol.* **7**:156–167.

Yasuda, N., and Kimura, M. (1973), A study of human migration in the Mishima district, *Ann. Hum. Genet.* **36**:313–322.

Yasuda, N., and Morton, N. E. (1967), Studies on human population structure, in *Proceedings of the Third International Congress of Human Genetics* (J. F. Crow and J. V. Neel, eds.), pp. 249–265, Johns Hopkins University Press, Baltimore.

Zanardi, P., Dell'Acqua, G., Menini, C., and Barrai, I. (1977), Population genetics in the province of Ferrara. I. Genetic distances and geographic distances, *Am. J. Hum. Genet.* **29**:169–177.

Zegura, S. (1975), Taxonomic convergence in Eskimoid populations, *Am. J. Phys. Anthropol.* **43**:271–284.

8

Distance Analysis and Multidimensional Scaling

J. M. LALOUEL

1. Introduction

1.1. Population Structure

A population consists of a collection of individuals presenting some common, prespecified characteristic, such as "living in a defined geographical area," or "speaking a given dialect." If the variability exhibited by individual members of this population for some traits is not random, but rather related to recognizable criteria defining subpopulations, this population may be differentiated. We shall concern ourselves with studies whose purpose is to reveal this underlying structure, as well as to attempt to make some inference concerning the process that led to that structure.

Having observations, quantitative or qualitative, on a sample of individuals from this population, one may proceed into the analysis of these data without *a priori* specification of a criterion for partition of this population into subpopulations. Identifying an underlying structure of differentiation consists then in finding such a partition on the basis of available observations. Various methods are available, generally referred to as "flat-clusters" methods, which will be briefly mentioned further, together with some relevant references.

We shall here restrict our attention to situations where some primary subdivisions are identified prior to the analysis of these data, whether geographical — as

J. M. LALOUEL • Population Genetics Laboratory, University of Hawaii, Honolulu, Hawaii. This work was supported in part by Grants GM 23498 and GM 17173 from the U.S. National Institutes of Health.

individuals tend to settle by groups rather than being dispersed over a geographical area — socio-cultural, linguistic, or other. The purpose of the analysis will be
to assess the significance of these primary subdivisions with regard to the differentiation of this population, and to identify possible secondary subdivisions or
groupings affecting population structure. Some understanding of the evolutionary
process having led to the observed differentiation may be obtained from the very
nature of the secondary subdivisions or groupings revealed, further analysis of
population structure involving evolutionary models (see Jorde, this volume),
and careful interpretation of analyses based on various data — anthropological
measurements, genetic markers, linguistic data, migration data, etc. — in the
light of the known ethnohistory.

1.2. The Concept of Distance

Each subpopulation may be characterized more succinctly by the distribution of these observations, or still more economically by parameters of these
distributions, such as means and variances, or possibly means alone. Consider
for the moment that only one trait was studied. In order to give an objective
measure reflecting the similarities or dissimilarities between subdivisions, an
analogy between similarity and proximity (or dissimilarity and distance) comes
naturally, as one can see by considering the following definition of distance:
for all pairs i,j of elements of a set E, we define a nonnegative element d_{ij}
such that

$$d_{ii} = 0$$

$$d_{ij} > 0, \qquad i \neq j$$

$$d_{ij} = d_{ji}$$

$$d_{ij} \leqslant d_{ik} + d_{kj} \tag{1.1}$$

More on the analogy between similarity and proximity can be found in Shepard
(1962) and Guttman (1968).

Were more than one trait considered, and were these traits independent,
the measure of dissimilarity sought should naturally be such that observed
differences for each trait be additive. A class of metric satisfying (1.1) as well as
this last condition is the class of L metrics, or metrics of Minkowski:

$$d_{ij} = \left(\sum_{k=1}^{m} | \bar{x}_{ik} - \bar{x}_{jk} |^c \right)^{1/c} \tag{1.2}$$

x_{ik} being the mean of the kth trait in the ith population. For $c = 1$, the "city
block metric" or "Manhattan distance" obtains, while the Euclidean distance is
defined for $c = 2$. The latter best corresponds to one's intuitive notion of
proximity in a continuous space, on the basis of measurements expressed as
real numbers, and has a very simple geometric interpretation: to m independent

traits, one associates m orthogonal directions defining a space where the ith subpopulation is represented by a point whose coordinates along those directions are given by the means $\bar{x}_{ik}$, $k = 1, \ldots, m$. The distance between two subpopulations i, j in that space is given by the length of the segment between points i and j, shortest path between i and j, invariant under rotation of the axes; this space is isotropic, and a given distance has the same interpretation, in terms of dissimilarity, along any directions.

To characterize dissimilarities between distributions of these m traits in subdivisions of the population by a distance measure based on mean differences alone would not, however, be in general appropriate: still assuming for the moment that these traits are independent, it is clear that, for a given mean difference, the degree of overlap of two distributions will depend on scale of measurement as well as spread of these distributions. Assuming that these traits have the same distribution law, this will be taken into account by a distance measure weighting squared differences of means by their corresponding variances, which also corresponds to weight each trait according to its amount of information (for example, see Kullback, 1968).

Consider now that the traits studied are not statistically independent. To neglect their covariations would introduce redundancy in the distance measure. Moreover, the m directions associated with m nonindependent traits are not orthogonal; to preserve isotropy, that is to give common significance to any distance between two populations along any direction of the space, a distance measure should take into account these covariations. This leads to defining the distance

$$d_{ij}^2 = \sum_{kl}^{m} v_{ij}^{kl}(\bar{x}_{ik} - \bar{x}_{jk})(\bar{x}_{il} - \bar{x}_{jl}) \tag{1.3}$$

or equivalently

$$d_{ij}^2 = (\bar{\mathbf{x}}_i - \bar{\mathbf{x}}_j)^T V_{ij}^{-1} (\bar{\mathbf{x}}_i - \bar{\mathbf{x}}_j) \tag{1.3'}$$

V_{ij}^{-1} being the inverse of the covariance matrix between these traits for subdivisions i and j. When more than two subpopulations are considered, simultaneous representation of all subpopulations in a same space requires definition of a common covariance matrix V norming that space, a point to which we shall return.

Assuming such a common covariance matrix, V, is used in (1.3'), a new system of orthogonal directions can be defined such that

$$d_{ij}^2 = (\bar{\mathbf{y}}_i - \bar{\mathbf{y}}_j)^T (\bar{\mathbf{y}}_i - \bar{\mathbf{y}}_j) \tag{1.4}$$

identical to (1.3'), the new variables $\bar{y}_{ik}$ being independent and having equal unit variances.

In general, not all individuals of the population will have been observed, but rather a sample will have been drawn from this population. This will contribute sampling errors to estimates of means and variances-covariances. Sampling corrections may be applied in estimating distances, although this source of variation is often neglected. In any event, for distances between samples to best reflect distances between subpopulations, careful planning of the sampling procedures is required. Sampling design extends beyond the scope of this presentation, and one may refer to classic texts on the subject (e.g., Hansen, Hurwitz, and Madow, 1953; Cochran, 1963). Let us only mention that, because in most instances characteristics of the whole population are to be estimated as well as that of its subdivisions, and generally subdivisions are of unequal sizes, an appropriate sampling for distance analysis will often consist in drawing randomly and independently individuals from each subdivision in such a way that sample sizes be proportional to the sizes of these subdivisions, the sampling rate being a function of cost of sampling as well as acceptable sampling errors determined *a priori*.

1.3 The Scope of This Chapter

The calculation of distances raises problems of statistical estimation, particularly with regard to the estimation of some common covariance matrix V. Distributional assumptions will be required and will clearly differ according to whether the traits are quantitative or qualitative. Particular emphasis, in the latter case, will be put on the analysis of genetic markers, and we shall distinguish distance measures based on minimal genetic assumptions from other measures implying an evolutionary model, where an attempt is made to estimate some biological measure of similarity or dissimilarity.

We shall thereafter consider multidimensional scaling methods that can be applied to distance matrices for exposure purposes.

Much of this presentation is based on a doctoral dissertation (Lalouel, 1975) where similar topics were considered in extensive details. This paper provided us with the opportunity of presenting some essential aspects of this work, and it is therefore hoped that the reader will not interpret frequent reference to this work as self-indulgence.

2. Distance Analysis

2.1. Quantitative Traits

Assume that observations have been made on individuals drawn from a population where n primary subdivisions are recognized *a priori*, observations on each individual consisting of measurement of m traits. The two most widely used distance measures we shall consider here both rest on the assumption that these m traits are normally distributed. Such an assumption should be validated in practice, possibly by testing for the existence of significant skewness and kurtosis; were either to be significant, important methological decisions have to be done with respect to recognition of outliers or transformation to normality.

2.1.1. CRL Index of Pearson

The Coefficient of Racial Likeness of Pearson (1926) rests on the assumptions that the m traits considered are normally and independently distributed with equal variance for each trait in all subdivisions. Denoting n_{ik} and $\bar{x}_{ik}$ the sample size and mean of the kth trait in the ith population, and s_k the estimation of the standard error of the kth trait obtained from both samples i and j,

$$\text{CRL}(i,j) = \frac{1}{m} \sum_{k=1}^{m} \frac{n_{ik} n_{jk}}{n_{ik} + n_{jk}} \left(\frac{\bar{x}_{ik} - \bar{x}_{jk}}{s_k} \right)^2 \tag{2.1}$$

is taken as a squared distance index between populations i and j. The analogy with t^2, where t follows a student distribution under the null hypothesis, is clear. For this index to be comparable for all pairs of subdivisions, some correction must be introduced, defining the "reduced" CRL or RCRL,

$$\text{RCRL}(i,j) = \frac{n_{i\cdot} + n_{j\cdot}}{n_{i\cdot} n_{j\cdot} m} \left[\sum_{k=1}^{m} \frac{n_{ik} n_{jk}}{n_{ik} + n_{jk}} \left(\frac{\bar{x}_{ik} - \bar{x}_{jk}}{s_k} \right)^2 - 1 \right] \tag{2.2}$$

with $n_{i\cdot} = \Sigma_k n_{ik}/m$, and it can be shown that

$$E\{\text{RCRL}(i,j)\} = \frac{n_{i\cdot} + n_{j\cdot}}{n_{i\cdot} n_{j\cdot} m} \sum_{k=1}^{m} \frac{n_{ik} n_{jk}}{n_{ik} + n_{jk}} \left(\frac{\mu_{ik} - \mu_{jk}}{\sigma_k} \right)^2 \tag{2.3}$$

μ_{ik} being the expectation of the kth trait in the ith population, and σ_k^2 the variance of the kth trait. Clearly, this index will be independent of sample sizes if $n_{ik} = n_{i\cdot}$, an assumption often made in distance analysis, as the general case of $n_{ik} \neq n_{il}$ raises additional estimation problems.

This index defines a Euclidean distance on standardized variables. The validity of its use depends on whether fundamental assumptions are satisfied or not. Normality and the assumption of equal variances within subdivisions may be tested prior to the analysis. The latter assumption, just as with the linear model of analysis of variance, will strictly be legitimate only for an analysis of local perturbations, i.e., for the analysis of the local differentiation of a population. More critical yet is the assumption of independence of the traits studied, generally invalidated in practice. The consequence of neglecting significant covariation between traits will be to introduce redundancy in the distance measure as well as anisotropy in the reference space where these distances are defined.

The use of such an index was justifiable prior to the advent of computers. In view of their now widespread availability, ease of computation is not an appropriate criterion to favor its use over more elaborate indices. Nullity of covariances between traits can be tested and, whenever not tenable, this hypothesis should be abandoned in favor of indices taking such covariances into account.

2.1.2. Mahalanobis Distance

A distance measure presented by Mahalanobis (1936) accounts for such covariation. It is assumed that the m traits studied follow, in each subpopulation, a multivariate normal distribution specified by the means $\{\mu_{ik}\}$ and covariances $\{w_{i,kl}\}$. Assuming furthermore that covariances within subdivision have same expectation, $\{w_{kl}\}$, define the distance index

$$d_{ij}^2 = \sum_{k,l=1}^{m} w^{kl}(\bar{x}_{ik} - \bar{x}_{jk})(\bar{x}_{il} - \bar{x}_{jl}) \tag{2.4}$$

or equivalently

$$d_{ij}^2 = (\bar{\mathbf{x}}_i - \bar{\mathbf{x}}_j)^T W^{-1}(\bar{\mathbf{x}}_i - \bar{\mathbf{x}}_j) \tag{2.4'}$$

Under the assumption of equal covariances within subdivisions, the best estimation of W is given by (Anderson, 1958: 248-250)

$$w_{kl} = \sum_{i=1}^{n} \sum_{\alpha=1}^{n_i} (x_{\alpha,ik} - \bar{x}_{ik})(x_{\alpha,il} - \bar{x}_{il}) \bigg/ \sum_{i=1}^{n} (n_i - 1) \tag{2.5}$$

where $x_{\alpha,ik}$ is the kth measurement on the αth individual in the ith subdivision, and $\bar{x}_{ik} = \Sigma_\alpha x_{\alpha,ik}/n_i$. This index can be alternately presented as the solution to the problem of optimal discrimination between groups (see Rao, 1948, 1952), and it has been shown to be proportional to "divergence" in the sense of information theory (see Kullback, 1968). The distance thus obtained effectively takes into account the amount of information contributed by each trait, while RCRL does not. Just as CRL relates to a t test of homogeneity between means, there is a simple relationship between Mahalanobis distance between two populations i and j and Hotelling T^2 statistics of homogeneity between mean vectors of these populations (see Rao, 1952, Chapter 7):

$$T^2 = n_i n_j d_{ij}^2/(n_i + n_j) \tag{2.6}$$

As usually calculated, using (2.4) and (2.5), Mahalanobis distance does not include a sampling correction. However, sampling bias for the case where $n_{ik} = n_i.,\forall k$, given by $m(n_i + n_j)/n_i n_j$ (see Rao, 1952: 364), may be safely neglected so long as sample sizes are large enough relative to the observed differentiation. This correction may also be neglected whenever such biases are of similar magnitude for all subdivisions.

Validation of underlying assumptions requires testing multinormality as well as equality of within-subdivision covariances, for which statistics are given in Anderson (1958, Chapters 9 and 10). If the former but not the latter hypothesis were satisfied, one may adopt either of two possible alternatives. One may decide to use such an index, in spite of significant heterogeneity of within-subdivision covariances, relying on the proven robustness of such an index under such deviations from assumptions, as well documented (Balakrishnan and Sanghvi, 1968; Sneath and Sokal, 1973). Alternatively, one may resort to statistics specifically allowing for unequal covariances. Of the various statistics proposed (Anderson and Bahadur, 1962; Reyment, 1962; Ito and Schull, 1964), that of Anderson and Bahadur should be preferred, although on the basis of numerical evidence only (Chaddha and Marcus, 1968). For two normal populations $N_1(\mu_1, \Sigma_1)$ and $N_2(\mu_2, \Sigma_2)$ with $\Sigma_1 \neq \Sigma_2$, a best linear discriminant, according to a minimax criterion, is given by

$$D^{*2} = \max_t \frac{2\mathbf{b}_t^T \delta}{(\mathbf{b}^T \Sigma_1 \mathbf{b})^{1/2} + (\mathbf{b}^T \Sigma_2 \mathbf{b})^{1/2}} \tag{2.7}$$

where

$$\mathbf{b}_t = [t\Sigma_1 + (1-t)\Sigma_2]^{-1} \delta \tag{2.8}$$

δ being the vector of mean differences for the two populations. Other relevant references on this subject are Bhattacharyya (1943), Kullback (1968), Matusita (1966), Adhikari and Joshi (1956), and Burnaby (1966). Clearly, however, each pairwise distance calculated as such is defined in a space with different norm, so that simultaneous representation in a common reference space is not feasible. Therefore, apart from situations where the problem is one of best discrimination between two groups or finding the most divergent pair of subpopulations, one may still choose to resort to Mahalanobis distance for purpose of description and exposure, especially when sample sizes are not too different.

2.2. Qualitative Traits

We shall in this section concern ourselves with the problem of calculating distance indices on the basis of data on genetic markers, restricting ourselves to regular phenotype systems in the sense of Cotterman (1953, 1969). We shall distinguish distance measures involving minimal biological assumptions, where the derivation of an index is primarily a problem in statistical estimation, from other measures that, in addition, involve some biological assumptions concerning the process having led to the present structure. However, some relevant points need to be considered prior to presenting available distance indices.

2.2.1. Preliminary Considerations on the Use of Genetic Markers in Distance Analysis

Data on genetic markers consists in identifications of the phenotypes exhibited by individuals at one or several loci. It is usual to base distance indices not on observed proportions of these phenotype themselves, but rather on gene frequencies estimated from these proportions, and all the distance measures presented here will be of this type, although it is worth noting that some indices based on proportions of observed phenotypes have also been proposed (e.g., Hedrick, 1971; Latter, 1973). For the geneticist, individuals are transient, being themselves the result of a sampling of gametes from a conceptually infinite gametic pool; in the absence of zygotic selection, gametic gene frequencies characterize the probability distribution of phenotypic observations. For codominant systems, this distribution is multinomial, provided panmixia within subdivisions is assumed. When there is dominance, knowledge of dominance relations will specify the distribution of the observations.

For distance analysis, a minimum set of genetic assumptions is required to specify the probability distribution of phenotypic observations: local panmixia within subdivisions; that gametes which led to procreation of individuals were conceptually drawn by Bernouilli trials in an "infinite" gametic pool (Malécot, 1966); no selection; and known dominance relations. Gene frequencies can then be estimated from phenotype frequencies by maximum likelihood, which, in addition, will also provide estimates of variances and covariances. It must be noted, however, that the validity of these assumptions should be checked in practice. In particular, for the assumption of local panmixia to be realistic, it is necessary that the primary subdivisions defined more or less correspond to true local panmictic units, that is, that secondary barriers within subdivisions be negligible. This assumption can be tested (Haldane, 1954), although with low power and, were subdivisions themselves significantly heterogeneous, an index of deviation from panmixia should be introduced, estimated from informative systems with respect to that parameter (see Yasuda, 1968).

Mention must be made at this point of two particular problems arising in connection with maximum-likelihood estimation of gene frequencies from random samples of phenotype, particularly with small samples or low sampling rate. Due to dominance effects, maximum likelihood will give no evidence for a recessive gene, although it may be present in the sample, so long as this gene is not necessary to explain a phenotypic class that cannot be accounted for by other allelic combinations, and in fact such an allele may well not be present in the population. Another difficulty is that, especially for systems involving a large number of loci, alleles present in a given subdivision may not be present in the sample drawn from it, and comparisons between subdivisions may thus lead to serious biases. This situation is particularly likely for systems such as Gm or HLA, presenting numerous alleles at low frequency, whenever the sampling rate in the population is low. Such biases can indeed be very serious, as shown by Ewens theory of sampling in a quasi-infinite series of alleles (Ewens, 1972). For distance analysis and study of population structure, a possible way to avoid such biases (Morton, 1973), consists in assuming that all alleles for which there is likelihood evidence from the sample pooled over subdivisions are also present within subdivisions, and apply to each sample from a subdivision only one cycle of gene counting, starting from gene frequencies estimated in the pooled sample. This was applied to a study of Lebanese population structure (Lalouel, Loiselet, Lefranc, Chaiban, Chashachiro, and Ropartz, 1975) for the Gm system on the ground that, although it will underestimate divergence between subdivisions with respect to such systems, it will avoid inferring false similarities and is compatible with the assumption of existence of some migration between subdivisions. Such an approach best applies to studies of local differentiation of a population, but its validity is questionable when studying populations so diverse and remote that no present day migration exists.

2.2.2. Distance Indices Based on Minimal Genetic Assumptions

These assumptions have been formulated in the previous section, being needed to specify phenotype probability distributions in terms of gene frequencies. Derivation of a distance index is considered solely as a problem in statistical estimation. Of many such indices presented in the literature, only the more widely used are discussed here.

2.2.2.1 Distance G^2 of Sanghvi. This was the first distance index specifically introduced for the purpose of analysis of genetic differences between populations, and Sanghvi's original paper (Sanghvi, 1953) also contributed quite interesting discussions on the purpose of distance analysis and the problems related to the study of genetic differences between populations.

Before computers became available, ease of computation was required, so that, just as Pearson's CRL was derived by analogy with a t^2 statistics, Sanghvi presented an index based on a contingency table χ^2 between pairs of populations characterized by their frequencies. Under the hypothesis of homogeneity, expected frequencies are given by marginal frequencies; assuming independence of the genetic systems considered, G^2 is defined by

$$G^2 = \sum_{r=1}^{s} \sum_{k=1}^{m_r} \left\{ \frac{(p_{irk} - \bar{p}_{rk})^2 + (p_{jrk} - \bar{p}_{rk})^2}{\bar{p}_{rk}} \right\} \bigg/ \sum_{r=1}^{s} (m_r - 1) \quad (2.9)$$

where $\bar{p}_{rk} = (p_{irk} + p_{jrk})/2$, and the rth system has m_r alleles. Division by degrees of freedom is not needed when all samples have been typed for the same set of genetic systems, and, being only concerned here with relative distances, G^2 can be defined alternatively as

$$G^2 = \sum_{r=1}^{s} \sum_{k=1}^{m_r} \frac{(p_{irk} - p_{jrk})^2}{\bar{p}_{rk}} \quad (2.10)$$

Although for a codominant system the probability density distribution of phenotypic observations is multinomial, it is not so when there is dominance, and in such case the best estimate of the mean gene frequencies in populations i and j pooled do not coincide with the means of the gene frequencies estimated separately in each sample; this bias may be particularly serious with small samples. Sample sizes are not taken into account in Sanghvi's original presentation, but this has been relaxed (Kurczynski, 1970). Steinberg, Bleuibtreu, Kurczynski, Martin, and Kurczynski (1967) have shown that G^2, so calculated, was proportional to (for one genetic system):

$$G^2 = \sum_{k=1}^{m-1} \sum_{l=1}^{m-1} s^{kl}(p_{ik} - p_{jk})(p_{il} - p_{jl}) \quad (2.11)$$

where

$$s_{kk} = \bar{p}_k(1 - \bar{p}_k), \qquad s^{kk} = \frac{1}{\bar{p}_m}, \qquad k = 1, \ldots, m-1$$

and

$$s_{kl} = -\bar{p}_k\bar{p}_l, \qquad s^{kl} = \frac{1}{\bar{p}_k} + \frac{1}{\bar{p}_m}, \qquad k \neq l = 1, \ldots, m = 1$$

that is, products of gene frequencies differences are weighted by the expected covariances of a multinomial distribution of which gene frequencies are the parameters.

The most serious restriction to the use of G^2 is that it is a measure based solely on the pair of populations i and j; addition of new populations will not modify indices already calculated; however, each pairwise distance has a distinct geometric interpretation, so that simultaneous representation of all pairwise distances may have little signification.

2.2.2.2. Distance B^2 of Balakrishnan. In order to express pairwise distances between n subdivisions in a common metric, thus allowing their simultaneous representation in a common reference space having a well-defined norm, some assumption is required to set up such a norm. Balakrishnan and Sanghvi (1968) introduced an analog of Mahalanobis distance for the discrete case such that products of gene frequency differences are weighted by a common variance-covariance matrix for all pairs of subdivisions. Its general form is

$$B_{ij}^2 = \sum_{r=1}^{s} B_{rij}^2 \tag{2.12}$$

where

$$B_{rij}^2 = \sum_{k=1}^{m_r-1} \sum_{l=1}^{m_r-1} s_r^{kl}(p_{irk} - p_{jrk})(p_{irl} - p_{jrl}) \tag{2.12'}$$

Two indices can be defined depending on how the common covariance matrix S_r is calculated. In both cases, it is assumed that within-subdivision covariances have the same expectation in all subdivisions. Depending on the type of data available, different estimates of S_r are proposed. Whenever phenotype information is available, for a given system r and a given population i, estimation of the within-subdivision covariance matrix S_{ir}, with a general element S_{irkl}, can be obtained simultaneously to that of gene frequencies by maximum likelihood, and the best estimation of S_r is given by

$$S_r = \sum_{i=1}^{n} n_{ir}^2 s_{irkl} \bigg/ \sum_{i=1}^{n} n_{ir} \tag{2.13}$$

When only gene frequency data are available, one must alternatively calculate the expected within-subdivisions covariances, assuming gene frequencies are parameters of a multinomial distribution:

$$s_{irkk} = p_{irk}(1 - p_{irk})/n_{ir} \tag{2.14}$$

$$s_{irkl} = -p_{irk}p_{irl}/n_{ir}, \qquad k \neq l$$

and S_r being estimated by

$$s_{rkl} = \sum_{i=1}^{n} n_{ir}^2 s_{irkl} \bigg/ \sum_{i=1}^{n} n_{ir} \qquad (2.14')$$

(2.12), (2.12'), and (2.13) define B_O^2 (O for "observed"), while (2.12), (2.12'), (2.14), and (2.14') define B_E^2 (E for "expected"). Clearly, B_O^2 should be preferred, and therefore used whenever phenotype data are available.

Another index presented by Balakrishnan and Sanghvi (1968), which they denoted G_C^2, uses also (2.12), (2.12'), but define S_r as

$$s_{rkk} = p_{rk}(1 - p_{rk})$$

$$s_{rkl} = -p_{rk}p_{rl}, \qquad k \neq l \qquad (2.15)$$

with

$$p_{rk} = \sum_{i=1}^{n} n_{ir} p_{irk} \bigg/ \sum_{i=1}^{n} n_{ir}$$

There is, however, little justification to favor (2.15) over B_O^2 or B_E^2, as using within-subdivisions as well as between-subdivisions covariation to weight products of gene frequency differences is not appropriate for best separation of subdivisions on the basis of their dissimilarities.

B_O^2 weights each system precisely according to its amount of information it allows simultaneous representation of all pairwise distances within subdivisions. It can be shown that this space is Euclidean and new variables with unit covariance matrix can be defined by projection on a new system of orthogonal coordinates, B_O^2 then obeying (1.4). This space is isotropic in the sense previously defined. Because of its analogy with a minimum discriminant, this index should best separate populations on the basis of their divergence. It is best suited for analysis of moderate, local differentiation of a population. This is so because covariances vary with gene frequencies and, for low frequencies, one can see from (2.14) that they are almost linear functions of gene frequencies. With increasing variability of gene frequencies between subdivisions, the hypothesis of equal covariances within subdivisions become less and less tenable, this all the more so for rare alleles. For widely differing populations, its use, as for Mahalanobis distance, can only be justified on the empirical ground of relatively greater robustness than other indices (Sanghvi and Balakrishnan, 1972).

2.2.2.3 The Distance of Edwards. This index differs conceptually from the previous ones in that it is based on an angular transformation of gene frequencies stabilizing the variances, first introduced by Fisher (see, for example, Fisher, 1958) for a binomial variable, and extended to the multinomial case by Bhattacharyya (1946). Independently of Bhattacharyya's work, Edwards and Cavalli-Sforza have used this transformation in the multinomial case to define an index of distance on the basis of gene frequencies (Cavalli-Sforza and Conterio, 1960; Edwards and Cavalli-Sforza, 1964). More rigorous justification of that index was presented in Edwards (1971) and Edwards and Cavalli-Sforza (1972).

For a codominant system with m alleles, expectations of gene frequencies are $\{p_{ik}\}$, with variances $\{p_{ik}(1-p_{ik})/n_i\}$, and covariances $\{-p_{ik}p_{il}/n_i\}$. To obtain distances in an isotropic space with variances-covariances constant and independent of gene frequencies, these authors argue that a nonlinear transformation is required, as the variance of some allele k is a nonlinear function of gene frequency. With the transformation

$$\sin^2\theta_k = p_k, \qquad k = 1,\ldots,m \qquad (2.16)$$

the new variables θ asymptotically have variances $\mathrm{var}(\theta_k) = 1/4n_i$ and covariances $\mathrm{cov}(\theta_k,\theta_l) = -\tan\theta_k \tan\theta_l/4n_i$. Hence the variances of the variables $\{\theta_k\}$ are only a function of sample sizes (in number of genes). The distribution of these new variables in this new space are approximately normal with spherical symmetry, the correlation between variables θ_k and θ_l being given by the cosine of the angle ϕ between axes corresponding to these variables, with $\phi = -\tan\theta_k \tan\theta_l$. Therefore covariances are appropriately taken into account, a point overlooked by Balakrishnan and Sanghvi (1968) and Kurczynski (1970). This corresponds to representing each population i on the $(1/2^m)$th part of the surface of a hypersphere with unit radius, the coordinates of the ith population on m orthogonal axes being given by $\{p_{ik}^{1/2}\}$, provided all samples are of equal size. The distance between two points i and j in this space is given by

$$d_{ij} = \arccos \sum_{k=1}^{m} (p_{ik}p_{jk})^{1/2} \qquad (2.17)$$

This distance clearly is not Euclidean, so that Edwards and Cavalli-Sforza (1964) initially proposed the chord approximation:

$$\mathrm{chord}(i,j) = \left[1 - \sum_{k=1}^{m} (p_{ik}p_{jk})^{1/2}\right]^{1/2} \qquad (2.18)$$

and some multiplier can be introduced to bound the domain on which these distances take their values. Another Euclidean approximation preserving as much as possible isotropy on the hypersphere consists in the stereographic projection on a plane tangent to the region of the hypersphere occupied by the points representing populations, defining the squared distance:

$$E_{ij}^2 = \frac{8[1 - \Sigma_k(p_{ik}p_{jk})^{1/2}]}{[1 + \Sigma_k(p_{ik}/m)^{1/2}][1 + \Sigma_k(p_{jk}/m)^{1/2}]} \qquad (2.19)$$

To obtain a distance measure on the basis of s independent genetic systems, one can then simply sum distances defined by E_{ij}^2 over systems as covariances have been taken into account.

Practical limitations to the use of such an index can be summarized as follows: use of such an index requires approximately equal sample sizes; the validity of this transformation being based on asymptotic results, it decreases with decreasing sample sizes; the effects of dominance deviations is not known; the transformation becomes of uncertain validity for gene frequencies lower than 0.10 (Gower, 1972); the stereographic projection may become an approximation of dubious value after summation over a large number of systems.

    2.2.2.4. Choice of Distance Measure for a Given Analysis. As we saw, all proposed indices have practical limitations, and no index appears definitely superior to all other irrespective of particular applications. In practice, choice of an index should be guided by careful considerations concerning the validity of required assumptions. Let us thus consider two extreme experimental conditions.

    In one instance, the study concerns the local differentiation of a population (or "microdifferentiation"). Subdivisions are likely to be small, limiting sample sizes, and most likely of unequal sizes, so that proportional sampling should be preferred over constant sample size; deviations from the assumption of equal covariances within subdivisions are not likely to be severe, and B_O^2 seems best adapted to the situation.

    For widely divergent populations, possibly not undergoing migration at the present time, there is no rigorous theoretical support in favor of any index. One may be guided by considerations of sample sizes and some judgement on the possible effect of violations of assumptions. If equal sample sizes can be realized without risking bias due to nonrepresentativeness of alleles present in a population, one may decide to use Edwards' distance E^2. When proportional sampling is required to reflect wide differences in population sizes, B_O^2 can be preferred. When some alleles are at very high or very low frequencies, we have seen that both E^2 and B_O^2 suffer, and choice of an index measure can hardly be justified on other grounds than sample size considerations.

2.2.3. Measures of Similarity and Dissimilarity Based on Genetic Models

    The indices that will be now considered depart from those previously presented in that they are based on both a genetic model and a statistical model of estimation. The assumptions embodied in the genetic model specify a probabilistic model of population evolution so that, in contrast with indices of the preceding section that merely purport to measure amounts of heterogeneity, some biological meaning may be attached to them. As a consequence, apart from describing similarities between populations, genetic indices may also provide some insight on the process having led to the present structure of differentiation. We shall concern ourselves here with three such models, attention being primarily directed to assumptions of the genetic models rather than the particular aspects of statistical estimation involved.

2.2.3.1. Bioassay of Kinship. This model was first introduced by Morton, Yee, Harris and Lew (1971). An alternate model of statistical estimation was presented later (Morton, 1975). Assumptions underlying the genetic model are better presented in Morton (1973a, c, 1975), Jacquard (1974), and Lalouel (1975).

Considering a subdivided population, it is assumed that all subdivisions originated from a common population of founders in a random manner with respect to the traits under study, so that the expectations of gene frequencies among founders of each subdivision coincide with expectations among the founders as a whole. Migration occurs between subdivisions and, although it is assumed that no differential immigration from neighbouring populations exists, random immigration from the outside may occur; this latter effect is assumed to be small in relation to exchanges between subdivisions. In addition, it is assumed that the effects of selection and mutation are small relative to these exchanges.

Under such a model, one expects covariation of gene frequencies to develop between subdivisions as a result of migration and random drift. If migration between subdivisions is important enough, one can expect that, by cumulating the information provided by a large series of independent genetic systems into a global index, the effect of random drift on this index should decrease in proportion of the number of systems studied.

As an index of genetic differentiation, Morton *et al.* (1971) proposed the probability of identity by descent, or kinship, of two random genes drawn in the same or two different subdivisions. If q_0 is the $m \times 1$ vector of gene frequencies of m alleles at a given locus among the founders, and q_i the corresponding vector of contemporary gene frequencies in the ith subdivision, the expected covariance between contemporary frequencies of the kth allele in subdivisions i and j is (Malécot, 1959, 1971, 1972)

$$E(q_{ik} - q_{0k})(q_{jk} - q_{0k}) = q_{0k}(1 - q_{0k})\phi_{ij} \qquad (2.20)$$

ϕ_{ij} being the probability of identity by descent of two random genes from i and j relative to the founding population. If the population has reached a stationary state, this probability coincides with the *a priori* probability of identity. It will be assumed that this probability has same expectation for all alleles of a given system as well as all systems under consideration, conditions for such assumptions to be fulfilled being discussed by Yasuda (1966) and Nei (1965), respectively.

These assumptions provide a genetic model allowing one to define a statistical model of estimation which relates allelic frequency correlations to probability of identity by descent; this holds, in expectation, for several genetic systems, and it should not be taken to imply that identity and isoaction are the same stochastic process.

It clearly appears, however, that in practice gene frequencies among founders q_0 cannot be estimated, although one can estimate contemporary frequencies of the population as a whole, q. Strictly speaking, one can only estimate what we shall call "relative kinship," such that

$$E(q_{ik} - q_k)(q_{jk} - q_k) = q_k(1 - q_k)\phi_{Rij} \qquad (2.21)$$

Estimates of relative kinship correspond to allelic correlations relative to contemporary gene frequencies in the population; Malécot (1973) designates as "pseudo covariances" such covariances expressed relative to regional means. It is therefore important to realize that, although the genetic model of bioassay of kinship is formulated in terms of probability of identity by descent, what is estimated from allelic frequencies are allelic correlations relative to contemporary population. These can be related to allelic correlations relative to founders through Wright's hierarchical model, and such correlations relative to founders are, over a large number of systems, estimates of probabilities of identity by descent.

For the purpose of describing relative similarity between subdivisions, estimates of relative kinship $\{\phi_{Rij}\}$ are satisfactory. However, in order to relate values of such estimates to kinship *a priori*, as can be done from migration data through Malécot's model (Malécot, 1950), one may resort to Malécot's model of isolation by distance by writing

$$\phi_R(d) = (1 - L)ae^{-bd} + L \qquad (2.22)$$

(Morton and Lalouel, 1973, Morton 1973b), which can be related to Wright's hierarchical model as follows: with S denoting subdivision, T the contemporary population, and A the set of all populations issued from founders of the present population, we can write

$$F_{SA} = \phi(d) = ae^{-bd}$$
$$F_{ST} = \phi_R(d) = (1 - L)ae^{-bd} + L \qquad (2.23)$$
$$F_{TA} = -L/(1 - L)$$

Estimates of relative kinship $\{\phi_{Rij}\}$ are measures of similarity from which various distance measures can be defined. The simplest consists in defining the genetic distance

$$d_{ij}^2 = \phi_{Rii} + \phi_{Rjj} - 2\phi_{Rij} \qquad (2.24)$$

the matrix of relative kinship $\{\phi_{Rij}\}$, in the absence of sampling correction being a matrix of scalar products relative to the origin ϕ_R, random kinship in the contemporary population; the role played by such matrices in multidimensional scaling will be considered later in this presentation. It will be clear that (2.24) is an appropriate distance index, all information on population structure inferred from gene frequencies being contained in the matrix $\{\phi_{Rij}\}$. Hybridity, defined as

$$\theta_{ij} = \frac{\phi_{Rii} + \phi_{Rjj} - 2\phi_{Rij}}{4 - 2\phi_{Rij} - \phi_{Rii} - \phi_{Rjj}} \tag{2.25}$$

a measure of genetic divergence introduced by Morton *et al.* (1971), also admits a biological interpretation, as well discussed by Jacquard (1973); its properties and intuitive interpretation are, however, less appealing than relative kinship itself.

Two different models of estimations have been proposed (Morton *et al.*, 1971; Morton, 1975) which, when considering a single genetic system, are analogous to Sanghvi's and Balakrishnan's indices of distance through (2.24), respectively. They differ from these indices in that similarity measures $\{\phi_{Rij}\}$ are estimated, as are their incorporation of sampling correction and their weighting over independent systems (Morton *et al.*, 1971), such that, rather than cumulating estimates of relative kinship $\{\phi_{Rij}\}$ over systems, these are weighted so as to have the same expectation for each system as well as over all systems.

These authors showed how estimates of relative kinship could also be obtained, under particular assumptions, from quantitative traits or isonymy, allowing derivation of a measure having same biological significance over various bodies of data.

Lastly, it is worth mentioning that, because of sampling corrections as well as weighting of estimates over systems, the matrix $\{d_{ij}^2\}$ obtained with (2.24) may not be positive definite, generally having some negative, although small, eigenvalues; this consideration is relevant for scaling purposes, as will be seen.

2.2.3.2. Harpending's Sample Kinship. Another index of genetic similarity closely related to $\{\phi_{Rij}\}$ was presented by Harpending and Jenkins (1972, 1973), who proposed as an estimate of the sample coefficient of relative kinship, for a given system, the quantity

$$r_{ij} = \sum_k \frac{(p_{ik} - \bar{p}_k)(p_{jk} - \bar{p}_k)}{\bar{p}_k(1 - \bar{p}_k)} \tag{2.26}$$

or covariances between standardized gene frequencies, where $\bar{p}_k$ is the weighted mean gene frequency of allele k. Substituting r_{ij} in (2.24) yields an index of genetic distance which bears some relationship with Sanghvi's distance. However, just as in bioassay of kinship or in Nei's model (presented further), a matrix of scalar products is first constructed, allowing averaging over genetic systems of quantities having the same expectations over systems, from which distances can be defined. We shall see later that a Euclidean representation can be obtained directly from such a scalar-product matrix, as was clearly understood by Harpending and Jenkins (1973).

2.2.3.3 The Model of Nei. Another model giving an index of genetic distance also related to a probability of gene identity was presented by Nei (1971, 1972, 1973). There has been some controversy and confusion in the literature with regard to this model and the model of bioassay of kinship, originating in the fact that, although both models are based on the concept of identity, they lead to somewhat different estimation formulas.

There is, however, no contradiction between these two models once it is realized that they are based on different definitions of allelism. In the model of bioassay of kinship, allelism is defined according to what could be referred to as a fixed allele model; it is assumed that a given number of recognizable alleles are present in the population under study, and that this population is at a stationary state of a stochastic process involving mutation-selection balance and migration, so that gene frequencies in the total population have constant expectation.

New developments of molecular genetics during the past decades allowed one to define a "finer" allelic relation based on observed structural gene differences at the codon level. Under such a definition of allelism, one is led to consider at a given locus a quasi-infinite series of alleles which, over a sufficiently long period of time, may vary in number as well as in frequency. For this variable-allele model, gene identity by descent coincides with structural identity (Kimura and Crow, 1964); that is, identity coincides with isoaction. With such a definition of allelism, and for two populations i and j characterized by their allelic frequencies at some locus $\{q_{ik}\}$ and $\{q_{jk}\}$, the probability of identity of two random genes drawn from the same population, say i, is

$$J_{ii} = \sum_k q_{ik}^2 \qquad (2.27)$$

and the probability of identity of two random genes drawn from each population is

$$J_{ij} = \sum_k q_{ik} q_{jk} \qquad (2.28)$$

If $\bar{J}_{ii}$, $\bar{J}_{jj}$, and $\bar{J}_{ij}$ are the arithmetic means of such probabilities for all loci under consideration, and defining $D_{ij(m)}$ the expected proportion of different genes in two random genomes from i and j, then

$$\begin{aligned} D_{mij} &= D_{ij(m)} - (D_{ii(m)} + D_{jj(m)})/2 \\ &= (\bar{J}_{ii} + \bar{J}_{jj} - 2\bar{J}_{ij})/2 \end{aligned} \qquad (2.29)$$

is a minimum estimate of net codon differences per locus between populations i and j. However, $D_{ii(m)}$, $D_{jj(m)}$, and $D_{ij(m)}$ being the proportion of different genes between two randomly chosen genomes, their variation is not additive. This led Nei to introduce another index, assuming that individual codon changes are independent and follow a Poisson distribution

$$D_{ij} = -\ln\{\bar{J}_{ij}/(\bar{J}_{ii}\bar{J}_{jj})^{1/2}\} \qquad (2.30)$$

D_{ij} is referred to as a "standard" estimate of net codon differences per locus (Nei, 1973). If the rate of gene substitution were not constant, D_{ij} would be an underestimate of net codon differences per locus; still another index, or maximum estimate of net codon differences per locus, would be more appropriate; it obtains as (2.30), substituting geometric means to arithmetic means $\bar{J}$.

Nei's presentation (1971, 1972, 1973) did not address the problem related to sampling within an infinite series of alleles that we already discussed. Which of Morton's or Nei's models best apply to a given situation is a matter of judging assumptions that are likely to be fulfilled. Allelic relation is based on different levels of observation. If fluctuations of gene frequencies in the total population may be considered negligible within subdivisions, which may be quite reasonable over relatively moderate times of evolution, as in the study of the local differentiation of a population, Morton's model may be used. When considering population differences over considerable times of separation, on the basis of electrophoretic differences as is typical of interspecies studies of variation, one may resort to Nei's model.

Rearranging (2.21) to write

$$\phi_{Rij} = E\left\{\left(\sum_k q_{ik}q_{jk} - \sum_k q_k^2\right) \middle/ \left(1 - \sum_k q_k^2\right)\right\}$$

Morton (1973d) defined the limiting kinship between populations i and j

$$\phi_{ij} = E\left\{\sum_k q_{ik}q_{jk}\right\} \tag{2.31}$$

relative to a gene pool corresponding to diverse organisms, containing a large number of alleles, none in polymorphic frequency ($\Sigma_k q_k^2 \to 0$), and proceeded to extend bioassay of kinship to molecular evolution and the variable-allele model.

2.2.3.4. The Phylogenic Model of Cavalli-Sforza and Edwards. This method (Edwards and Cavalli-Sforza, 1964; Cavalli-Sforza and Edwards, 1967) attempts to reconstruct the phylogeny of present day populations on the basis of contemporary observed gene frequency differences. This led these authors to specify an evolutionary process of population divergence. As in the preceding sections, attention will be restricted to the conceptual framework of such a model without consideration of problems in statistical estimation.

For a population evolving by drift alone, the gene frequency variance changes in time according to

$$\text{var}(p) = p(1-p)(1 - e^{-t/2N}) \tag{2.32}$$

p being the initial frequency, as shown by Kimura (1955), assuming gene frequencies are the parameters of a multinomial distribution. For the process of gene frequency change to be homogenous in time, gene frequency variances should be proportional to time t. In addition, to allow meaningful interpretation of gene frequency changes, new variables must be defined independent of their variances. The angular transformation already presented, $\sin^2\theta_k = p_k$, is such that the new variables $\{\theta_k\}$ are asymptotically normally distributed with variances

$t/8N$ independent of $\{p_k\}$. The space so defined being curvilinear, a Euclidean approximation, necessary to conform to a random process of Brownian motion, is obtained by stereographic projection, as seen earlier (Edwards, 1971).

The probability density of a point at distance d from its origin, under a random process of Brownian motion in this Euclidean space is, in any direction, defined by

$$\{1/\sigma(2\pi t)^{1/2}\}^m \exp(-d^2/2t\sigma^2) \tag{2.33}$$

Malyutov, Passekov, and Richov (1972) studied the same random process on the surface of the hyperspherical space itself, therefore doing without the Euclidean approximation; this however, does not generalize to several genetic systems.

For the evolution of several populations to be described by the same process in a common space, they must have effective sizes sensibly constant and of equal magnitude. Mutation and nonrandom variable selection are assumed negligible, no sudden population change nor migration are allowed. A random process of population subdivision is assumed: it is a Greenwood-Yule branching process. Populations originate from a common founding group and, at any time, any existing population may, with equal probability, split into two new populations such that these new populations be initially identical. No population may become extinct, and each population evolves randomly and independently at constant and equal rate.

Limitations of this model are the absence of migration, equal effective sizes, and constant rates of evolution; in most applications, one or several of these assumptions are likely to be seriously violated.

3. Multidimensional Scaling

We assume at this point that we dispose of pairwise indices of similarities or dissimilarities between subdivisions of a population, calculated on the basis of individual observations. To allow interpretation of similarity in terms of proximity, such indices must necessarily satisfy metric properties; this, however, does not imply that an index of dissimilarity must necessarily be a Euclidean or a Minkowski metric, as we shall present further a class of methods that operate on rank order.

However, interpretation of proximities implied by the matrix of pairwise indices of similarities or dissimilarities may be quite simplified by a low-dimensional, Euclidean approximation, where the n subdivisions are represented by n points whose interdistances best approximate, according to some specified criterion, the calculated similarities or dissimilarities.

In the following, various methods allowing to obtain such an approximation are presented that apply to symmetric matrices of similarities and dissimilarities. Some similar methods that apply to nonsymmetric matrices of measures of functional association will be considered thereafter. Lastly, methods allowing comparisons of several such low-dimensional approximations will be presented, followed by a brief discussion of hierarchical cluster methods.

3.1. Multidimensional Scaling of Symmetric Matrices of Similarities or Dissimilarities

3.1.1. Principal Coordinates Analysis and Its Relation to Principal Component Analysis

3.1.1.1. Recall of Some Relevant Results of Linear Algebra. Useful to the present discussion are the following classical results, of which proof can be found in any standard textbook on linear algebra.

Theorem 1. Any real symmetric matrix can be decomposed in spectral form.

Theorem 2. The eigenvalues of a real symmetric matrix are real.

Theorem 3. The eigenvectors of a real symmetric matrix associated to two different eigenvalues, and expressed on an orthonormal base, are orthogonal.

Theorem 4. If S is a real symmetric matrix, there exists a nonsingular orthogonal matrix B such that $B^T S B$ be diagonal.

Theorem 5. A real symmetric matrix is positive definite if all its eigenvalues are positives.

Theorem 6. A real symmetric matrix is positive semidefinite if all its eigenvalues are nonnegatives.

Theorem 7. Any positive definite or semidefinite matrix S can be factorized as $S = CC^T$.

Theorem 8. An orthogonal transformation $\mathbf{y} = C\mathbf{x}$ of a random vector $\mathbf{x}$ leaves invariant the generalized variance and the sum of the variances of elements of $\mathbf{x}$.

3.1.1.2. Principal Components Analysis. There is widespread confusion in the literature on distance analysis and population structure, between principal components and related linear methods of projection or multidimensional configuration into a space of lower dimensionality. As introduced by Hotelling (1933) and used in multivariate statistics, the principal components of a random vector can be thus defined: denote $\mathbf{x}$ a $m \times 1$ random vector such that $E(\mathbf{x}) = 0$

and $E(\mathbf{x}\mathbf{x}^T) = \Sigma$. There exists an orthogonal linear transformation

$$\mathbf{y} = B^T\mathbf{x} \tag{3.1}$$

such that the covariance matrix of $\mathbf{y}$ be $E(\mathbf{y}\mathbf{y}^T) = \Lambda$, where Λ is a diagonal matrix whose diagonal elements, satisfying $\lambda_1 \geqslant \lambda_2 \geqslant \cdots \geqslant \lambda_m \geqslant 0$ are the roots of the characteristic polynomial $|\Sigma - \lambda I|$. The rth column of B, $\mathbf{b}_r$, satisfies $(\Sigma - \lambda_r I)\mathbf{b}_r = 0$. The rth element of $\mathbf{y}$, $y_r = \mathbf{b}_r^T\mathbf{x}$, has greatest variance of all linear combinations without correlation with $y_1, \ldots, y_{r-1}$. $\mathbf{y}$ is the vector of principal components of $\mathbf{x}$. Theorem 8 states that $|\mathbf{y}\mathbf{y}^T| = |B^T\mathbf{x}\mathbf{x}^T B| = |\mathbf{x}\mathbf{x}^T|$ and $\text{tr}(B^T\mathbf{x}\mathbf{x}^T B) = \text{tr}(\mathbf{x}\mathbf{x}^T)$, hence the generalized variance of the vector of principal components, $\mathbf{y}$, is equal to that of $\mathbf{x}$, and the sum of the variances of the principal components is equal to the sum of the variances of the elements of $\mathbf{x}$.

Therefore a given principal component, y_r, is a *scalar*, and the vector $\mathbf{b}_r$ such that $y_r = \mathbf{b}_r^T\mathbf{x}$, gives the weights attributed to each variable x_s in their linear combination producing y_r. The purpose of principal components analysis is, having m correlated random variables $x_1, \ldots, x_m$, to approximate them by a few number of independent variables obtained as linear combinations of the elements of $\mathbf{x}$, while accounting by this process for as much as possible of the total variance of the original variables. The first principle component, y_1, has greater variance than all others and explains a proportion $\lambda_1 / \Sigma_{i=1}^m \lambda_i$ of the total variance. For more details on this method, a good reference is Anderson (1958).

3.1.1.3. Spatial Configuration Associated with Positive or Semi-Positive Definite Matrix. Consider a real symmetric matrix S of order n. From theorems recalled in a previous section, we know it can be decomposed into spectral form: $S = V\Lambda V^{-1}$ where V is an orthogonal matrix such that $V^{-1} = V^T$ and $V^T V = I$. In practical situations where S is some matrix calculated on the basis of $m > n$ observations, one can assume without loss of generality that all eigenvalues are distinct.

If the matrix S is positive definite, then all its eigenvalues are positive. Defining $C = V\Lambda^{1/2}$, S can be written as $S = CC^T$. To the matrix C one can associate a configuration of n points in R^n, the coordinates of the ith point being given by the ith row of C. The square of the length of the vector from the origin to the ith point is defined by the quadratic form $\Sigma_{k=1}^n c_{ik}^2 = \Sigma_{k=1}^n \lambda_k v_{ik}^2$, and the scalar product of two vectors is defined by $\Sigma_{k=1}^n c_{ik}c_{jk} = \Sigma_{k=1}^n \lambda_k v_{ik}v_{jk}$. The distance between two points i and j in this space is defined by

$$
d_{ij}^2 = \sum_{k=1}^n (c_{ik} - c_{jk})^2
$$
$$
= \sum_{k=1}^n c_{ik}^2 + \sum_{k=1}^n c_{jk}^2 - 2\sum_{k=1}^n c_{ik}c_{jk} \tag{3.2}
$$

These distances can be expressed in terms of the elements of the matrix S, as we have $s_{ij} = \Sigma_k c_{ik} c_{jk}$, and therefore

$$d_{ij}^2 = s_{ii} + s_{jj} - 2s_{ij} \qquad (3.3)$$

One clearly conceives that a configuration C of n points in Euclidean space can always be represented in $n-1$ dimensions; it is also evident that this configuration is invariant under a change of origin leaving unaltered the interdistances. This was shown in a more general context by Young and Householder (1938), whose results served as a basis for Torgerson (1958) to represent n points in an $n-1$ dimensional space. This author showed that, to express the distance between two points j and k relative to their distances from point i, one writes

$$d_{jk}^2 = d_{ij}^2 + d_{ik}^2 - 2d_{ij}d_{ik} \cos \theta_{jik} \qquad (3.4)$$

hence

$$d_{ij}d_{ik} \cos \theta_{jik} = \tfrac{1}{2}(d_{ij}^2 + d_{ik}^2 - d_{jk}^2) \qquad (3.5)$$

defining the matrix of scalar products B_i with general element $b_{jk} = d_{ij}d_{ik} \cos \theta_{jik}$; these scalar products can be expressed as the function of coordinates of the n points relative to origin at point i $\{a_{jk}\}$, where $B_i = AA^\tau$, of order n and rank $n-1$ as a consequence of Young and Householder's results and our assumptions.

It is clear, however, that such a representation in $n-1$ dimensions can be obtained in various ways, depending on which point is chosen as origin. Alternately, another solution consists in choosing as origin the barycenter of the n points in n dimensions, which Torgerson (1958) favored. Schönemann (1970a) showed that reduction of an n-dimensional configuration to $n-1$ dimensions could be done by applying an oblique projection to the matrix of squared pairwise distances $D^{(2)}$ of general element d_{jk}^2. The matrix B_i can be rewritten as

$$B_i = (J\mathbf{d}_i^{(2)\tau} + \mathbf{d}_i^{(2)}J^\tau - D^{(2)})/2 \qquad (3.6)$$

where $\mathbf{d}_i^{(2)}$ is the ith row of $D^{(2)}$ and J an $n \times 1$ vector of unit elements. Defining the oblique projection operator

$$Q_m = I - J\mathbf{b}_m^\tau$$

with

$$J^\tau \mathbf{b}_m = 1 \qquad (3.7)$$

and writing $B_i = A_i A_i^\tau$, translation to a new origin is given by

$$A_m = Q_m A_i \qquad (3.8)$$

A_m giving coordinates of the n points relative to a new origin whose coordinates in the previous reference set of coordinates are given by $g_m^\tau = \mathbf{b}_m^\tau A_i$. The matrix of scalar products, B_m, is given by

$$B_m = A_m A_m^\tau = Q_m B_i Q_m^\tau = -Q_m D^{(2)} Q_m^\tau / 2 \qquad (3.9)$$

A solution with origin at point i is given by choosing $\mathbf{b}_i^\tau = (0, \ldots, 1, \ldots, 0)$, the unit element being the ith element of $\mathbf{b}_i$. A solution with the origin as the barycenter of the n points in the original space is given by choosing Q_c defined by $b_c^\tau = (1/n, \ldots, 1/n)$. This has the effect of defining A_c by subtracting the column means from each row of A_m:

$$a_{cjk} = a_{mjk} - a_{m \cdot k}$$

so that column sums of A_c are zero; therefore A_c is of rank $n - 1$, hence $B_c = A_c A_c^\tau = - Q_c D^{(2)} Q_c / 2$ is of rank $n - 1$. We shall see that this choice of Q_c defines the method of principal coordinates (Gower, 1966).

For a configuration $\mathbf{C}$ of n points in an n-dimensional Euclidean space defined by their coordinates A_m with respect to some origin m, defining the matrix of scalar products $B_m = A_m A_m^\tau$, finding the least-squares approximation of rank one to B_m consists in finding a translation on each axis such that

$$a_{mik} = v_k + e_k$$

or in matrix notation $\qquad\qquad A_m = J v^\tau + E$ $\qquad\qquad$ (3.10)

The solution $\mathbf{v}$ is that vector which minimizes tr $E^\tau E$, yielding

$$\mathbf{v} = \frac{A_m^\tau J}{n} \qquad\qquad (3.11)$$

The ith element of $\mathbf{v}$ is therefore $a_{\cdot i}$, mean of the ith column of A_m, and $A_c = A_m - J v^\tau = Q_c A_m$, A_c and Q_c as previously defined. This demonstrates the optimal property of projecting the configuration $\mathbf{C}$ in an $(n - 1)$-dimensional space with origin as the barycenter of $\mathbf{C}$ in the original n-dimensional space (Lalouel, 1975).

3.1.1.4. *Principal Coordinates Analysis.* Gower's method of principal coordinates (Gower, 1966) essentially consists in the following. For a positive definite matrix of pairwise distances, D, calculate the matrix of scalar products relative to the barycenter of the n-dimensional configuration $\mathbf{C}$ implied by D:

$$B_c = - Q_c D^{(2)} Q_c / 2 \qquad\qquad (3.12)$$

and find the spectral decomposition of B_c:

$$B_c = A_c A_c^\tau = V \Lambda V^{-1} \qquad\qquad (3.13)$$

The best linear approximation to $\mathbf{C}$ in a least-squares sense, in an s-dimensional space ($s \leqslant n - 1$) is obtained by orthogonal projection of B_c into this subspace, where scalar products are defined by

$$b_{sij} = \sum_{k=1}^{s} \lambda_k v_{ik} v_{jk} = \sum_{k=1}^{s} u_{ik} u_{jk} \qquad\qquad (3.14)$$

λ_k being the kth largest eigenvalue of B_c, v_k its associated eigenvector, and $u_{ik} = \lambda_k^{1/2} v_{ik}$. The distance between i and j in this subspace is given by

$$d_{sij} = b_{sii} + b_{sjj} - 2 b_{sij} \qquad\qquad (3.15)$$

Conversely, the configuration **C** associated with a positive definite matrix of similarity, S, is such that

$$d_{ij}^2 = s_{ii} + s_{jj} - 2s_{ij} \tag{3.16}$$

and a lower-dimensional approximation can be obtained similarly by defining (3.12), and so on. As shown by Gower (1966), and as should be apparent from the previous section, this is equivalent to carrying out a principal components analysis on the coordinates a_{cik} of the original configuration after "centroid adjustment," or placement of the origin at the barycenter of the original configuration. Defining the *dispersion* on each axis,

$$d_k^2 = \sum_{ij} \lambda_k (v_{ik} - v_{jk})^2 \tag{3.17}$$

and writing $h_k = \Sigma_i v_{ik}$, we have $d_k^2 = 2\lambda_k(n - h_k^2)$. For the matrix B_c, we have $\Sigma_i v_{ik} = 0$, and therefore the proportion of the total dispersion accounted for by the first s axes, eigenvalues being arranged in order of decreasing value, is given by

$$\sum_{k=1}^{s} \lambda_k \bigg/ \sum_{k=1}^{n} \lambda_k \tag{3.18}$$

this is the proportion of the sum of squared distances accounted for by this representation, and defines its optimality: for s fixed, (3.18) is maximum, in a least-squares sense, given a linear method based on orthogonal projection is used.

For a matrix $D^{(2)}$ already centroid adjusted, the operator Q_c has no effect in (3.12) and one could define $B_c = -D^{(2)}/2$. For a matrix that is not positive definite but present at some small negative eigenvalues, as may happen, for example, when sampling corrections are applied in calculating a Mahalanobis distance matrix, this still allows one to give a Euclidean approximation in a lower-dimensional space, although the optimality of (3.18) does not hold any more.

Clearly, this method applies to many matrices of similarity, as they are quite often obtained as a product MM^τ, where M is an $n \times m$ matrix, which is the case, for example, with Guttman scales (Guttman, 1941).

3.1.2. A Method Based on a Criterion of Maximum Correlation

For the purpose of best approximating interdistances of an n-dimensional configuration **C** of n points as specified by a distance matrix D, there seems no particular reason to restrict oneself to the linear operation of an orthogonal projection, nor to choose as best criterion maximizing the proportion of the total sum of squared distances accounted for in the low-dimensional representation. Another possible method (Lalouel, 1975) is presented here.

Consider a matrix of distances $\{d_{ij}\}$ of order n, not necessarily Euclidean, to which an approximation in an s-dimensional space is sought ($s < n$). The criterion retained is that Euclidean distance in the s-dimensional space, $\{d_{sij}\}$, be in maximum correlation with distances $\{d_{ij}\}$. If both matrices are centroid adjusted and given the same norm, this maximum will correspond to the minimum of

$$\sum_{ij} e_{ij}^2 = \sum_{ij} (d_{sij} - \hat{d}_{sij})^2 \tag{3.19}$$

where $\hat{d}_{sij} = ad_{ij} + b$, a and b being obtained by solving the regression $d_{sij} = ad_{ij} + b + e_{ij}$, and distances $\{d_{ij}\}$, $\{d_{sij}\}$ being given the same norm.

An iterative solution can be obtained as follows. It is known that it is more efficient to find a minimum of a quadratic function of the unknowns rather than a function such as the correlation $R(d_{ij}, d_{sij})$. Therefore we have resorted to Guttman's two-phase iterative method, yielding the algorithm: the matrix D is centroid adjusted and normed such that $\Sigma_{ij}d_{ij}^2 = n$; given some initial trial values or some current values of the coordinates of the n points in s dimensions $\{x_{ik}\}$, $k = 1, s$, $\{d_{sij}\}$ are obtained, centroid adjusted, and given the same norm as the $\{d_{ij}\}$; elements $\{\hat{d}_{sij}\}$ are obtained by linear regression of $\{d_{sij}\}$ on $\{d_{ij}\}$; now coordinates $\{x_{ik}^+\}$ are obtained by reducing $f = \Sigma_{ij}(d_{sij} - \hat{d}_{sij})^2$ by one step of steepest descent $x_{ik}^+ = x_{ik} - \partial f/\partial x_{sik}$, where $\partial f/\partial x_{ik} = \Sigma_{ij}(d_{sij} - \hat{d}_{sij})(x_{ik} - x_{jk})(\delta_{ki} - \delta_{kj})d_{ij}^{-1}$ and δ_{ki} is Kronecker's symbol. This procedure rapidly yields a maximum of the correlation $R(d_{sij}, d_{ij})$ and the corresponding solution $\{x_{ik}\}$. Extensive numerical experience, some of which is published (Lalouel, 1975, Lalouel and Langaney, 1976), led us to favor this approach over the method of principal coordinates, as it is efficient and better preserves interdistances.

3.1.3. Nonmetric Multidimensional Scaling of a Symmetric Matrix

Nonmetric multidimensional scaling methods originated with considerations by Shepard (1958) on the isomorphism of constraints governing measures of similarities or association and the metric axioms. The concept of nonmetric multidimensional scaling was introduced by Shepard (1962), seeking to relate distances with similarities or dissimilarities by a monotonic relation.

> The proposition has already been tendered that similarity is interpretable as a relation of proximity; this immediately suggests that the structure we are seeking in data of this kind is a spatial structure. Certainly we usually think that a greater degree of proximity implies a smaller distance of separation. If some monotonic transformation of the proximity measure could be found that would convert these implicit distances into explicit distances, then we should be in a position to recover the spatial structure contained only latently in the original data.

As originally presented, the method lacked a rigorous formulation. Ulterior work by various authors, particularly Kruskal (1964a, b), Guttman (1968), Young (1970), and Lingoes (1971), gave to nonmetric multidimensional scaling a sound theoretical basis, with well-defined monotonic loss functions, efficient algorithms, guarantee of existence of a solution in $s \leqslant n - 2$ dimensions, and demonstration of the power of rank information to recover quantitative information provided by the data.

　　3.1.3.1. Monotonicity; Definition of Loss Functions. Consider we have calculated a matrix of coefficients of dissimilarity C between n subdivisions. We shall also assume that all pairwise elements c_{ij} were calculated and that $c_{ij} \neq c_{kl}$ for all $i, j = 1, \ldots, n$, with $i \neq j$, $k \neq l$. The method is not in fact restricted to such assumptions, introduced here only to simplify the presentation.

　　To find a Euclidean representation of these dissimilarities in s dimensions $(s \leqslant n - 2)$, a condition of monotonicity is introduced: for all $i \neq j$ and $k \neq l$ corresponding to two distinct elements of C, distances d_{ij} and d_{kl} in s dimensions (dropping the subscript s) should be such that whenever

$$c_{ij} < c_{kl}$$

then, as much as possible,

$$d_{ij} < d_{kl} \tag{3.20}$$

　　In order to give an objective measure of the extent to which this monotonic condition is violated, which could then be minimized to obtain some optimal solution $\{d_{ij}\}$, a function of monotonic adjustment must be defined. Such an objective measure was first proposed by Kruskal (1964a). Rank the M elements c_{ij}, $i < j$, in increasing order of magnitude, identifying this order by an additional subscript:

$$c_{i_1 j_1} < c_{i_2 j_2} < \cdots < c_{i_M j_M} \tag{3.21}$$

and then arrange the distances associated to these coefficients according to these subscripts

$$d_{i_1 j_1} < d_{i_2 j_2} < \cdots < d_{i_M j_M} \tag{3.22}$$

which can be graphically represented (Fig. 1). In Fig. 1a, we note there is perfect monotonic correspondence between dissimilarities and distance, that is, (3.22) also constitutes a monotonic increasing sequence. On the other hand, this is no more so in Figs. 1b and 1c, with no more perfect monotonic relation between the sequences (3.21) and (3.22). Just as in classic problems of parametric curve fitting, an objective measure of departure from monotonicity will be a function of these deviations. For a solution not to be affected by any monotonic transformation of the $\{c_{ij}\}$, as only their ranks are used for scaling, deviations should not be measured along the dissimilarity axis. Similar to parametric least-squares fitting, some expected values of distances $\{d_{ij}^*\}$ must be defined such that

$$d_{i_1 j_1}^* \leqslant d_{i_2 j_2}^* \leqslant \cdots \leqslant d_{i_M j_M}^* \tag{3.23}$$

and a function of deviations from monotonicity will be expressed in terms of squared differences $\{(d_{ij} - d_{ij}^*)^2\}$. Formal definitions of such "rank images" $\{d_{ij}^*\}$ were given by Kruskal (1964a) and Guttman (1968); they are here only "described" in Figs. 1b and 1c, corresponding to Kruskal's and Guttman's

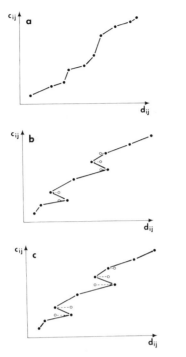

FIGURE 1. Illustrative examples of monotone adjustment of distances $\{d_{ij}\}$ to dissimilarity coefficients $\{c_{ij}\}$. (a) perfect monotone fit; (b) Kruskal's measure of departure from monotonicity; (c) Guttman's rank images.

"rank images," respectively. One can clearly see, for example, how these $\{d_{ij}^*\}$ obtain in Fig. 1c by permutations of the elements $\{d_{ij}\}$ such that these elements are arranged in increasing order of magnitude.

Objective measures of deviation from monotonicity can then be defined. Kruskal defined the Stress coefficient

$$S = \frac{\{\Sigma_{i<j}(d_{ij}-d_{ij}^*)^2\}^{1/2}}{\{\Sigma_{i<j}d_{ij}^2\}^{1/2}} \qquad (3.24)$$

while Guttman defines the coefficient of monotonicity

$$m = u(vw)^{-1/2} \qquad (3.25)$$

where $u = \Sigma_{i<j}d_{ij}d_{ij}^*$, $v = \Sigma_{i<j}d_{ij}^{*2}$, and $w = \Sigma_{i<j}d_{ij}^2$, and the "alienation"

$$a = (1-m^2)^{1/2} \qquad (3.26)$$

Kruskal and Guttman definitions differ with respect to the treatment of tied values among the $\{c_{ij}\}$, the latter better allowing untying of tied values. We have written computer programs incorporating both approaches, which also differ with respect to the numerical procedure retained for obtaining of a solution. Both minimize a loss function [either (3.24) or (3.26)] iteratively and, although giving in general rather similar results, our numerical experience favors the latter approach. Goodness of fit is assessed by the final value of (3.24) or (3.26) obtained.

   3.1.3.2. On the Use of Nonmetric Multidimensional Scaling. The ability of rank order information to convey the metric information contained in the data was particularly investigated by Shepard (1962) and Young (1970). Shepard showed that, for true two-dimensional Euclidean configurations, the correlation between such distances and distances obtained by sole utilization of their rank in nonmetric scaling increased rapidly with the number of points, n, being almost unity for n greater or equal to 10. Young (1970), through the definition of an index of metric determinacy, showed numerically that, when the degree of freedom ratio $F = \{n(n-1)/2\}/\{s(n-1) - s(s-1)/2\}$ exceeded 2, recovery of metric information using rank information was almost perfect. This translates into the practical limitation that one cannot expect quasiperfect recovery of metric information of any configuration for which F is lower than 2, such as $n < 8$ and $s = 2$, for example. This, however, should not be taken to imply that any configuration for which F exceeds 2 can be quasiperfectly recovered by nonmetric scaling.

   One cannot stress too strongly the usefulness of nonmetric methods in multidimensional scaling. Because of the nonlinear operation applied to the original data to obtain a low-dimensional approximation, one can expect in general that less dimensions may be needed to obtain such an approximation with this method than with the method of principal coordinates. Allowing missing values in the matrix of similarity or dissimilarity coefficients enlarges considerably the field of application of this method, as does the fact that it may be applied also to non-Euclidean metrics. Because no metric relations between pairwise measures of similarity or dissimilarity and distances in the representation is assumed, it is possible to recover a mapping function by fitting *a posteriori* $\{c_{ij}\}$ to $\{d_{ij}\}$. An example of nonmetric scaling with missing values and *a posteriori* recovery of mapping functions can be found in Lalouel (1977). Lastly, it is worth mentioning that nonmetric methods can be used for a much larger variety of problems and data than considered here, as can be seen in Shepard, Romney, and Nerlove (1972).

   3.1.3.3. Which Method to Use. On the basis of our experience, for purpose of representation of proximities implied by indices of similarity or dissimilarity, one should certainly favor the use of the nonmetric method, unless n is small in relation to s. When applied to distance indices, an index of the metric distortion induced by this operation can be calculated, such as the correlation between original distances and distances in the representation; whenever some predetermined tolerance is not met, or when the degree of freedom ratio is lower than 2, our method of maximum correlation may be preferred. Our experience is that these two methods lead to rather similar results, while principal co-ordinates analysis may yield quite discrepant results for the same dimensionality.

3.2. Multidimensional Scaling of Asymmetric Matrices

3.2.1. Conceptual Framework

We shall concern ourselves here with the following problem: we wish to interpret similarity, affinity, interaction, or association between all pairs of element i and j belonging to two distinct sets I and J ($i = 1, 2, \ldots, n; j = 1, 2, \ldots, m$) in terms of proximities between two sets of n and m points in a joint space. We may also have in addition some measures of similarity or dissimilarity (in a very general sense) between elements belonging to the same set, although this possibility will be ignored in most of the present discussion. The modality and nature of such observations are numerous. For example, we may have, for each of n individuals, an $m \times m$ matrix of "individual preferences" relating all pairs of m objects, each element of the matrix, corresponding to a pairwise comparison, being equal to one or zero according to whether the row element is preferred over the column element or not. We shall not concern ourselves here with these types of data, although of quite great interest; multidimensional scaling methods appropriate to such data are given in Carroll (1972), Schönemann and Wang (1972), Wang, Schönemann, and Rusk (1975).

Our attention will be restricted to situations where an $n \times m$ matrix $\{s_{ij}\}$, $i \in I$ and $j \in J$, of similarity, dissimilarity, affinity, association, interaction, or correlation between elements belonging to distinct sets has been obtained. Observations may consist of frequencies of m traits in n populations or in the outcomes of n trials, measures of preferences of n individuals for m stimuli, input–output relationships, etc. Another type of data which may conceptually be so interpreted consists in number or probabilities of transition from one state to another (or possibly the same) state, or some measure of functional association between all pairs of n elements. Although in such situations there exists formally only one set of n objects, the measure of "association" between pairs of elements is no more symmetric (in general $s_{ij} \neq s_{ji}$); to such measures one could associate a graph with n vertices and oriented paths linking them such that to the path from i to j is associated a weight reflecting directed flow along it. It therefore comes naturally that, for the purpose of representing graphically the dynamic of such relationships, one may define two sets of n points I and J to represent inflows and outflows. This is the situation we shall concern ourselves with here, although the very much greater variety of problems that can be similarly addressed, as pointed out, should be kept in mind. Such dynamic data may concern migration, social contacts, economic exchanges, etc. The representation sought, given such measures of oriented, functional associ-ation, will consist in $2n$ points in some common space, each element (say, population) being represented by two points, inflow and outflow points, such that the distance from the outflow point i to inflow point j reflects the amount of flow, or exchanges from i to j.

The scaling model for such types of data is the "unfolding model" of Coombs (1964), originally formulated in terms of individuals' preferences. Having measures of preference of n individuals for m objects, $\{s_{ij}\}, i \in I, j \in J$, such that the ith row indicates the preferences expressed by individual i for each of the m objects, a conceptual scale of preference for individual i is obtained by arranging objects on this scale, relative to some origin, such that proximities from this origin relate to the preference judgments $s_{ij}, j = 1, \ldots, m$. The origin on each scale is the individual "ideal point." It is assumed that all these preference judgments reflect proximities between m points representing the objects in an s-dimensional space. The scaling problem consists then in inferring these proximities between m objects from individual scales of preference, and such that, in this space relating perceived similarities between objects from preference judgments, each individual ideal point is also represented such that its distance to each object reflect that individual's preferences.

Various methods have been proposed for this multidimensional scaling problem. Early methods lacked efficiency (Coombs, 1958; Bennet, 1956; Bennett and Hays, 1960; Hays and Bennett, 1961; Coombs and Kao, 1955). More efficient methods have more recently been introduced (Schönemann, 1970b; Schönemann and Wang, 1972; Wang, Schönemann, and Rusk, 1975; Carroll, 1972, which includes many other references; Young 1972). Three methods we used in Lalouel and Langaney (1976) to study the dynamics of migration exchanges will be briefly considered here.

3.2.2. Measure of Functional Association

Having data on the number $\{n_{ij}\}$ of migrants from subdivision i to subdivision j of a population of n subdivisions, we calculate the matrix $\{p_{ij}\}$ of probabilities of transition from i to j. This matrix describes direct flows from i to j between all pairs of subdivisions. It is clear, however, that an appropriate measure of functional association $\{f_{ij}\}$ should take into consideration, in the network of migration exchanges, direct flows between two points as well as indirect flows through other points, so as to reflect appropriately the connexity of the network of exchanges. In a first-order Markovian process, a useful composite measure of oriented interaction between two subdivisions that takes into account direct as well as indirect flows is the mean first passage time f_{ij} from i to j. This can readily be computed from the transition matrix $\{p_{ij}\}$ (see Lalouel and Langaney, 1976, or Kemeny and Snell, 1960; a better method to obtain these mean first passages times was given by Meyer, 1978). Such a measure of functional association was used in a social context by Beshers and Lauman (1967) and by Brown and Horton (1971) to study migration in New York State.

Having obtained $\{f_{ij}\}$, we seek a representation in an s-dimensional Euclidean space where each population i is represented by two points, a row point i_R and a column point i_C such that for any two subdivisions i and j, the distance between points i_R and i_C reflects the functional association f_{ij} from i to j, while the distance between points j_R and i_C reflects the functional association f_{ji} from j to i. Proximities between points i_R, j_R or i_C, j_C should then reflect the similarity of patterns of outflows and inflows, respectively, for i and j.

3.2.3. The Metric Unfolding Method of Schönemann

This method applies to the case where functional association may be measured in terms of Euclidean or quasi-Euclidean distances in r dimensions $(r \leqslant n, m)$. We seek, in a low-dimensional space of s dimensions $(s \leqslant r)$, a representation of $n + m$ row and column points (with $m = n$ in the particular situation we are considering here) such that distances in this new space best approximate original distances in a least-squares sense. We refer here to Schönemann (1970b) for further details.

3.2.4. Nonmetric Method

Our experience is with the method of Torgerson and Young (1967) and Young (1970). Distances sought in a lower space $\{d_{ij}\}$ are obtained from measures of functional association $\{f_{ij}\}$, not necessarily Euclidean, through a criterion of maximum monotonicity. The nonmetric method presented earlier for the symmetric case extends naturally to the present situation by assuming that only an $n \times m$ submatrix, part of an $(n + m) \times (n + m)$ matrix, is available, and similarly obtaining estimates of coordinates of $n + m$ points in s dimensions through the Torgerson and Young (1967) method and the optimization method of Davidon, Fletcher, and Powell (Davidon, 1959; Fletcher and Powell, 1963).

Additional constraints could be incorporated by also calculating the matrices of correlations between rows of $\{f_{ij}\}$ and that of correlation between columns of $\{f_{ij}\}$ finding coordinates of $n + m$ points in s dimensions by minimizing a linear combination of three alienation coefficients, no metric relationships being implied between these three matrices (Lingoes, 1970). Our experience was that this led to less satisfactory representations, possibly because of imposing too many constraints on the desired representation (Lalouel and Langaney, 1976).

3.2.5. Maximum Correlation Criterion

Just as for the symmetric case, we presented a method where the $\{d_{ij}\}$ in the s-dimensional space are obtained by maximizing their correlations with functional associations $\{f_{ij}\}$ (Lalouel, 1975; Lalouel and Langaney, 1976). Experience shows that the latter two methods give similar results (Fig. 2), while the method of Schönemann should give generally somewhat less satisfactory solutions, in terms of representation of proximities, because of its restriction to the use of a linear operation.

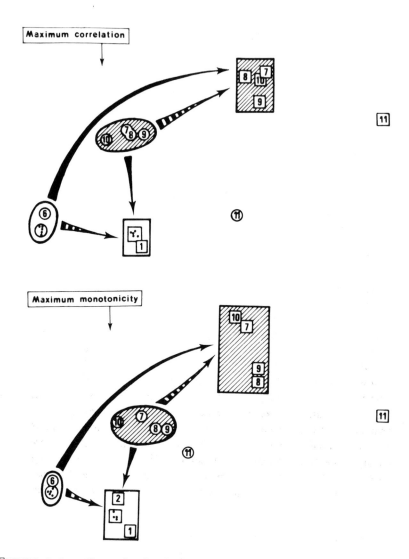

FIGURE 2. Intervillage migration in Senegal. Two-dimensional representations of mean first passage times. Circles correspond to outflow points, squares to inflow points. Top: Using a criterion of maximum correlation, alienation = 0.144, correlation = 0.993; Bottom: using a criterion of maximum monotonicity, alienation = 0.060, correlation = 0.988. Villages 1 to 6 and 7 to 11 belong to two distinct ethnic groups.

3.3. Simultaneous Analysis of Several Matrices of Similarity or Dissimilarity

3.3.1. Simultaneous Representation of Two Configurations by Rotation to Maximum Congruence

Consider that we wish to compare two configurations **A** and **B**, each referring to n points corresponding to same entities, both defined in a Euclidean space of the same dimensionality. These configurations are specified by their matrices of coordinates A and B, both $n \times s$. Correlation between interdistances of points of each configuration will give a measure of the relative similarity of these configurations. However, as with the analysis of residuals, one may be interested in assessing individual departures from the general trend of association and obtaining a graphical representation of the departures.

This can be done by resorting to the Schönemann (1966) and Schönemann and Carroll (1970) method of fitting one matrix to another under choice of a dilation, a translation, reflection of the axes, and a rotation to maximize congruence between both representations, as suggested by Lalouel (1973), with some natural simplifications we introduced. Assume we fit matrix B to matrix A by finding the least-squares solution of

$$B = cAT + Jg^{\tau} + E \qquad (3.27)$$

where B and A are $n \times s$ matrices of coordinates, c a scaling factor of dilation, **g** an $s \times 1$ translation vector, J an $n \times 1$ vector of unit elements, T an $s \times s$ orthogonal matrix, and E an $n \times s$ matrix of residual. Setting the partial derivatives of (3.27) to zero, T obtains by Eckart-Young decomposition (1936), $c = \text{tr } S^{\tau}T/rA^{\tau}QA$, and $q = (B - cAT)^{\tau}J/n$, where $S = A^{\tau}QB$ and Q is the oblique projection operator $I - JJ^{\tau}/n$. A symmetric measure of fit invariant to whether B is fitted to A or A to B is given by

$$e_s = \text{tr } E^{\tau}E(\text{tr } A^{\tau}QA/\text{tr } B^{\tau}QB)^{1/2}/ns \qquad (3.28)$$

However, when comparing two representations whose scales of measurement are different, assuming one is only interested in similarity of relative interdistances, it seems natural to compare A and B by reference to a common norm and placing their centroid at the origin, so that $\text{tr } A^{\tau}A = \text{tr } B^{\tau}B = \text{tr } A^{\tau}QA = \text{tr } B^{\tau}QB = n$, say, (3.27) reduces to

$$B = AT + E \qquad (3.29)$$

and we introduced, as measure of fit, the correlation

$$r_c = 1 - (se_s/2) \qquad (3.30)$$

e_s being defined by (3.28) with some simplification; r_c is the correlation between

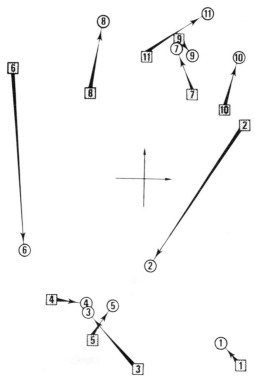

FIGURE 3. Intervillage migration in Senegal. Simultaneous representation of kinship predicted from migration data (circles) and geographical locations (squares). Maximum correlation: 0.980; correlation between coordinates of the two configurations, $r_c = 0.811$.

coordinates of the final representations (Lalouel, 1973, 1975), which is maximized by this procedure. Examples of applications can be found in Workman, Harpending, Lalouel, Lynch, Niswander, and Singleton (1973), Lalouel and Morton (1972), or Lalouel and Langaney (1976) (Fig. 3).

3.3.2. Search for Factors Common to Several Distance Matrices

Consider having obtained m matrices of pairwise coefficients of similarity or dissimilarity between n subdivisions of a population based on m distinct sets of observations, and assume that for each such matrix we define a transformation leading to a distance matrix between n points of a multidimensional configuration.

In order to give a simultaneous description of m such matrices, we postulate that, underlying the structure associated to each matrix, there exist a small number s of factors common to all sets of observations that may account for a large proportion of the observed differentiation. The method of Carroll and Chang (1970), originally intended for the analysis of individual perception of differences between pairs of n stimuli, can be applied to the present problem. These assumptions lead to the formulation that, for each set i $(i = 1, \ldots, m)$ of observations

$$d_{ijk}^2 = \sum_{t=1}^{s} w_{it}(x_{jt} - x_{kt})^2 + e_{ijk} \tag{3.31}$$

the elements $\{x_{jt}\}$ being the coordinates of each subdivision j on each common axis t, $j = 1, \ldots, n$, $t = 1, \ldots, s$, $\{w_{it}\}$ being weights on each axis t for each set of observations, $i = 1, \ldots, m$, and $\{e_{ijk}\}$ being residuals. From previous considerations, this model can alternately be formulated in terms of scalar-products matrices

$$b_{ijk} \cong \sum_{t=1}^{s} w_{it} x_{jt} x_{kt} \tag{3.32}$$

If for each matrix $D_i^{(2)}$ we define the matrix of scalar products B_i with (3.12), then the mean of the elements of each such matrix is equal to zero, and from this it follows that the sum of its squared elements will be proportional to the total variance of these elements. If each matrix is given equal weight, for example by making all such variances equal to one, to (3.22) we can substitute the model

$$b_{ijk}^* = \sum_{t=1}^{s} w_{it} x_{jt} x_{kt} \tag{3.33}$$

where $b_{ijk}^* = b_{ijk}/(\Sigma_{jk} b_{ijk}^2)^{1/2}$. A least-squares solution can be obtained (Carroll and Chang, 1970) through use of the method of nonlinear iterative least squares of Wold (1966). As in (3.33) $\{w_{it}\}$ and $\{x_{jt}\}$ are defined up to a diagonal non-singular transformation, the final solution is scaled such that $x_t^T x_t = 1$ for $t = 1, \ldots, s$, so that each w_{it} reflects the extent to which the tth factor accounts for the variation observed with the ith set of observations. For each matrix B_i, the proportion of the sum of squares explained by these factors is given by

$$f_i = 1 - \sum_{jk} (b_{ijk} - \hat{b}_{ijk})^2 \tag{3.34}$$

where $\hat{b}_{ijk} = \Sigma_t w_{it} x_{jt} x_{kt}$ is the s-dimensional approximation to b_{ijk} according to the model (3.33), recalling that $\Sigma_{jk} b_{ijk}^2 = 1$. An application to three matrices of distances based on anthropometrics, genetic markers, and shared cognate frequences in Micronesia was given in Lalouel (1975).

3.4. Cluster Analysis

We shall only briefly outline here the rationale of a broad class of descriptive methods generally referred to as methods for cluster analysis, as the variety of methods belonging to this class, in terms of axiomatic approach as well as computing algorithms, defy any significant presentation within the limited scope of the present paper.

The aim of such methods, as opposed to those already presented, is primarily to identify a discrete rather than continuous structure underlying the data. A partition of the data into discrete groups is sought, on the basis of similarity or dissimilarity between sampling units concerning a number of discrete or continuous traits, and broad categories of methods can be distinguished according to whether the partition sought is of a hierarchical nature or not.

3.4.1. Flat-Cluster Methods

Such methods seek a partition of sampling units (whether individuals or subpopulations) into several, generally mutually exclusive, classes, although some methods often so classified generate overlapping clusters (see Jardine and Sibson, 1971). Most of these methods require, as an initial step, definition of a measure of similarity or dissimilarity in a continuous space, often a Euclidean metric (for example, Rohlf, 1970); a partition into a given number of classes is then obtained through an algorithm minimizing a loss function defined so as to maximize some measure of intraclass similarity, often through some criterion involving covariances within and among groups. This problem has received considerable attention, often developing on the work of Rubin (1967); useful references in this respect are Jardin and Sibson (1971) and Hartigan (1975), together with some numerical comparisons presented by Maronna and Jacovkis (1974).

3.4.2. Hierarchical Clustering

Another class of clustering methods generate instead a hierarchical partition, most often yielding a representation of similarities having a tree structure. Numerous methods have been developed for that purpose, often classified on the basis of the method, numerical procedure, or nature of the algorithm used. The multiplicity of such methods, together with the frequent lack of a rigorous axiomatic approach, has often left potential users in disarray as to what method should be used in a given situation. We found useful guidance, in this respect, in the axiomatic approach of Jardine and Sibson (1971) from which, on the basis of rigorous definition of an ultrametric distance, together with definition of a number of conditions that such a method should satisfy, the well-known method of "minimum single linkage" receives rigorous foundations. Other useful references in this respect are again Sneath and Sokal (1973) and Hartigan (1975), the latter providing the user with numerous computer implementations.

3.4.3. General Considerations on Clustering Methods

The use of cluster analysis cannot be reduced to technical considerations about the choice of a method for some application, as can be seen in Sneath and Sokal (1973), a master reference on the theory and practice of numerical taxonomy. The very purpose of taxonomic classification on the basis of phenetic resemblance has often been confused with that of methods explicitly attempting phylogenic reconstructions. The rigorous definition of taxonomic units, measures of similarity or dissimilarity, the interpretation of classification generated, deserve considerable attention on the part of the user. In many instances where such methods are applied to continuous measurements or continuous variables derived from discrete observations, such as frequencies of polymorphic characters, it is probably fair to say that the purpose of the analysis is not any more one of classification or inference of a discrete structure, but rather one of data reduction, as it is often true that, when a large number of units are considered, the insight provided by a continuous representation of structure may be slight. Hierarchical clustering methods are often used to in fact define a nonhierarchic partition for a given level of similarity or dissimilarity. This can only be useful for setting an hypothesis to be submitted to further investigation and testing, whether by discriminant analysis, statistical tests of heterogeneity, or specific model building.

4. Envoi

All the methods discussed here are only of a descriptive nature, essentially data reduction and exposure. Although they may provide insight regarding relationships between present-day populations, the ultimate goal of most studies resorting to such methods should be to obtain some knowledge about the process having led to the present structure. The usefulness of descriptive methods will be greatly enhanced if they lead to design of further experiments, hypothesis testing, as well as model building, methods of inference from which they are too often dissociated.

References

Adhikari, B. P., and Joshi, D. D. (1956), Distance, discrimination et résumé exhaustif, Pub. Inst. Stat. Univ. Paris. 5:57–74.

Anderson, T. W. (1958), *Introduction to Multivariate Statistical Analysis*, New York, Wiley,

Anderson, T. W., and Bahadur, R. R. (1962), Classification into two multivariate normal distributions with different covariance matrices, *Ann. Math. Stat.* 33:420–431.

Balakrishnan, V., and Sanghvi, L. D. (1968), Distance between populations on the basis of attribute data, *Biometrics* 24:859–865.

Bennett, J. F. (1956), Determination of the number of independent parameters of a score matrix from the examination of rank orders, *Psychometrika* 21:383–393.

Bennett, J. F., and Hays, W. L. (1960), Multidimensional unfolding determining the dimensionality of ranked preference data, *Psychometrika* 25:27–43.

Beshers, J. M., and Laumann, E. O. (1967), Social distance: A network-approach, *Am. Sociol. Rev.* 32:225–236.

Bhattacharyya, A. (1943), On a measure of divergence between two statistical populations defined by their probability distributions, *Bull. Calc. Math. Soc.* **35**:99–109.

Bhattacharyya, A. (1946), On a measure of divergence between two multinomial populations, *Sankhyā* **7**:401–406.

Brown, L. A., and Horton, F. E. (1971), Functional distance: an operational approach, *Geog. Anal.* **3**:76–83.

Burnaby, T. P. (1966), Growth-invariant discriminant functions and generalized distances, *Biometrics* **22**:96–110.

Carroll, J. D. (1972), Individual differences and multidimensional scaling, in *Multidimensional Scaling* (R. N. Shepard, A. K. Romney, and S. B. Nerlove, eds.), pp. 105–155, Seminar Press, New York.

Carroll, J. D., and Chang, J. J. (1970), Analysis of individual differences in multidimensional scaling via an *N*-way generalization of "Eckart-Young" decomposition, *Psychometrika* **35**:283–319.

Cavalli-Sforza, L. L., and Conterio, F. (1960), Analisi della fluttuazione di frequenze geniche nella populazione della val Parma, *Atti Assoc. Genet. Ital.* **5**:333–344.

Cavalli-Sforza, L. L., and Edwards, A. W. F. (1967), Phylogenetic analysis models and estimation procedures, *Evolution* **21**:550–570.

Chaddha, R. L., and Marcus, L. F. (1968), An empirical comparison of distance statistics for populations with unequal covariance matrices, *Biometrics* **24**:683–694.

Cochran, W. (1963), *Sampling Techniques*, Wiley, London.

Coombs, C. H. (1958), Psychological scaling without a unit of measurement, *Psych. Rev.* **57**:148–158.

Coombs, C. H. (1964), *A Theory of Data*, Wiley, New York.

Coombs, C. H., and Kao, R. C. (1955), Nonmetric factor analysis, Department of Engineering Research Bulletin No. 38, University of Michigan, Ann Arbor.

Cotterman, C. W. (1953), Regular two allele and three allele phenotype systems, *Amer. J. Hum. Genet.* **5**:193–235.

Cotterman, C. W. (1969), Factor-union phenotype systems, in *Computer Applications in Genetics* (N. E. Morton, ed.), pp. 1–18, University of Hawaii Press, Honolulu.

Davidon, W. C. (1959), Variable metric method for minimization, A.E.C. Research and Development Report, No. ANL-5990.

Eckart, C., and Young, G. (1936), The approximation of one matrix by another of lower rank, *Psychometrika* **1**:211–218.

Edwards, A. W. F. (1971), Distances between populations on the basis of gene frequencies, *Biometrics* **27**:873–881.

Edwards, A. W. F., and Cavalli-Sforza, L. L. (1964), Reconstruction of evolutionary trees, *Publs. Syst. Assoc.* **6**:67–76.

Edwards, A. W. F., and Cavalli-Sforza, L. L. (1972), Affinity as revealed by differences in gene frequencies, in *The Assessment of Population Affinities in Man* (J. S. Weiner and J. Huizinga, eds.), Oxford University Press, London.

Ewens, W. J. (1972), The sampling theory of selectively neutral alleles, *Theor. Popul. Biol.* **3**:87–112.

Fisher, R. S. (1958), *Statistical Methods for Research Workers*, 13th ed., Oliver and Boyd, Edinburgh.

Fletcher, R., and Powell, M. J. (1963), A rapidly convergent descent method for minimization, *Computer J.* **6**:163–168.

Gower, J. C. (1966), Some distance properties of latent root and vector methods used in multivariate analysis, *Biometrika* **53**:325–338.

Gower, J. C. (1972), Measures of taxonomic distance and their analysis, in *The Assessment of Population Affinities in Man* (J. S. Weiner and J. Huizinga, eds.), pp. 1–24, Oxford University Press, Oxford.

Guttman, L. (1941), The quantification of a class of attributes: A theory and method for scale construction, The prediction of personal adjustment, Social Science Research Council, New York.

Guttman, L, (1968), A general nonmetric technique for finding the smallest coordinate space for a configuration of points, *Psychometrika* 33:469–506.

Haldane, J. B. S. (1954), An exact test for randomness of mating, *J. Gen.* 52:631–635.

Hansen, M. H., Hurwitz, W. N., and Madow, W. G. (1953), *Sample Survey Methods and Theory* (2 vols.), Wiley, New York.

Harpending, H., and Jenkins, T., 1972, !Kung population structure, in *Genetic Distance*, (J. F. Crow, ed.), Plenum Press, New York.

Harpending, H., and Jenkins, T. (1973), Genetic distances among southern African populations, in *Method and Theories of Anthropological Genetics*, (M. H. Crawford and P. L. Workman, eds.), University of New Mexico Press, Albuquerque.

Hartigan, J. A. (1975), *Clustering Algorithms*, Wiley, New York.

Hays, W. L., and Bennett, J. F. (1961), Multidimensional unfolding: determining configuration from complete rank order preference data, *Psychometrika* 26:221–238.

Hedrick, P. W. (1971), A new approach to measuring genetic similarity, *Evolution* 25: 276–280.

Hotelling, H. (1933), Analysis of a complex of statistical variables into principal components, *J. Educ. Psychol.* 24:417–411, 498–520.

Ito, K., and Schull, W. J. (1964), On the robustness of the T_0^2 test in multivariate analysis of variance when variance-covariance matrices are not equal, *Biometrika* 51:71–82.

Jacquard, A. (1973), Distances généalogiques et distances génétiques, *Cah. Anthropol. Ecol. Hum.* 1:11–125.

Jacquard, A. (1974), *The Genetic Structure of Populations*, Springer-Verlag, Berlin.

Jardine, N., and Sibson, R. (1971), *Mathematical Taxonomy*, Wiley and Sons, London.

Kemeny, J. C., and Snell, J. L. (1960), *Finite Markov Chains*, Van Nostrand, Princeton, New Jersey.

Kimura, M. (1955), Random genetic drift in a multi-allelic locus, *Evolution* 9:419–435.

Kimura, M., and Crow, J. F. (1964), The number of alleles that can be maintained in a finite population, *Genetics* 49:725–738.

Kruskal, J. B. (1964a), Multidimensional scaling by optimizing goodness of fit to a nonmetric hypothesis, *Psychometrika* 29:115–129.

Kruskal, J. B. (1964b), Nonmetric multidimensional scaling: A numerical method, *Psychometrika* 29:115–129.

Kullback, S. (1968), *Information Theory and Statistics*, Wiley, New York.

Kurczynski, T. W. (1970), Generalized distance and discrete variables, *Biometrics* 26: 525–534.

Lalouel, J. M. (1973), Topology of population structure, in *Genetic Structure of Populations*, (N. E. Morton, ed.), pp. 139–149, University of Hawaii Press, Honolulu.

Lalouel, J. M. (1975), Differentiation locale d'une population; aspects méthodologiques et applications, Thèse de Doctorat es Sciences, Université Pierre et Marie Curie, Paris (535 pp.).

Lalouel, J. M. (1977), Linkage mapping from pairwise recombination data, *Heredity* 38:61–77.

Lalouel, J. M., and Langaney, A. (1976), Analysis of inter-villages matrimonial migrations among the Bedik and Niokholonko of Sénégal, *Amer. J. Phys. Anthropol.* 45:453–466.

Lalouel, J. M. Loiselet, J., Lefranc, G., Chaiban, D., Chashachiro, L., and Ropartz, C. (1975), Genetic differentiation among Lebanese communities, *Acta Anthropogenetica* 1:15–33.

Lalouel, J. M., and Morton, N. E. (1972), Bioassay of kinship in a South American Indian population, *Amer. J. Hum. Genet.* **25**:62–73.

Latter, B. D. H. (1973), Measures of genetic distance between individuals and populations, in *Genetic Structure of Populations*, (N. E. Morton, ed.), pp. 27–37, University of Hawaii Press, Honolulu.

Lingoes, J. C. (1970), A general nonparametric method for representing objects and attributes in a joint metric space, in *Les comptes rendus du Colloque International sur l'emploi des ordinateurs en archéologie: Problèmes sémiologiques et mathématiques*, (J. C. Gardin, ed.), pp. 277–298, CNRS, Marseille.

Lingoes, J. C. (1971), Some boundary conditions for a monotone analysis of symmetric matrices, *Psychometrika* **36**:195–203.

Mahalanobis, P. C. (1936), On the generalized distance in statistics, *Proc. Natl. Inst. Sci. India* **2**:49–55.

Malécot, G. (1950), Quelques schémas probabilistes sur la variabilité des populations naturelles, *Ann. Univ. Lyon Sci. Sect. A* **13**:37–60.

Malécot, G. (1959), Les modèles stockastiques en génétique de population, *Publ. Inst. Statist. Paris* **8**:173–210.

Malécot, G. (1966), *Probabilités et Hérédité*, INED, Travaux et Documents, Cahier No. 47, P.U.F., Paris.

Malécot, G. (1971), Génétique des populations naturelles dans le case d'un seul locus. I. Evolution de la fréquence d'un gène. Etude des variances et covariances, *Ann. Génét. Sélect. Anim.* **3**:255–280.

Malécot, G. (1972), Génétique des populations naturelles dans le case d'un seul locus. II. Etude de coefficient de parenté, *Ann. Génét. Sélect. Anim.* **4**:385–409.

Malécot, G. (1973), Parenté, mutations et migrations, *Ann. Génét. Sélect. Anim.* **5**:333–361.

Maltyutov, M. B., Passekov, V. P., and Richkov, Y. F. (1972), On the reconstruction of evolutionary trees of human populations resulting from random genetic drift, in *The Assessment of Population Affinities in Man*, (J. S. Weiner and J. Huizinga, eds.), pp. 48–71, Oxford University Press, London.

Maronna, R., and Jacovkis, P. M. (1974), Multivariate clustering procedures with variable metrics, *Biometrics* **30**:499–505.

Matusita, K. (1966), A distance and related statistics in multivariate analysis, in *Multivariate Analysis. I* (P. R. Krishnaiah, ed.), pp. 187–200, Academic Press, New York.

Meyer, C. D. (1978), An alternative expression for the mean first passage matrix, *Lin. Alg. Appl.* **22**:41–47.

Morton, N. E. (1973a), Kinship and population structure, in *Genetic Structure of Populations* (N. E. Morton, ed.), pp. 66–69, University of Hawaii Press, Honolulu.

Morton, N. E. (1973b), Isolation by distance, in *Genetic Structure of Populations* (N. E. Morton, ed.), pp. 76–77, University of Hawaii Press, Honolulu.

Morton, N. E. (1973c), Kinship bioassay, in *Genetic Structure of Populations* (N. E. Morton, ed.), pp. 158–162, University of Hawaii Press, Honolulu.

Morton, N. E. (1973d), Kinship and molecular evolution, in *Genetic Structure of Populations*, (N. E. Morton, ed.), pp. 263–267, University of Hawaii Press, Honolulu.

Morton, N. E. (1975), Kinship, information, and biological distance, *Theor. Popul. Biol.* **7**:246–255.

Morton, N. E., and Lalouel, J. M. (1973), Bioassay of kinship in Micronesia, *Amer. J. Phys. Anthropol.* **38**:709–720.

Morton, N. E., Yee, S., Harris, D. E., and Lew, R. (1971), Bioassay of kinship, *Theor. Popul. Biol.* **2**:507–524.

Nei, M. (1965), Variation and covariation of gene frequencies in subdivided populations, *Evolution* **19**:256–258.

Nei, M. (1971), Identity of genes and genetic distance between populations, *Genetics* 68:347.

Nei, M. (1972), Genetic distance between populations, *Am. Nat.* 105:385–398.

Nei, M. (1973), The theory and estimation of genetic distance, in *Genetic Structure of Populations* (N. E. Morton, ed.), pp. 45–51, University of Hawaii Press, Honolulu.

Pearson, K. (1926), On the coefficient of racial likeness, *Biometrika* 18:105–117.

Rao, C. R. (1948), The utilisation of multiple measurements in problems of biological classification, *J. R. Stat. Soc.* 10:159–203.

Rao, C. R. (1952), *Advanced Statistical Methods in Biometric Research*, Wiley, New York.

Reyment, R. A. (1962), Observations on homogeneity of covariance matrices in paleontologic biometry, *Biometrics* 18:1–11.

Rohlf, F. J. (1970), Adaptive hierarchical clustering schemes, *Syst. Zool.* 19:58–82.

Rubin, J. (1967), Optimal classification into groups an approach for solving the taxonomy problem, *J. Theor. Biol.* 15:103–144.

Sanghvi, L. D. (1953), Comparison of genetical and morphological methods for a study of biological differences, *Am. J. Phys. Anthropol.* II:385–404.

Sanghvi, L. D., and Balakrishnan, V. (1972), Comparison of different measures of genetic distance between human populations, in *The Assessment of Population Affinities in Man* (J. S. Weiner and J. Huizinga, eds.), pp. 25–36, Oxford University Press, London.

Schönemann, P. H. (1966), A general solution of the orthogonal procrustes problem, *Psychometrika* 31:1–10.

Schönemann, P. H. (1970a), Fitting a simplex symmetrically, *Psychometrika* 35:1–21.

Schönemann, P. H. (1970b), On metric multidimensional unfolding, *Psychometrika* 35:349–366.

Schönemann, P. H., and Carroll, R. M. (1970), Fitting one matrix to another under choice of a central dilation and a rigid motion, *Psychometrika* 35:245–255.

Schönemann, P. H. and Wang, M. M. (1972), An individual difference model for the multidimensional analysis of preference data, *Psychometrika* 37:275–309.

Shepard, R. N. (1958), Stimulus and response generalization: Tests of a model relating generalization to distance in psychological space, *J. Experim. Psychol.* 55:509–523.

Shepard, R. N. (1962), The analysis of proximities: Multidimensional scaling with an unknown distance function. I, *Psychometrika* 27:125–140.

Shepard, R. N., Romney, A. K., and Nerlove, S. B. (1972), *Multidimensional Scaling: Theory and Applications in the Behavioral Sciences* (2 vols.), Seminar Press, New York.

Sneath, P. H. A., and Sokal, R. R. (1973), *Numerical Taxonomy* Freeman, San Francisco.

Steinberg, A. G., Bleuibtreu, H. K., Kurczynski, T. W., Martin, A. O., and Kurszynski, E. M. (1967), Genetic studies on an inbred human isolate, *Proceedings of the 3rd International Congress on Human Genetics* (J. F. Crow and J. V. Neel, eds.), pp. 267–289, Johns Hopkins University Press, Baltimore.

Torgerson, W. S. (1958), *Theory and Methods of Scaling* Wiley, New York.

Torgerson, W. S., and Young, F. W. (1967), TORSCA, FORTRAN IV program for Shepard-Kruskal multidimensional scaling analysis, *Behav. Sci.* 12:498.

Wang, M. P., Schönemann, P. H., and Rusk, J. G. (1975), A conjugate gradient algorithm for the multidimensional analysis of preference data, *Multivar. Behav. Res.* 10:45–79.

Wold, H. (1966), Estimation of principal components and related models by iterative least squares, *International Symposium of Multivariate Analysis, Dayton, Ohio, 1965* (P. R. Krishnaiah, ed.), pp. 391–420, Academic Press, New York.

Workman, P. L. Harpending, H., Lalouel, J. M., Lynch, C., Niswander, J. D., and Singleton, R. (1973), Population studies on southwestern Indian tribes. Papago population structure: a comparison of genetic and migration analyses, in *Genetic Structure of Populations* (N. E. Morton, ed.), pp. 166–194, University of Hawaii Press, Honolulu.

Yasuda, N. (1966), The genetical structure of northeastern Brazil, Ph.D. thesis, University of Hawaii, Honolulu.

Yasuda N. (1968), Estimation of the inbreeding coefficient from phenotype frequencies by a method of maximum likelihood scoring, *Biometrics* **24**:915–935.

Young, F. W. (1970), Nonmetric multidimensional scaling: recovery of metric information, *Psychometrika* **35**:455–475.

Young, F. W. (1972), A model for polynomial conjoint analysis algorithms, in *Multidimensional Scaling*, Vol. I (R. N. Shepard, A. K. Romney, and S. B. Nerlove, eds.), pp. 68–104, Seminar Press, New York.

Young, G., and Householder, A. S. (1938), Discussion of a set of points in terms of their mutual distances, *Psychometrika* **3**:19–22.

9

Pedigree Analysis of Complex Models

C. CANNINGS, E. A. THOMPSON, and M. SKOLNICK

1. Introduction

A basic component of any analysis of genetic data on members of a pedigree is the probability that, conditional on the structure of their pedigree and the model for the trait, a set of individuals will have certain phenotypes or genotypes. Risk probabilities required in genetic counseling problems (Binet, Sawyer, and Watson, 1958; Murphy, 1970; Chase, Murphy, and Bolling, 1971) may be computed as the ratio of two such probabilities. An ancestral likelihood is such a probability and may be computed under assumed ancestral genotype combinations (Thompson, Cannings, and Skolnick, 1978a). If the genetic model for the trait is known, the probability is the likelihood function enabling us to infer genealogical structure (Thompson, 1976a). If the genealogy is known, this same probability may be expressed as the likelihood for the genetic model assumed in the computation (Elston and Stewart, 1971). Elston and Stewart (1971) developed a recursive algorithm for the computation of probabilities on pedigrees and discussed its application to the problem of inferring genetic models. Heuch and Li (1972), following the theory of Hilden (1970), and Smith (1976) developed similar algorithms; they also discussed their use in

C. CANNINGS ● Department of Probability and Statistics, University of Sheffield, Sheffield, England and Department of Medical Biophysics and Computing, University of Utah, Salt Lake City, Utah.   E. A. THOMPSON ● Department of Medical Biophysics and Computing, University of Utah, Salt Lake City, Utah, and King's College, Cambridge, England. M. SKOLNICK ● Department of Medical Biophysics and Computing, University of Utah, Salt Lake City, Utah.   This project was supported in part by National Institutes of Health Research Grant CA-16573, awarded by the National Cancer Institute, Public Health Services/DHEW.

genetic counseling problems. However, both the structure of the pedigree and the class of models were restricted in these approaches. Lange and Elston (1975) and Cannings and co-workers (Cannings, Thompson, and Skolnick, 1976; Cannings, Thompson, and Skolnick, 1978) (the 1978 paper will be referred to in text as CTS) generalized the peeling logic of Elston and Stewart (1971) to pedigrees of arbitrary size and complexity, at least in theory.

Relatively simple models are usually used for the inference of genealogical relationship (e.g., paternity testing: Chakraborty, Shaw, and Schull, 1974), for the estimation of genealogical structure, for risks for individuals or for ancestral genotypes. However, inferring the mode of inheritance of a specific characteristic requires some consideration of complex genetic systems (at least as alternative hypotheses), as well as the possible effects of environmental components and interactions. This paper will demonstrate the generality of the models that fall within the scope of the theorems of CTS; it will also illustrate a method for deriving the basic recursions required. This is achieved by partitioning an individual's node into a collection of nodes, which correspond to the various genetic and environmental effects determining the phenotype and which are transmittable to any offspring. A diagrammatic representation of this "model structure" assists in the selection of an appropriate set of recursions.

The CTS method already permits consideration of age- and sex-dependent differences in the expression of genotypes (see also Elston and Yelverton, 1975), and a minor extension of this method will allow some models of assortative mating to be included. In addition, the complexities introduced by incorporating linear models that were outside the scope of the previous methods are dealt with here. (A brief discussion was presented by Cannings, Thompson, and Skolnick, 1979.)

Two distinct methods have evolved for inferring complex modes of inheritance. Morton (1974; Rao, Morton, and Yee, 1974, 1976) has developed a method for estimating genetic and environmental correlations on nuclear family data by path analysis (Wright, 1921), whereas the analysis of pedigree data has focused on estimating complex modes of genetic transmission (Elston and Yelverton, 1975). Rao, Morton, and Yee (1976) stress the dichotomy between the estimation of complex nonlinearities of a genetic model and the estimation of environmental effects which may be represented as additive components. Morton and Rao (1978) and Elston and Rao (1978) have also presented a dichotomy of methods as a dichotomy of models for the genetic and environmental factors underlying a set of phenotypic observations.

However, the ability to estimate a common-sib environment, for example, is not the prerogative of analysis of nuclear family data. Both the additive effects of environmental correlations and the correlations imposed by assortative mating, for example, are within the scope of pedigree analysis. These linear effects, together with the additive genetic effects (i.e., a polygenic component) or nonlinear major-gene effects, or both, can be included within the framework of a single pedigree analysis algorithm, and the inclusion of all these effects is not beyond the bounds of computational feasibility (Cannings, Thompson, and Skolnick, 1979; Boyle and Elston, 1979). The power of a pedigree structure to resolve these components, and to distinguish alternative models of environmental and genetic effects, remains to be investigated. However, Elston and Rao (1978) note that any analysis of a genetic model has greater power where the information on the complete structure of a pedigree can be utilized. This has also been demonstrated in the case of linkage by Thompson, Kravitz, Hill, and Skolnick (1978). By bringing such models within the framework of pedigree analysis, we hope (1) to unify the theory of computation of probabilities on pedigrees, (2) to increase the power of current procedures for estimating modes of inheritance from currently available genetic data, and hence (3) to improve both genetic counseling and genealogical inference, and (4) to provide some merging of genetic and epidemiological analyses.

2. Synopsis

We present here the general theory for computing the Pr{observations| model and pedigree} for pedigrees which are in theory of arbitrary size and complexity. This algorithm permits the incorporation of any mode of transmission (whether genetic or otherwise), assortative mating, common environmental components, and linear models. These results follow directly from the two theorems presented in Section 5.3 of CTS. Despite the generality added by the new results, some simplification of the theorems is achieved.

First, we derive the basic theory (Section 3). Then, to provide a proper setting and to emphasize the scope of models permitted by this theory, we review some of the forms which the functions involved can take (Section 4). Section 5 presents recursions for a few models, both to illustrate the scope allowable and to provide the reader with an opportunity to see how the theory may be translated into specific sets of recursions. It should be noted that the particular set of recursions chosen is in a sense arbitrary. Problems of optimization arise and are discussed in Section 6.1, although the results obtained so far are fairly limited. We address some questions concerning the use of probabilities in an inferential setting (Section 6.3) and review the data analyses that have been made with this method. A glossary of all the notations is provided as an appendix.

3. General Theory

The derivation of the appropriate recurrence relations for complex models will be presented in a general form. The derivation of recurrences by CTS was developed in two contexts, (i) for zero-looped pedigrees and (ii) for complex pedigrees (the latter including the former as a particular case). The models used in these derivations involved transmission, penetrance, and random mating and, as such, encompassed many of the standard genetic models (linked and X-linked loci, polygenic, mixed, etc.). On the other hand, assortative mating, linear models for the determination of the phenotypes, and environmental correlations between pairs of relatives, such as sibs and parent—offspring, were excluded. We shall prove that all these additional factors can be handled; and, in fact, the two theorems presented by CTS can be easily extended to these more complex models.

The model structure introduced by adding these new factors involves changing a zero-loop model to a looped model. For example, the introduction of a common-sib environment creates a loop for the phenotypes of each pair of sibs, since these are now each joined to a parental node (through transmission) and to a common-sib node C (illustrated in Fig. 4). The graph of the model, called a *model structure diagram*, may be drawn by using the nodes involving the smallest set of relatives on which it can be represented. For example, if we are dealing with a major-gene model, we require only the parents and a single offspring, but if a common-sib environment is required, two offspring will be necessary. In practice it may be easier to represent the whole nuclear family or a larger structure where needed.

The complete representation of the model and pedigree can be achieved by embedding the model structure diagram within the pedigree. However, in a zero-loop pedigree this will be unnecessary, because explicit recursions can be derived without specifying the actual pedigree.

First, we must describe the various components of a model structure diagram, and then relate these to the theorems of CTS. A slight change in the nature of the nodes is required from the previous concept that each node corresponded to an individual or a pair of individuals: Specifically, we now associate with each node a random variable $(\mathbf{I};\mathbf{A})$. For a vector (list) of individuals $\mathbf{I}$ and a vector of attributes $\mathbf{A}$ (some subset of phenotype, genotype, observation, etc.), $(\mathbf{I};\mathbf{A})$ is defined as the complete set of pairs of individuals and attributes contained in $\mathbf{I}$ and $\mathbf{A}$, respectively. Each arc represents the probabilistic relationship between the random variables at the ends of that arc. The probability functions are given in Table 1. We shall use directed arcs to indicate the temporal direction implicit in the process being represented. A requirement of all graphs used is that no chains (directed cycles) should exist. The directed arcs also have a probabilistic interpretation: Suppose we have a node $(\mathbf{I};\mathbf{A})$, and the set of arcs into the node have $(\mathbf{I}_j;\mathbf{A}_j), j = 1, 2, \ldots, k$ at the other ends. Then we can specify $P\{(\mathbf{I};\mathbf{A})|(\mathbf{I}_j;\mathbf{A}_j), j = 1, 2, \ldots, k\}$ without reference to any other arcs or nodes. Further, this will not be true for any other set of arcs unless it contains all of $(\mathbf{I}_j;\mathbf{A}_j)$, $j = 1, 2, \ldots, k$. To do this we introduce a set of arcs and their appropriate probability (PROB) functions

Table 1. The Arcs, Associated PROB Functions, and Descriptions of Functions for Model Structure Diagrams

Name of probability function	Notation for arc	Description
TRANS	———→——	genetic or environmental transmission function
PEN	———▷——	probability of a phenotype given a genotype
OBS	———D——	function to assure consistency between the observation and the age-specific phenotype
INIT	——▷▷——	initial genotype probabilities
ASSORT	——▷▷——	scale factor to correct mating frequency for assortative mating
LINCOMP	———▶——	linear components contributing to phenotype
COMMON	——▷▷——	common environmental components
JOIN	———≫——	combination of information from two nodes onto one
SPLIT	———≫——	division of information from one node onto two or more
COND	———≫——	incorporation of information from one node onto another

(see Table 1). As an example we may consider a child and his parents, and their genotypes. Now $P\{$child's genotype | parents' genotypes$\}$ is simply an element of the transmission function, whereas the specification of $P\{$parents' genotypes | child's genotype$\}$ requires information on the parents' genotype frequencies, based on population frequencies

In order to show how recurrence relations are derived, we proceed via the CTS theory, which associates each node in H (the total graph) with a single individual, or with a couple; but implicitly the genotype is also associated with that node. The basic rules for peeling require that (i) we have some set $(Q - F)$ of nodes that have already been removed, (ii) we have a split set F [i.e., any chain joining a node in $(Q - F)$ to one in $(H - Q)$ contains at least one element of F], on which we have defined a function synthesizing all the information on $(Q - F)$ (R function), and (iii) we have $(Q^1 - F^1)$ and F^1 similarly structured to $(Q - F)$

and F, with $(Q - F) \subset (Q^1 - F^1)$ and $Q \subset Q^1$. Then Theorem 1 of CTS specifies an operation giving a new R function, defined on F^1, and condensing the information on $Q^1 - F^1$. This progression from (Q,F) to (Q^1, F^1) is called peeling. The recurrence equation given in the theorem is

$$R((Q^1, F^1); i) = \sum_j \left(\prod_X \text{PEN}(\cdot | j) \right) \left(\prod_{X \downarrow \theta} R(\cdot; j) \right) \text{TRANS}(Q^1 - (Q - F); j) R((Q, F); j) \tag{3.1}$$

where $X = (Q^1 - F^1) - (Q - F)$ (X being the set of nodes peeled off in this recursion), $X \downarrow \theta$ is the set of originals in X, and $\text{TRANS}(Q^1 - (Q - F); j) = P\{Q^1 - (Q - F) \equiv j | (Q^1 - (Q - F)) \downarrow \equiv j\}$, that is, the probability that the nodes which have now entered consideration for the first time, or which are being finally eliminated, take the appropriate values given all the ancestors amongst them (see CTS). TRANS is a probabilistic function of the type discussed above and is associated with specific arcs, and PEN can be made to be so by introducing into our representation a phenotype node and by defining PEN on that arc. In addition, we change our previous approach slightly by removing $R(\cdot | j)$, which accounted for the population values for original ancestors, and replacing them by a looped arc (illustrated in Fig. 2) joining an original to itself. Such arcs have the function INIT defined on them. INIT(G) is simply the probability that an individual has genotype G. Accordingly, we may rewrite the recurrence as

$$R((Q^1, F^1); i) = \sum_j R((Q, F); j) \prod_N \text{PROB}(j; i) \tag{3.2}$$

where N is the set of arcs which have been removed, and $\text{PROB}(j; i)$ takes the appropriate value on each arc (i.e., TRANS, PEN, INIT, etc.). The summation is over all j consistent with i and the observations. If we introduce an additional node corresponding to the actual observation W, with an arc joining this to phenotype Z, this will ensure consistency. The appropriate arc function OBS will be a Dirac δ-function (i.e., 1 if $Z = W$; 0 elsewhere) subscripted by the identity of the individual involved. Expressions (3.2) and (3.1) are equivalent, but in some ways (3.2) is easier to handle, at least now that all probabilities are associated with arcs.

In terms of our new notation, our basic rule requires that a node $(\mathbf{I}; \mathbf{A})$ can only be peeled onto a node $(\mathbf{I}^*; \mathbf{A}^*)$ if all the nodes connected to $(\mathbf{I}; \mathbf{A})$ other than $(\mathbf{I}^*; \mathbf{A}^*)$ have been previously peeled off or are peeled off in the current operation. Denoting by "$'$" a new R function,

$$R'(\mathbf{I}^*; \mathbf{A}^*) = \sum_{(\mathbf{I}; \mathbf{A}) - (\mathbf{I}^*; \mathbf{A}^*)} R(\mathbf{I}; \mathbf{A}) R(\mathbf{I}^*; \mathbf{A}^*) f((\mathbf{I}; \mathbf{A}), (\mathbf{I}^*; \mathbf{A}^*)) \tag{3.3}$$

where $(\mathbf{I}; \mathbf{A}) - (\mathbf{I}^*; \mathbf{A}^*)$ denotes all those random variables in $(\mathbf{I}; \mathbf{A})$ that are not in $(\mathbf{I}^*; \mathbf{A}^*)$, $f((\mathbf{I}; \mathbf{A}), (\mathbf{I}^*; \mathbf{A}^*))$ is the function associated with the arc joining $(\mathbf{I}; \mathbf{A})$ and $(\mathbf{I}^*; \mathbf{A}^*)$; summation is over all values of the random variables $(\mathbf{I}; \mathbf{A}) - (\mathbf{I}^*; \mathbf{A}^*)$ consistent with the values of $(\mathbf{I}^*; \mathbf{A}^*)$. We may also rewrite Theorem 2 of CTS: Suppose $(\mathbf{I}_1; \mathbf{A}_1)$ and $(\mathbf{I}_2; \mathbf{A}_2)$ are disjoint, and $(\mathbf{I}^1; \mathbf{A}^1)$ is a "combination" of them, as per CTS: Then

$$R((\mathbf{I}^1;\mathbf{A}^1);i) = \sum R((\mathbf{I}_1;\mathbf{A}_1);j)R((\mathbf{I}_2;\mathbf{A}_2);j)f((\mathbf{I}_1;\mathbf{A}_1)\cup(\mathbf{I}_2;\mathbf{A}_2),(\mathbf{I}^1;\mathbf{A}^1))$$

where Σ is over all random variables in $(\mathbf{I}^1;\mathbf{A}^1) - \{(\mathbf{I}_1;\mathbf{A}_1)\cup(\mathbf{I}_2;\mathbf{A}_2)\}$. Thus we see that additional factors can be added provided they can be properly associated with an arc. We will discuss this in detail for three specific factors: original frequencies (Section 4.3), assortative mating (Section 4.4), and linear models (Section 4.5).

The genotype frequencies of the original ancestors in the pedigree were incorporated in CTS at the stage that those individuals were peeled. In the spirit of our new approach, we have required all functions (in this case genotype frequencies) to be associated with an arc. Accordingly, we have drawn an arc from each original to the same original (i.e., a loop). This arc has associated with it a function $\mathrm{INIT}(\cdot)$; this will be a probability or a density depending on the model considered.

The addition of assortative mating is made similarly by adding a single loop to a node which contains all the phenotype/genotype information on a married pair. The function

$$\mathrm{ASSORT} = \frac{P\{\text{pairs' phenotype}\}}{P\{\text{males' phenotype}\}P\{\text{females' phenotype}\}}$$

is a simple scale factor which corrects the mating frequency from the value in the denominator (under random mating) to that for the assortative mating model. If the population is to mate at random, then the arc may be omitted.

The addition of a linear model requires a slight modification. Suppose we have a linear model, where the phenotype $Z = A_1 + A_2 + \cdots + A_k + B_1 + B_2 + \cdots + B_l + E$, components $A_1,\ldots,A_k$ are determined by transmission, $B_1,\ldots,B_l$ are independently determined components common to more than one individual (not necessarily the same set of individuals in each case), and E is an independent contribution. This section of the model is illustrated in Fig. 1, where "$\cdot$" denotes a specific individual. The components of the linear model are connected to Z by a set of arcs, on which $\mathrm{PROB} = 1$.

In order to peel a model that includes linear components, a new type of node, represented by a rectangular box, is introduced. This box indicates that the attribute in that box is the result of the sum of the inputs. Accordingly, during the peeling process, the removal of some components requires that the remainder of Z be regarded as the sum of the unpeeled components. Thus, referring to Fig. 1, suppose that we wish to proceed by first peeling off $(\cdot;A_1)$, supposing A_i's are continuous variables, then we compute

$$R(\cdot;Z-A_1)\int R(\cdot;A_1)R(\cdot;Z)dA_1$$

We might now peel off other A_i components in a similar way. In general

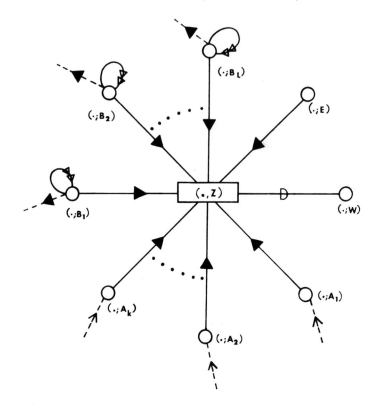

FIGURE 1. Nodes with arcs to Z, the phenotype.

we have

$$R(\cdot;Z - \Sigma - A_i) = \int R(\cdot;A_i)R(\cdot;Z - \Sigma)dA_i$$

where Σ denotes the sum of all A's previously removed.

The removal of the B_i's requires that we hold a joint function on the nodes to which it is joined, or that other information has already been collapsed onto the $(\cdot;B_i)$. In the latter case, the above recursion can be applied immediately. In the former, we would compute

$$R((\cdot;Z - \Sigma - B_i),(*;Z^* - \Sigma^* - B_i)) = \int R(\cdot;B_i)R((\cdot;Z - \Sigma),(*;Z^* - \Sigma^*))dB_i$$

where $*$, Z^*, and Σ^* are defined for the other individual connected to $(\cdot;B_i)$, in an analogous manner to $\cdot$, Z, and Σ. A similar recurrence occurs for $(\cdot;A_i)$ if it is to be peeled onto a joint set of nodes. The distribution of the B_i's is introduced by the function on the looped arcs at B_i. The distribution of E can be included on the arc to the rectangular box.

Finally, we comment on the arc joining $(\cdot;W)$ to the rectangular box: This arc has a function which has arguments Z and W, and accordingly it must be peeled before any of the A's, B's, or C (common-sib environment) are removed, for if any of these have been peeled, Z is no longer defined, and the function in question cannot be used.

All nodes are initially labeled with value unity with the exception of the W nodes. These are labeled with unity if no actual value is available (i.e., no observation has been made on the associated individual), or with a δ-function that takes the value 1 for the specific observation, but is 0 elsewhere.

4. Specific Models

The components required to specify a model are the probability functions on the arcs of the model structure diagram. These are presented in Table 1 with the symbols used in structure diagrams and brief descriptions. We now need to discuss these components in relation to some specific models.

4.1. Transmission Functions

The transmission function, TRANS, specifies the conditional probability of an offspring attribute, given the corresponding attributes of the parents. Usually we will have transmission of one or more genotypic components, but we may also have a direct transmission of phenotype, such as in a cultural model, or the transmission of a common-sib environment, or both.

4.1.1. Simple Transmission Models

Some examples of simple transmission models have already been given in CTS. For a single autosomal locus with alleles $a_1 \ldots a_k$, we have for offspring T of father Y and mother X

$$\text{TRANS}((T; a_m a_n) | (Y; a_i a_j), (X; a_i' a_j'))$$

$$= \text{coefficient of } a_m a_n \text{ in } \tfrac{1}{4}(a_i + a_j)(a_i' + a_j')$$

For an X-linked locus, separate transmission functions must be specified for the male (haploid) and female (diploid) offspring. We have

$$\text{TRANS}((T; a_m a_n) | (Y; a_i), (X; a_i' + a_j')) = \text{coefficient of } a_m a_n \text{ in } \tfrac{1}{2}(a_i' + a_j')a_i$$

for female T, and

$$\text{TRANS}((T; a_m) | (Y; a_i), (X; a_i' a_j')) = \text{coefficient of } a_m \text{ in } \tfrac{1}{2}(a_i' + a_j')$$

for male T.

Where several genetic components are transmitted independently, the joint transmission probability is the product of the separate transmissions; this applies whether we are considering the transmission of essentially identical components,

such as several unlinked loci, or the transmission of a major genotypic component or a polygenic component or environmental components. For n linked loci,
however, we must have a joint transmission probability: Denoting the haplotype
vectors by $\mathbf{a_1}$ and $\mathbf{b_1}$ for the mother, $\mathbf{a_2}$ and $\mathbf{b_2}$ for the father, and $\mathbf{a_3}$ and $\mathbf{b_3}$ for
the offspring, we have

$$\text{TRANS}((T; \mathbf{a_3 b_3})|(X; \mathbf{a_1}, \mathbf{b_1}), (Y; \mathbf{a_2 b_2}))$$

$$= \text{coefficient of } \mathbf{a_3}, \mathbf{b_3} \text{ in } \left[\sum_{\nu} P(\nu)\nu(\mathbf{a_1}, \mathbf{b_1})\right], \left[\sum_{\nu} P(\nu)\nu(\mathbf{a_2}, \mathbf{b_2})\right]$$

where ν is any of the two offspring chromosomes formed by crossovers between
each pair of parental chromosomes. Thus all possible recombination patterns are
represented; the $P(\nu)$ are the probabilities of each recombination pattern, which
may be simply the product of the recombination or the nonrecombination
probabilities between adjacent loci. However, they may be more complex and
include the possibility of positive or negative interference. For separate chromosomes, we have the product of the separate TRANS functions, and a similar
expression may be given for the X chromosome.

4.1.2. Polygenic Transmission

A second class of models are those of polygenic transmission where the
phenotype of an individual is taken to be a continuous variable resulting from
a large number of additive gene effects. It is assumed that the number of such
genes is sufficiently large that effects of individual genes are essentially not
observable. Specifically one assumes that the phenotype of the offspring $(T;P)$
is a linear combination of the mother's genotype $(X;P)$, the father's genotype
$(Y;P)$, and a sampling effect ζ. In general, if we suppose that the contributions
to male and female offspring are unequal, we take

$$(T;P_f) = \lambda(X;P) + (1-\lambda)(Y;P) + \zeta_f, \qquad \lambda \in [0, 1]$$

where subscript f denotes that T is female, and

$$(T;P_m) = (1-\mu)(X;P) + \mu(Y;P) + \zeta_m, \qquad \mu \in [0, 1]$$

where m denotes that T is male, it being assumed that ζ_f and ζ_m are independent
of parental genotypes and that the offspring values are conditionally independent,
given the parental values.

The choice of λ and μ enables us to encompass a wide range of models,
e.g., (i) if $\lambda = \mu = \frac{1}{2}, \zeta_f = \zeta_m$, we would have the autosomal-type polygenic model;
(ii) $\lambda = \frac{1}{2}$, $\mu = 0$, a sex-linked type; (iii) $\lambda = 1$, $\mu = 0$, a cytoplasmic type. We
note that the precise genetic mechanism is not specified. Karlin formalizes and
extends the multifactorial models of inheritance and their basic convergence
properties (Karlin, 1979).

The transmission function, one for males and one for females, are specified by

$$\text{TRANS}((T_m;P)|A_m,A_f) = f_m(Y - A_m)$$

where T_m is a male offspring with polygenic component P, $A_m = (1 - \mu)(X;P) + \mu(Y;P)$, and $f_m(Y - A_m)$ is the density function for ζ_m; a similar expression holds for $\text{TRANS}((T_f;P)|A_m,A_f)$. Note that we list both A_f and A_m in the function although only one is strictly relevant. This is done because both A_f and A_m are defined at the parental node and because all PROB functions are defined to relate all the variables at either end of the arc in question.

Another useful approach is to consider the polygenic component as the sum of independent discrete effects at a number of different loci. A discretized version of polygenic transmission was given in CTS and has been used by Thompson and Skolnick (1977). However, their version of discretized polygenic transmission did not operate separately on the parental contributions of the separate loci, but on the combined parental value. A more satisfactory approach would be to consider each multilocus genotype and to multiply the transition probabilities over the independent loci, as described above.

The TRANS function may be used to specify the transmission of environmental factors in addition to genetic factors. C, the contribution of common-sib environment to the phenotype of the offspring, may be dependent on the same factor in the parental sibships (C_X and C_Y). Thus, we might have

$$\text{TRANS}(C|C_X,C_Y) = \phi\left[\frac{C - \frac{1}{2}(C_X + C_Y)}{\sigma}\right]$$

where ϕ is the standard Normal density for some specified or unknown, and to-be-estimated, standard deviation σ. In the model structure diagrams, a "JOIN" arc will connect the parental common-sib nodes to a contribution node, whose value is $\frac{1}{2}(C_X + C_Y)$, and this node may be connected to the offspring common-sib node by an arc carrying the TRANS function. This transmission of a common environmental factor is not to be confused with common-environment contributions *common* to parents and offspring, or to more remote relatives such as cousins or uncle—nephew: Nontransmitted common environments are single random variables which may be eliminated from the split-set on which an R function is held, when the phenotype of the last individual involved is incorporated, via some population distribution. A transmitted environment will instead be replaced by those components on which its distribution depends, via the TRANS factor.

4.1.3. Models of Cultural Evolution

Models of cultural inheritance have been considered by Cavalli-Sforza and Feldman (1973a, b). Direct transmission of components of phenotype may also be incorporated via a TRANS function that connnects parental and offspring phenotypic nodes. In general, this may require us to calculate joint functions over several components of phenotype, particularly if the transmission is not only via parents but also through elder sibs and more remote relatives. However, simple models may be handled readily; Cannings, Thompson, and Skolnick (1978) illustrate one example of direct transmission of a discrete phenotype.

Another simple model was considered by Cavalli-Sforza and Feldman (1973a); a child of genotype G has phenotype

$$A = f_G(Z_X, Z_Y) + \epsilon$$

where ϵ is a random variable with mean 0 and variance σ^2, Z_X, Z_Y are the parental phenotypes, and f_G specifies the genotype-dependent response to these phenotypes. Thus we shall have to consider the transmission from the joint parental phenotype–genotype combination to an offspring phenotype–genotype. Specifically, for this model we have for child T with genotype G and phenotype Z

$$\text{TRANS}((T; G, Z)|(X; G_X, Z_X),(Y; G_Y, Z_Y))$$

$$= g(Z - f_G(Z_X, Z_Y))\text{TRANS}(G|G_X, G_Y)$$

where $\text{TRANS}(G|G_X, G_Y)$ denotes the Mendelian segregation matrix and g the density function of random noise ϵ. In the case where f_G is a linear function, the equilibrium variances of and covariances between random pairs of individuals have been obtained (Cavalli-Sforza and Feldman, 1973a). These may be used to give the probabilities for the originals in the pedigree (see Section 4.3). Although Cavalli-Sforza and Feldman consider only the case of a single-locus autosomal model, the genotypes G may be any discrete genotypes for which the segregation matrix can be given. As pointed out by these authors, the model reduces to a simple genetic model if $f_G(Z_X, Z_Y)$ is a constant a_i, and to a direct phenotypic model alone if f_G is independent of G.

Although specific contributions from more remote relatives can be incorporated (see Section 5.6), the concept of a "group" effect (Cavalli-Sforza and Feldman, 1973b) poses problems for pedigree analysis, since all members of the pedigree are presumably concurrently members of the group. One way in which such an effect could be incorporated would be to assume an equilibrium value for the duration of the period of the pedigree, and assume that the group is sufficiently large so that values of the trait within the pedigree have no effect on this group mean. In this case the effect is simply a constant stabilizing factor that can be incorporated into the transmission. The model of Cavalli-Sforza and Feldman (1973b) does not include genotypic transmission; the only TRANS arc is the one that connects parent to offspring phenotype, and the function on this arc is expressed as

$$\text{TRANS}((T;Z)|(X;Z_X),(Y;Z_Y)) = g\left[\frac{Z - \lambda Z_0}{(1-\lambda)} - (\mu Z_Y + (1-\mu)Z_X)\right]$$

where Z_0 is the equilibrium group mean, λ the parameter "G" of Cavalli-Sforza and Feldman (1973b), g the density function of the random variations, which may be dependent on the sex of the child, and μ and $(1-\mu)$ are the male and female parental contributions, denoted by P_1, P_2 by Cavalli-Sforza and Feldman. The equilibrium means and variances derived by Cavalli-Sforza and Feldman (1973b) may be used to assign probabilities for the original members of the pedigree. If the density functions g are Normal, the equilibrium distribution will also be Normal.

The transmission functions of the selection model of Feldman and Cavalli-Sforza (1976) are readily specified, but a problem arises as the selection component is confounded with the pedigree structure. Family size and age at death provide information about selection. If the ages at death are available and the type of selection is viability, we may incorporate the effect of selection into penetrance functions and pedigree structure; that is, the size of each nuclear family conveys no further information. Feldman and Cavalli-Sforza (1976) give transmission probabilities in their Table 1. In some simple cases, equilibria may be derived and may be used for original ancestors.

4.2. Penetrance Functions

The penetrance function expresses the conditional probability of a phenotypic component, given the corresponding genotypic component, i.e.,

$$\text{PEN}((\cdot;Z)|(\cdot;G)) = \text{PROB} \{Z|G\}$$

In many cases there will be a single genetic component, so that Z will be the phenotype, and G the genotype. In other cases we may have both multiple genotypic and phenotypic components, and the PEN function will accordingly be multivariate. In some models, separate PEN functions may be determined for individual genotype–phenotype component pairs, and the total phenotype may then be determined as a simple function of these phenotypic components.

Environmental and age effects may also be incorporated. We list a variety of important models:

(i) One Locus, Two Alleles (A_1, A_2), Two Phenotypes. Suppose we label the phenotypes 1 and 2. We have

$$\text{PEN}(1|G) = 1 - \text{PEN}(2|G)$$

Table 2 gives the penetrance functions for a number of simple models.

(ii) Generalized Major-Gene Model. In this model we again postulate a major gene with two alleles; however, the expression of the genotype as a phenotype is by way of a distribution. Thus we define

$$\text{PEN}(Z|G) = f_G(Z)$$

which is a density function. A variety of special cases have been treated which assume that $f_G(Z)$ are normal densities. In particular, Elston, Namboodiri, Glueck, Fallat, Tsang, and Leuba (1975) have taken the $f_G(Z)$'s to be normals with the same variances but with different means. Kravitz and co-workers

Table 2. Penetrance Functions for Some Simple Single-Locus Models

Genetic model	PEN(1|G)		
	A_1A_2	A_1A_2	A_2A_2
Recessive	1	0	0
Dominant	1	1	0
Partially penetrant dominant	α	α	0
Partially penetrant recessive	α	0	0
Partially penetrant heterozygote	1	α	0
General	α	β	α

(Kravitz, Skolnick, Edwards, Cartwright, Cannings, Amos, Carmelli, and Baty, 1978; Kravitz, Skolnick, Cannings, Carmelli, Baty, Amos, Johnson, Mendell, Edwards, and Cartwright, 1979) have considered a model with arbitrary means and variances.

(iii) Age-, sex-, and time-dependent effects. Many quantitative traits, such as the levels of lipids and proteins, are dependent on age and sex. Other traits, such as pyloric stenosis and stuttering, show different rates in males and females. These differences are thought to be caused by differential penetrance in the sexes (Kidd and Spence, 1976; Kidd and Records, 1979). It is important that models of this kind be formulated so that we can compare these alternative modes of inheritance.

Further complications in penetrance can be introduced by cyclic variation. Some protein levels vary with the time of day, the degree of activity, or by the foods and drinks that have been consumed. Others, especially estrogens and the other hormones related to ovulation, vary according to the phase of the menstrual cycle. Penetrance functions that incorporate these effects need to be constructed for a thorough analysis of these variables.

One method of correcting for age-specific penetrance is by performing a regression on age. Another approach would be to incorporate age into a penetrance function, permitting one to make the age correction dependent on genotype and also to analyze the age correction simultaneously with the other parameters of the model. The way in which this would be done would depend on the exact way in which the age effects occurred.

In certain cases we may wish to introduce a specific stochastic process for penetrance with age; the parameter of that model would have some meaningful biological interpretation. One such model is the multi-hit model (Knudson, 1973) where it is assumed that each "hit" occurs as a Poisson process, and the disease has its onset when some specific collection of n hits has occurred. These hits may be envisioned as chance somatic mutations or recombinations. Then $P(t) = \Pi_{i=1}^{n}(1 - e^{-\lambda_i t})$, where λ_i are the Poisson rates for the independent hits, and $P(t)$ is the probability an individual has the disease at age t. Both n and the λ_i may be genotype specific. Another example is the steady-state-rate process (Johnson, Eyring, and Stover, 1974), suggested as a model for the process of aging and reflecting both biological and environmental factors.

(iv) Threshold Models. Liability thresholds (Falconer, 1965) can be included in pedigree analysis as penetrance functions. In some instances, one cannot measure a quantitative trait, but must analyze data on a discrete phenotype. For example, one might have a pedigree with cholesterol values on living members, but a dichotomized cause of death on deceased members. A threshold must be incorporated into the model in order to analyze jointly the cause of death and cholesterol data. Several thresholds, such as age-dependent thresholds, can also be incorporated.

4.3. Population Frequencies for Individuals

In the peeling procedure, it is necessary to assign appropriate genotypic probabilities to the original ancestors in the pedigree. It will often be both convenient and economic to assume Hardy–Weinberg proportions, at least during preliminary analysis. One can then either assume some specific set of gene frequencies or estimate these jointly with the other parameters of the model. On the other hand, it will often be desirable to relax the assumption of Hardy–Weinberg values and to accomodate more realistic assumptions.

If Hardy–Weinberg values are not taken, then one may allow complete freedom for the genotype frequencies or introduce some model of population structure which generates the genotype frequencies as a function of a few parameters. It is necessary to adopt this latter approach in complex models for there will be too many genotypes, although the former approach is clearly possible in one-locus, two-allele models, for example.

Supposing then that some model is assumed which may either specify these genotypes as a function of some parameters directly, or it may do so through the equilibrium properties of some population process. It is important to ensure that the population process being used does not invalidate the peeling procedure adopted. For example, a selection model may be assumed. Selection is a process which may affect not only the prior original genotype probabilities, but also the relative chances that an individual has offspring, and hence the form of the pedigree. With regard to the former aspect, we must again derive the equilibrium genotype probabilities as functions of the parameters of the assumed selection model. Although the pedigree structure is taken as given, the latter factor may be taken into account through age at death or, if this is not known, through the distribution of offspring and the conditioning which it imposes on age at death. Where the selection mechanism operates through mortality, age at death is an important part of the phenotype and enters into the penetrance functions of the peeling procedure.

So far, the question of genotypic probabilities has been discussed with reference to characteristics determined by a finite number of loci, but the same applies to a polygenic trait or to the polygenic component of a trait for which a mixed model is assumed. Again, the equilibrium densities of the metric trait must be determined in terms of the transmission parameters. (In the Normal case these will be the equilibrium mean and variance.) Once this is done, the unknown parameters may be incorporated into the peeling procedure and estimated by likelihood analysis of the pedigree.

For example, using the model discussed in Section 4.1.2, suppose ζ_f has mean 0 and variance σ_f^2, ζ_m has 0 and σ_m^2, then it is easy to show that at equilibrium [assuming that $(X;P)$ and $(Y;P)$ are uncorrelated for mates] we have

$$\text{var}(P_f) = \frac{(1-\mu)^2 \sigma_f^2 + (1-\lambda)^2 \sigma_m^2}{(1-\mu^2)(1-\lambda^2) - (1-\lambda)^2 (1-\mu)^2}$$

with a similar expression for males (convergence to this value is assured since $\lambda, \mu \in [0, 1]$). The means are equal at equilibrium, the precise value depending on earlier conditions. Accordingly, if we estimate the means and variances of P_f and P_m from population data, we can fix σ_f^2 and σ_m^2 initially. If population data are not available, we shall need to add these parameters to those to be estimated. We shall, of course, need to assume a specific distribution when peeling. In particular, a Normal distribution for the variables ζ_f and ζ_m would lead to Normal distributions for P_f and P_m.

When $\lambda = \mu$, and $\sigma_m^2 = \sigma_f^2 = \sigma^2$ in the above equation, we have the classical result $\text{var}(P_m) = \text{var}(P_f) = 2\sigma^2$. Where the polygenic model is defined via the additive effects of a set of independent equally contributing loci, we note that this relation between the variances derives directly from the stationary assumption of the model (Fisher, 1918).

A different situation arises when founders are of diverse origin. This is true for the pedigree of Tristan da Cunha, which has very few original ancestors and is accurately known (Roberts, 1968). In analyzing the genetic data for this population, it is simplest to assign Hardy–Weinberg prior probabilities to the original founders and then estimate a single-founder allele frequency (Thompson, 1978). However, the founders are actually of diverse ethnic origin, and genotype probabilities incorporating some Wahlund variance would probably be more appropriate. For many loci there were probably more homozygotes amongst the founders than is suggested by a Hardy–Weinberg assumption on the basis of an overall allele frequency. Incorporating such a Wahlund factor increases the probability of current phenotypic data observed on the pedigree, although for no characteristic has the increase been "significant" in view of the extra degree of freedom.

Last, we must discuss the incorporation of linkage disequilibrium in models with linkage. For illustrative purposes, consider several loci: Supposing that an association has been found between the phenotypes determined by the individual loci, it is important to use this information in pedigree analysis. Possible causes of association are selection (with or without genetic linkage) or a transient phenomenon resulting from drift or population admixture, and perhaps maintained by linkage. In the cases of linkage and selection, and of transience involving linkage, the maintenance of an association is more likely if the linkage is tight. Thus association is suggestive of tight linkage. Further it is important to condition the initial genotype frequencies to reflect the association.

4.4. Assortative Mating

It has been pointed out by various investigators that the correlation between spouses is highly relevant to the interpretation of family data. Humans do not mate completely at random, and it is obvious that the choice of mates can affect the genetic structure of a pedigree. Nonrandomness in the pairing may result from external influences, such as geographic isolation and enforced marriage patterns, or from the internal preferences of individuals belonging to similar social groups (i.e., social homogamy) within the population. In genetic analysis, we are interested only in these effects on the phenotypic and genetic correlations.

It is assumed that mating occurs with respect to phenotype. Let the function $P(X, Y)$ denote the joint equilibrium density distribution of fertile matings of a female type X and a male type Y. Similarly, $P(X)$ and $P(Y)$ are the equilibrium density distributions in the population. In the following, various models are presented, and explicit expressions for $P(X, Y)/P(X) P(Y)$ are given; recall that this is the ASSORT function that enters the recursions for R functions.

(i) Monogenic Models. We consider one-locus diallelic traits producing three genotypes, AA, Aa, and aa. A two-phenotype model, where A is dominant to a, was considered by O'Donald (1960). A parameter α $(0 \leqslant \alpha \leqslant 1)$ denotes the fraction of dominant (or recessive) females preferring to mate with their own kind; thus $1 - \alpha$ is the fraction of A or aa females mating at random. The genotypic distribution at equilibrium is given by

$$P(AA) = u = p - \tfrac{1}{2}v$$

$$P(Aa) = v = -(1 - \alpha)p^2 + p\left[(1 - \alpha)^2 p^2 + 4(1 - \alpha)q\right]^{1/2}$$

and

$$P(aa) = w = q - \tfrac{1}{2}v$$

where p and q are the allele frequencies which remain unchanged with time. There are three phenotypic mating pairs: $\bar{A} \times \bar{A}$ (where $\bar{A}$ denotes the dominant phenotype), $\bar{A} \times aa$, and $aa \times aa$. For these, the equilibrium ASSORT function becomes

$$P(\bar{A}, \bar{A})/(P(\bar{A}))^2 = 1 + \alpha w/(u + v)$$

$$P(\bar{A}, aa)/P(\bar{A})P(aa) = 2(1 - \alpha)$$

and

$$P(aa, aa)/(P(aa))^2 = 1 + \alpha(u + v)/w$$

The two parameters of the model are α and p. Further, both parameters can sometimes be estimated from population data, and thus in some situations may be fixed in pedigree analysis. There are thus no more parameters here than in a model of arbitrary population–genotype frequencies with no assortative mating. For example, we may already know the parameters for this trait but be interested in its linkage to some other.

A similar model, with no dominance but with genotype-dependent preferences for homogamy, was considered by Karlin and Scudo (1969). Let the degrees of assortment for the three genotypes, AA, Aa, and aa, be described by α, β, and γ, respectively. Thus a fraction α of the aa female type mates with the same type, while the remaining fraction mates at random, β and γ being defined in a similar way.

In the symmetric case $\alpha = \gamma < \beta$, the interior equilibrium simplifies to

$$\hat{u} = \hat{w} = \frac{1}{2(2-\alpha)}, \qquad \hat{v} = \frac{1-\alpha}{2-\alpha} \qquad \text{with } p = q = \tfrac{1}{2}$$

Thus the equilibrium genotype distribution is independent of the parameter β. The equilibrium ASSORT function is given in Table 3. The parameters α, β of assortment, and the allele frequency p, determine the functions required for pedigree analysis.

Sewall Wright (1921) expressed the effect of nonrandom mating on the genotype frequencies in terms of a single parameter, which we denote by f:

$$P(AA) = u = p^2 + fpq$$

$$P(Aa) = v = 2pq(1-f)$$

$$P(aa) = q^2 + fpq$$

The parameter f is the correlation between uniting gametes, and for an additive trait is related to the parental correlation ρ by $f = \rho/(2-\rho)$ (Li, 1955: 131). For positive f we thus have an increased tendency for matings between like types. This form of population genotype frequencies may arise outside the context of assortative mating [for example, in deviations from Hardy–Weinberg amongst the founders of a pedigree, resulting from admixture (see Section 4.3)]. In the symmetric and nonselective mating schemes considered by Stark (1977), the parameter f will reflect the deviations from random mating due to assortment. The preference scheme is that proposed by Penrose (1933) and Stanton (1946), and the equilibrium ASSORT function is given in Table 3. With respect to likelihood calculations, the relevant parameters in this model are f (or ρ) and p.

(ii) Assortative Mating with a Major-Gene Model. Wagener (1976) analyzed a model in which assorting is on the basis of phenotype, that phenotype being determined by a single diallelic locus with each genotype specifying a distribution for its corresponding phenotype. The preference function is symmetric and proportional to the distance between the phenotypic values of the mates.

Table 3. Examples of Equilibrium Assortment Functions which can be Incorporated in Pedigree Analysis

Phenotype (genotype) pair	ASSORT function	
	Model of Karlin and Scudo (1969)	Model of Wright (1921). Stark (1977)
$AA \times AA$	$1 - \alpha + \dfrac{\alpha}{2(2 - \alpha)}$	$1 + \dfrac{f}{p^2(p + fq)^2} = 1 + \dfrac{f}{p(p + fq)^2}$
$AA \times Aa$	$2 - \alpha - \beta$	1
$AA \times aa$	$\dfrac{1 - \alpha}{2(2 - \alpha)^2}$	$1 - \dfrac{f}{(p + fa)(q + fp)}$
$Aa \times Aa$	$1 - \beta + \dfrac{\beta(1 - \alpha)}{2 - \alpha}$	1
$Aa \times aa$	$2 - \alpha - \beta$	1
$aa \times aa$	$1 - \alpha + \dfrac{\alpha}{2(2 - \alpha)}$	$1 + \dfrac{fp}{q(q + fp)^2}$

Iterative equations for the genotype frequencies are given, but no specific expressions for the equilibrium values are given for the general case. In a particular case, however, it will be possible to use these iterative equations (her Eq. 8) to produce the appropriate values.

(iii) Assortative Mating with a Polygenic Model. The above sections have considered the effect of assortative mating only for the case of a single locus. In this section, the relevant expressions appropriate for the polygenic model will be presented. Recently, there has been considerable controversy (Vetta and Smith, 1974; Bulmer, 1977; Vetta, 1977a, b) about the processes underlying the assortative mating models, but our concern here is only with equilibrium conditions so we do not need to concern ourselves with that controversy.

Suppose, following Fisher (1918) and Wilson (1973), we introduce assortative mating via a Normal preference function. Specifically, suppose that if the mating densities for males and females at maturity are $p(x)$ and $q(y)$, respectively, then the density of matings of type (x, y) is taken to be $r(x, y)$ where

$$r(x, y) = \frac{p(x)q(y)S(x, y)}{\int\int p(x)q(y)S(x, y)\,dx\,dy}$$

and where $S(x, y)$ is a bivariate Normal function [as defined by Wilson's Eq. (1.3)].

Under a polygenic mating scheme, i.e., by using a large number of contributing loci and assuming (i) that there is no genetic–environment interaction, (ii) that environmental deviations are Normal with means zero and independent over individuals, Wilson has derived the equilibrium distribution [her Eqs. (1.23) and (1.24)]. Equilibrium for Fisher's model is given by his Eqs. (XXV) and (XXVIa).

4.5. Linear Models

The essence of a linear model has been specified in Section 1. The phenotype of each individual is supposed to be determined by the sum of a variety of contributions, namely,

$$Z = A_1 + A_2 + \cdots + A_k + B_1 + B_2 + \cdots + B_l + E$$

where the A's are transmitted components, the B's are components that are common with some other set of individuals, and E is an environmental contribution specific to that particular individual. It is assumed that the complete set of B's and E's for all the individuals in the pedigree are mutually independent of each other and of the A's.

In this paper we shall use, for illustrative purposes, a model with a single B component, namely a common-sib environment (Figs. 4–6) and one with both a common-sib environment and an uncle–nephew common environment (Fig. 7). A variety of models of this type have been treated by, amongst others, Wright (1921), Morton (1974), Rao, Morton, and Yee (1974, 1976), and these all fall within the scope of the present method, although our treatment of assortative mating will be done through a preference function rather than through a linear component.

4.6. The Observation

In the model structure diagrams, we have separated the phenotype Z, as determined by genotype and environment, from the observation W of that phenotype. In practice, the phenotype may be comprised of several characteristics. Some of these may be of direct relevance in mating preferences, but in other cases the ASSORT function may express a correlation induced by mating dependence on some other character. Many phenotypes change with age; from the evolutionary point of view, the relevant phenotype is that at marriage which may have been influenced by common childhood environment. For unobserved individuals, this is the only relevant component. However, the phenotype we actually observe may be at any age and may have been influenced by environment subsequent to marriage. This influence may be genotype dependent.

Thus there may be several relevant phenotype values, even for a single trait in a single individual. In addition, for age-dependent traits, age at marriage may also be a relevant aspect of the phenotype. Any observation, if made, is an age-specific observation, and the function OBS ensures consistency with the age-specific phenotype of the individual:

$$\text{OBS}(Z; W) = \delta(Z - W) = \begin{cases} 1 & \text{if } Z = W \\ 0 & \text{otherwise} \end{cases}$$

The initial R function on the observation made is

$$R(\cdot; W) = \begin{cases} 1 & \text{if no observation is made} \\ 1 & \text{if observation } W \text{ is made} \\ 0 & \text{if any other observation is made} \end{cases}$$

For unmarried individuals, this current age-specific phenotype may be the only relevant component, and we shall be interested only in age-dependent penetrances with respect to the component. For other individuals, we shall require both the age of marriage and the current observation to be part of the phenotype. These will have some bivariate genotype-dependent distribution, given by genotype-specific, age-dependent penetrance functions.

5. Recursions

In this section we shall, via standard examples, demonstrate how the peeling recursions are derived from the model structure diagram. For ease of presentation, we shall present these models in the context of a pedigree without genealogical loops. (The model structure diagram of course has loops; see Section 3.) There is no difficulty in the extension to looped pedigrees; the same general formulas apply. However, formulas become cumbersome and for this reason will not be presented in detail. A simple example is discussed in Section 5.5.

As discussed by CTS, a zero-loop pedigree is most readily peeled by nuclear families. In most of the complex models in this paper, a nuclear family remains a sufficient unit for the representation of the model in a structure diagram. In such cases, at every stage except the final likelihood calculation, there will exist at least one nuclear family which is peripheral; that is, it is connected to the remainder of the pedigree by a *pivot* individual. The pivot may be an offspring who is a parent, offspring, or both, in other families. This peripheral family may then be analyzed and removed from the pedigree structure, the formation being expressed as a function on the attributes of the pivot. We introduce the notion of the upper and lower sections of an individual in a zero-loop pedigree, as defined by CTS. The upper section of an individual is the set of those individuals connected to him in the genealogy via his parents, including all his ancestors, all his ancestors' descendents who are not his own, and all individuals related to his ancestors' other spouses. The lower section consists of that part of the genealogy connected to him via his spouses, including all his descendents and all his spouses' relatives. An individual who has been used

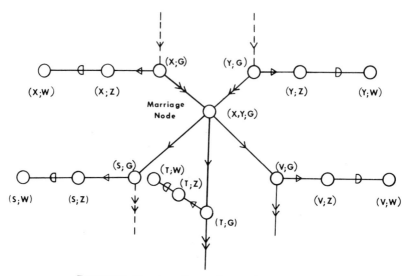

FIGURE 2. Structure diagram for a major-gene model.

as a pivot may have had his upper section peeled to him, or he may have that part of his lower section resulting from one or more of his spouses peeled to him. For a more rigorous presentation and a formal definition of the marriage node graph, the reader should consult CTS; for a less formal presentation of a similar methods, see Smith (1976).

We can simplify our presentation by including only simple penetrance functions. The complications of age-dependent penetrances, involving complex functions on the W–Z arc, and the retention of age and life-history information as part of the phenotype, will not be included. The function OBS is thus a δ-function (Section 5.3). However, the inclusion of complex effects, as discussed in Section 4, involves no theoretical difficulties.

5.1. Major Gene

Fig. 2 shows the diagram for a simple major-gene model for a single nuclear family that is assumed to be part of a zero-loop pedigree. This is effectively a marriage node graph (as defined by CTS), but we have added nodes here to represent the phenotype (Z) and a possible observation (W) for each individual, as described in Section 1, so that all components of the recurrence equations may be represented by a function, f, on an arc of the graph. As before, we shall denote previously derived R functions on attributes $\mathbf{A}$ of individuals $\mathbf{I}$ by $R(\mathbf{I}; \mathbf{A})$ and the R function resulting from the peeling recursion by $R'(\cdot; \cdot)$.

Using Fig. 2, we may apply Eq. (3.3) to derive the following recursions. Peeling an observation on any individual to the phenotype node of the same, we have

(i) $(\cdot;W) \rightarrow (\cdot;Z)$ ($\cdot$ denotes X, Y, S, T, or V)

(This notation denotes that for any specific individual we have input functions on observation W, and an output function on phenotype Z.) We thus have

$$R'(\cdot;Z) = \sum_W R(\cdot;W)R(\cdot;Z)\text{OBS}(Z;W)$$

where
$$R(\cdot;W) = \begin{cases} 1 & \text{if individual is not observed or observed to be } W \\ 0 & \text{otherwise} \end{cases}$$

In this case, all this operation does is to require consistency of observation and phenotype and will, in practice, usually be combined implicitly with the following operation. Now peeling phenotype to genotype, we have

(ii) $(\cdot;Z) \rightarrow (\cdot;G)$ ($\cdot$ denotes X, Y, S, T, or V)

$$R'(\cdot;G) = \sum_Z R(\cdot;G)R(\cdot;Z)\text{PEN}(Z|G)$$

incorporating the expression of phenotype. The genotype of any offspring may be peeled to the genotype combination of the parents, provided all other nodes connected to this offspring's genotype node have been previously peeled. We then have

(iii) $(\cdot;G) \rightarrow (X, Y;G)$ ($\cdot$ denotes S, T, or V)

$$R'(X, Y;G) = \sum_{(\cdot;G)} R(X, Y; G)R(\cdot;G)\text{TRANS}((\cdot;G)|(X,Y;G))$$

where TRANS is the segregation probability of the offspring genotype, conditional on the parental genotype combination. When all sections of the pedigree connected to Y via his parents have been peeled, the node $(Y;G)$ can be peeled to the genotype combination $(X, Y; G^*)$ by

(iv) $(Y;G) \rightarrow (X, Y; G^*)$

$$R'(X, Y;G^*) = R(X, Y; G^*)R(Y; G)$$

the function on this arc being 1. The effect of this recursion is to weight each term of any previously derived function on combination G^* by the term of the previously derived $R(Y; G)$ consistent with G^*, the "summation" being over this single term. If all offspring have been peeled, we may then reduce the information onto the final node $(X; G)$ of this nuclear family by

(v) $(X, Y; G^*) \rightarrow (X; G)$

$$R'(X;G) = \sum_{(X,Y;G^*)} R(X, Y; G^*)R(X;G)$$

again the arc function being 1. Alternatively, the nodes $(X; G)$ and $(Y; G)$ may both be peripheral, after peeling off the relevant Z and W, and both may be peeled to the node $(X, Y; G^*)$ by two applications of recursion (iv). In this case one offspring (e.g., V) may be connected to other nuclear families via his spouse and offspring, and we may complete the peeling of this nuclear family by peeling $(X, Y; G^*)$ to $(V; G)$ by the recurrence

(vi) $(X, Y; G^*) \rightarrow (V; G)$

$$R'(V; G) = \sum_{G^*} R(X, Y; G^*)R(V; G)\mathrm{TRANS}(V; G \mid X, Y; G^*)$$

where TRANS is as in operation (iii).

These six operations are directly analogous to the four of Cannings, Thompson, and Skolnick (1976). We have expanded them here, peeling only a single arc in each operation, in order to facilitate the extension to more complex models.

5.2. Major Gene with Assortative Mating

Next we extend this model to include assortative mating (Fig. 3). Because assortment is an operation on the joint parental phenotype, the phenotypes must be retained in a marriage node $(X, Y; G, Z)$, and arcs connecting the separate $(X; G)$, $(Y; G)$, $(X; Z)$, and $(Y; Z)$ to this node are required; the assortment arc operates on this central node. Despite this complication, we see from Fig. 3 that the genotype node of an individual remains a split-set and, hence, for a zero-loop pedigree, we may peel by nuclear families, retaining finally a function $R(\cdot; G)$ on the pivot member of the family; however, at intermediate stages, we shall require joint functions on phenotype Z and genotype G. For clarity we have introduced an additional node $(X, Y; G)$, eliminating the joint parental phenotype, since it is only through genotype that parents transmit to offspring.

We have operation (i) above for any individual. For an offspring whose marriage node has already been peeled, we have also

(ii') $(\cdot; Z) \rightarrow (\cdot; G)$

$$R'(\cdot; G) = \sum_{Z} R(\cdot; G)R(\cdot; G, Z)\mathrm{PEN}(Z \mid G)$$

where now previous R functions may sometimes be joint on both Z and G, since both enter into the offspring marriage node. However, this cannot be performed for parental individuals, since the nodes $(X; Z)$ and $(Y; Z)$ are connected both to a marriage node and a genotype node.

For any nonpivot offspring, we have then also operation (iii), and for non-pivot parent Y, we have a slight generalization of (iv):

(iv') $(X; G, Z) \rightarrow (X, Y; G, Z)$

$$R'(X, Y; G^*, Z^*) = R'(X, Y; G^*, Z^*)R(Y; G, Z)\text{PEN}(Z \,|\, G)$$

again the summation reducing to a single weighting factor, but the factor PEN now enters into the equation, since it is at this stage that this arc disappears.

For simplicity, we now separate the two cases of offspring pivot (e.g., V) and parent pivot X. In the latter case, all offspring may be peeled by operation (iii), and we have a function $R(X, Y; G)$ which may then be peeled to the marriage node, simply by incorporating parental phenotypes:

$$R'(X, Y; G, Z) = R(X, Y; G, Z)R(X, Y; G)$$

again simply weighting each item of our function on $(X, Y; G, Z)$ given by (iv'). Eliminating the assortment arc, we have also a weighting operation,

$$R'(X, Y; G, Z) = R(X, Y; G, Z)\text{ASSORT}(X, Y; Z)$$

Note that ASSORT is a function of the phenotypes of X and Y.

Then analogously to (v), we have

$$(\text{v}') \quad R'(X; G, Z) = \sum_{(X, Y; G, Z)} R(X, Y; G, Z)R(X; G, Z)$$

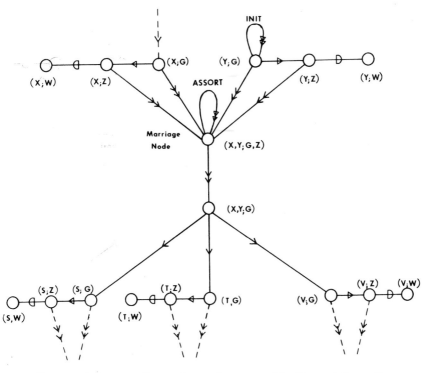

FIGURE 3. Structure diagram for a major-gene model with assortative mating.

and finally we eliminate the PEN arc by the equation (ii′) already defined above; which in this instance becomes $R'(X; G) = \Sigma_Z R(X; G, Z)R(X; G)\text{PEN}(Z \mid G)$. The previous R function $R(X; G)$ in this recursion will usually be 1, unless other sections of the pedigree have been previously peeled to X, via his parents. The derived function $R'(X; G)$ will be that required as input in peeling the nuclear family in which X is an offspring. In the event that X has several spouses, we shall derive a function $R(X; G, Z)$ via (v) resulting from all sections of the pedigree connected through these spouses, only finally eliminating the phenotype Z of X, since this is a relevant component in each of his marriages.

Where V is the pivot of the family, we reverse the above elimination of arcs. Since X is nonpivot, we have

$$(\text{iv}') \quad R'(X, Y; G, Z) = R(X, Y; G, Z)R(X; G, Z)\text{PEN}(Z \mid G)$$

and then, eliminating the ASSORT arc

$$R'(X, Y; G, Z) = R(X, Y; G, Z)\text{ASSORT}(X, Y; Z)$$

and reducing the random variable of the R function to genotypes alone,

$$R'(X, Y; G) = \sum_{(X, Y; Z)} R(X, Y; G, Z)R(X, Y; G)$$

where now $R(X, Y; G)$ will be the R function derived via (iii) from all nonpivot offspring. Finally we may apply (vi), as in the simple case, to obtain a function $R(V; G)$ which incorporates all information from the upper section of V.

5.3. Polygenic with Assortative Mating and Common-Sib Environment

We shall now extend our genetic model to include the linear effects of a common-sib environment. The phenotype is assumed to be continuous and is the sum of the polygenic genetic component (P), a common-sib component (C), and an environmental component (E) (Fig. 4). $Z = P + C + E$, and as described in Section 1, we use a rectangular node to denote this relationship. In this example we shall assume the single genetic component P to be subject to polygenic transmission only, although it could equally be a major gene. The mixed model is treated in Section 5.4. We shall again assume that Y is the male parent and X the female, and that genetic transmission is through linear combination:

$$A = \alpha P_Y + (1 - \alpha)P_X$$

where P_X, P_Y are the P values of X and Y (Section 4.1.2). For simplicity we assume α to be the same for both sons and daughters.

Because the derivation of recurrences by the elimination of single arcs becomes overly detailed with more complex models, we shall present them here as they would more normally be used in practice. Our previous examples have

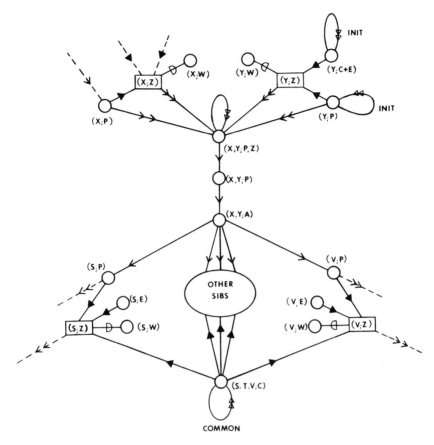

FIGURE 4. Model structure diagram for polygenic inheritance with assortative mating and common-sib environment.

introduced the method in sufficient detail so that several operations may now be combined without confusion. Since we are considering a continuous trait, with continuous underlying genetic transmission, we shall write our sums as integrals. Further, we note that the individual Y in Fig. 4 is represented as an original without sibs. Thus her polygenic value derives from the population distribution, calculated in the INIT function, while her common-sib environmental variance may be combined to a single variable $C + E$, with a distribution also determined by the population values.

Further, we restrict our attention to the case where all distributions are Normal, since in this case analytic recursions for the R functions are feasible (Section 5.7). Thus C is $N(0, \sigma_C^2)$ and E is $N(0, \sigma_E^2)$, this environmental density taking the place of PEN. For an offspring, P is $N(A, \sigma_P^2)$ where A is the weighted parental value as defined above. INIT(P) is normal with population mean P_0 and

and an equilibrium variance

$$\bar{\sigma}_P^2 = \sigma_P^2/2\alpha(1-\alpha)\rho$$

where ρ is the genotypic parental correlation, induced by assortative mating (Section 4.4). We see from the diagram that pairs of attributes (P, Z) form split-sets on which it will be convenient to define R functions, as also does the pair (A, C), which will enable us to peel each offspring in turn. For each non-pivot offspring we have the recursion

(i*)　　$(\cdot; P, Z) \to (X, Y; A, C)$　　　($\cdot$ denotes S, T, or V)

$R'(X, Y; A, C)$

$$= R(X, Y; A, C) \int \int R(\cdot; P, Z)\phi\left(\frac{P-A}{\sigma_P}\right) \phi\left(\frac{Z-P-C}{\sigma_E}\right) \{\delta_.(Z-W)\} dZ dP$$

where ϕ denotes the $N(0, 1)$ density and, for convenient notation, we view C as an attribute of pair (X, Y). This operation combines previous operations (i), (ii), and (iii). Operation (i) results in the term

$$\delta_.(Z - W) = \begin{cases} 1 & \text{if } Z = W, \text{ the observation on the offspring individual} \\ 0 & \text{otherwise} \end{cases}$$

Operation (ii) provided for the incorporation of PEN which is replaced by the $N(0, 1)$ density of $(Z-P-C)/\sigma_E$, while the TRANS of (iii) is replaced by the $N(0, 1)$ density of $(P-A)/\sigma_P$. For the first offspring peeled, the INIT function $R(X, Y; A, C) = 1$.

　　If all offspring are nonpivot, we may then eliminate the arc INIT(C) to give

(ii*)　　$(X, Y; A, C) \to (X, Y; A)$

$$R'(X, Y; A) = R(X, Y; A) \int \phi\left(\frac{C}{\sigma_C}\right) R(X, Y; A, C) dC$$

[The previous function $R(X, Y; A)$ will again be 1, but is included for completeness of the general theory.] And since $A = \alpha P_Y + (1-\alpha)P_X$, we may peel the central arcs to obtain

(iii*)　　$(X, Y; A) \to (X, Y; P, Z)$

$$R'(X, Y; P, Z) = R(X, Y; P, Z)R(X, Y; A = \alpha P_Y + (1-\alpha)P_X)$$

where the function $R(X, Y; P, Z)$ will again be 1, unless the parents have already been peeled to this central marriage node, and the second is our function derived in (ii*). Thus $P = (P_X, P_Y)$ is restricted to values for which $\alpha P_Y + (1-\alpha)P_X = A$.

　　Peeling Y to this same marriage node we have, recalling Y is an original,

(iv*)　　$(Y; W)$ and $(Y; Z) \to (X, Y; P, Z)$

$$R'(X, Y; P, Z) = R(X, Y; P, Z)\phi\left(\frac{P_Y - P_0}{\bar{\sigma}_P}\right)\phi\left[\frac{Z - P_Y}{(\sigma_E^2 + \sigma_C^2)^{1/2}}\right]\delta_Y(Z - W)$$

since $Z - P_Y = E + C$ is $N(0, \sigma_E^2 + \sigma_C^2)$ and P_Y is $N(P_0, \bar{\sigma}_P^2)$. Finally, we may peel the marriage node to pivot X, incorporating the observation on X and the assortment, obtaining

(v*) $(X; W) \to (X, Y; P, Z)$

$$R'(X; P, Z) = R(X; P, Z) \iint\limits_{(Y; P, Z)} \{\text{ASSORT}(X, Y; Z)R(X, Y; P, Z)\delta_X(Z - W)\}dPdZ$$

where the initial function $R(X; P, Z)$ will be 1 unless previous nuclear families have already been peeled to X.

If offspring V is the pivot, we derive the function $R(X, Y; A, C)$ using operation (i*) above, for all nonpivot offspring. The contribution to $R(X, Y; P, Z)$ from Y is also as above. The contribution from the now nonpivot (but also nonperipheral) parent X must incorporate any previous R function on $(X; P, Z)$ from other sections of the pedigree, and we have

$$R'(X, Y; P, Z) = R(X, Y; P, Z)R(X; P, Z)\delta_X(Z - W)$$

and, incorporating the ASSORT arc,

$$R'(X, Y; P, Z) = R(X, Y; P, Z)\text{ASSORT}(X, Y; Z)$$

Eliminating $Z = (Z_X, Z_Y)$, we have

$$R'(X, Y; P) = \iint\limits_{(X, Y; Z)} R(X, Y; P, Z)dZ_X dZ_Y$$

and transforming $P = (P_X, P_Y)$ to the single reproductive value, we have

$$R'(X, Y; A) = \iint\limits_{A = \alpha P_Y + (1 - \alpha)P_X} R(X, Y; P) \, dP_X dP_Y$$

(that is, effectively, a single, not a double, integral). This may be combined with our previous function, on $(X, Y; A, C)$:

$$R'(X, Y; A, C) = R(X, Y; A, C)R(X, Y; A) \qquad [(X, Y; A) \to (X, Y; A, C)]$$

Recall that C was regarded as an attribute of (X,Y) for notational convenience; more correctly it is an attribute of the sibs. Thus we now have a function defined on A and C that incorporates all information relevant to V and, moving from split-set $(X, Y; A)$ and $(S, T, V; C)$ to $(V; P)$ and $(S, T, V; C)$, and eliminating the single TRANS arc, we have

$$R'(V; P, C) = \int_A R(X, Y; A, C)\phi\left(\frac{P - A}{\sigma_P}\right)dA \qquad [(X, Y; A) \to (X, Y; A, C)]$$

the previous R function on $(V; P, C)$ being 1. Finally, eliminating C and incorporating any observation on V, we have

$$R'(V;P,Z) = R(V;P,Z) \int R(V;P,C) \phi\left(\frac{C}{\sigma_C}\right) \phi\left(\frac{Z-P-C}{\sigma_E}\right) \delta_V(Z-W) dC$$

$$[(V;P,C) \to (V;P,Z)]$$

This provides us with a function on attributes (P, Z) of V, incorporating all information in V's upper section, to be used as the initial R function for analysis of the nuclear family in which V is a parent.

In the case where the sex-specific parental contributions to sons and daughters differ, some modifications are necessary, e.g., in place of (i^*) above, we could substitute two operations, the first for peeling sons; the second for peeling daughters; (ii^*) would be replaced by

$$R'(X, Y; A_f, A_m) = R(X, Y; A_f, A_m) \int \phi\left(\frac{C}{\sigma_C}\right) R(X, Y; A_f, C) R(X, Y; A_m, C) dC$$

where A_f and A_m are the parental contributions to females and males.

5.4. General Mixed Model

We complete our examples of models with a discussion of the mixed model with assortative mating and common-sib environment; this diagram is shown in Fig. 5, and the recursions are analogous to those discussed in Section 5.3. However, we now present two complications: Even where all distributions are Normal, the nonlinearities of the major-gene contribution result in an R function which is no longer of Normal form. It is instead a mixture of Normals, the number of components being equal to the number of possible major-genotype combinations on the pedigree. It will thus normally be necessary to polychotomize. The second problem is that the polygenic and major-gene contributions contribute to Z in slightly different ways, and it is therefore necessary to partition these components into separate nodes.

We see from the diagram that the natural split-set of attributes for a single individual in a zero-loop pedigree is the triple (G, P, Z) of major-genotype, the polygenic value, and the phenotype. In peeling the successive offspring of a nuclear family, we shall use the triple (G^*, A, C), the major-genotype parental combination, the combined polygenic value of the pair, and the value of the common-sib component. Thus the peeling operations will be directly analagous to those of Section 5.3, except that peeling an offspring becomes conditional on $(X, Y; G)$ and, in eliminating no longer relevant major-gene components, we have summation in place of integration. We have

$$Z = M_G + P + C + E$$

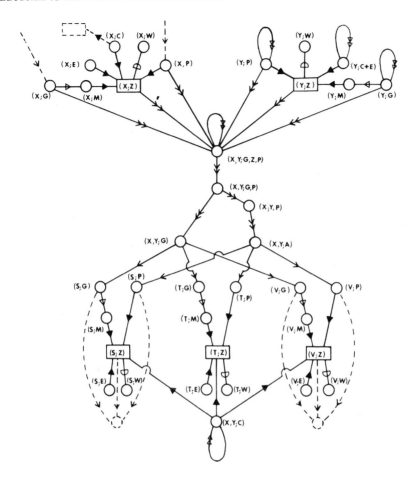

FIGURE 5. Mixed model with assortative mating and common-sib environment.

where P, C, and E are as before and M_G, the major-genotype contribution for genotype G, is $N(\mu_G, \sigma_G^2)$. Thus equation (i*) becomes

$$R'(X, Y; G^*, A, C) = R(X, Y; G^*, A, C)$$

$$\times \sum_G \int_M \int_Z \int_P \left\{ R(\cdot; G, P, Z)\phi\left(\frac{P-A}{\sigma_P}\right)\text{TRANS}(G \,|\, G^*)\delta\,(Z-W) \right.$$

$$\times \left. \phi\left(\frac{Z-P-C-M}{\sigma_E}\right) \phi\left(\frac{M-\mu_G}{\sigma_G}\right)\right\}dPdMdZ$$

where G^* is the parental major-genotype combination, G the offspring genotype, M the resulting offspring contributions, and the remaining variables as before.

Equations (ii*) and (iii*) are unchanged except by the inclusion of the parental genotype combination G^* in all R functions. Equation (iv*) becomes

$$R'(X, Y; G^*, P, Z) = R(X, Y; G, P, Z)\phi\left(\frac{P_Y - P_0}{2\sigma_P}\right)\phi\left[\frac{Z - P_Y - \mu_G}{(\sigma_E^2 + \sigma_C^2 + \sigma_G^2)^{1/2}}\right]\delta_Y(Z - W)$$

where now the phenotype Z for an original with polygenic value P_Y and genotype G is

$$N(P_Y + \mu_G, \sigma_E^2 + \sigma_C^2 + \sigma_G^2)$$

and (v*) becomes

$$R'(X; G, P, Z) = R(X; G, P, Z)\sum_{(Y; G, P, Z)}\iint\{\text{ASSORT}(X, Y; Z)R(X, Y; G, P, Z)\delta_X(Z - W)\}dPdZ$$

In the case of peeling down, the first five recursions require only the extra inclusion of the major genotypes in all R functions. (The major-gene *contribution* M to X will have already been incorporated at a previous stage.)

The sixth equation becomes

$$R'(V; G, P, C) = \sum_{G^*}\int_A R(X, Y; G^*, A, C)\text{TRANS}(G \mid G^*)\phi\left(\frac{P - A}{\sigma_P}\right)dA$$

and the final one, incorporating the major-gene contributing to V (see above comment regarding X), becomes

$$R'(V; G, P, Z) = R(V; G, P, Z)\int_C R(V; G, P, C)\phi\left(\frac{C}{\sigma_C}\right)\delta_V(Z - W)\phi\left[\frac{Z - P - C - \mu_G}{(\sigma_E^2 + \sigma_G^2)^{1/2}}\right]dC$$

since $Z - P - C = M + E$ is $N(\mu_G, \sigma_E^2 + \sigma_G^2)$ for a given genotype G.

5.5. Looped Pedigrees

The peeling recursions have been presented for the peeling of nuclear families as in a zero-loop pedigree. Each family has been assumed to have a pivot, all other members being peripheral at the current peeling stage. However, precisely the same formulation holds for looped pedigrees, except that R functions must now be held jointly on the attributes of several individuals. This set of attribute nodes must constitute a pedigree split-set. The simplest looped pedigree, a sib mating, is presented in Fig. 6 for the polygenic model with assortative mating and common-sib environment. R functions must now be held jointly on the set $(S, V; P, Z)$, the genotype and phenotype of the pair of sibs S and V. However, the recursions are essentially unaltered, all resulting, as before, from repeated application of Eq. (3.3). Since the offspring J of S and V has no sibs, the variables C and E may be combined to a single "$C + E$" variable which gives an $N(0, \sigma_C^2 + \sigma_E^2)$ contribution to the phenotype Z. For

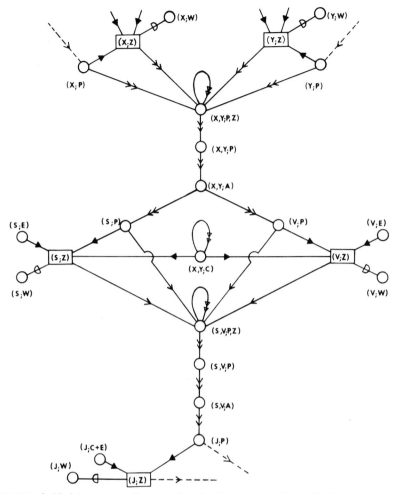

FIGURE 6. Model structure diagram of a sib–sib marriage (S and V) for the polygenic model with assortative mating and with a common-sib environment.

peeling upwards to X, a suitable sequence of recursions would thus be

(1) $(J; W)$ and $(J; C + E) \rightarrow (J; Z, P)$

(2) $(J; Z, P) \rightarrow (J; P)$

(3) $(J; P) \rightarrow (S, V; P, Z)$ [via intervening nodes]

(4) $\begin{cases} (V; W) \text{ and } (V; E) \rightarrow (V; P, Z) \\ (S; W) \text{ and } (S; E) \rightarrow (S; P, Z) \end{cases}$

(5) $(S, V; P, Z) \rightarrow (X, Y; A, C)$ [incorporating also last two derived functions]

(6) $(X, Y; A, C) \rightarrow (X, Y; P, Z)$

(7) $\begin{cases} (Y; P, Z) \rightarrow (X, Y; P, Z) \\ (X, Y; P, Z) \rightarrow (X; P, Z) \end{cases}$ [incorporating ASSORT]

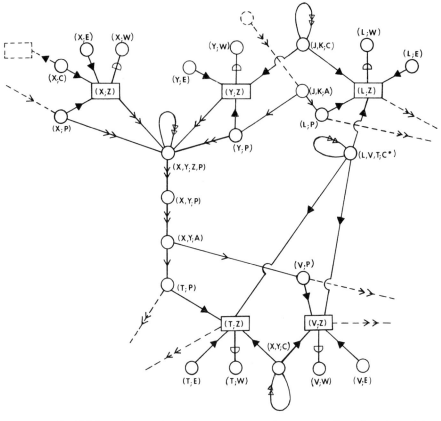

FIGURE 7. Addition of an uncle–nephew common environment to the polygenic model with assortative mating and with a common-sib environment.

Looped pedigrees are discussed more fully in CTS and Thompson (1977). The principles underlying the derivation of peeling sequences are the same as previously discussed. Given the sequence, the explicit recursions are similar to those for zero-loop pedigrees.

5.6. An Uncle–Nephew Common Environment

An example that illustrates a situation for which our R function must involve individuals who are not all in the same nuclear family is shown in Fig. 7. Here we have added to the model of Section 5.3 an extra linear component, namely, a common uncle–nephew environmental contribution C^* that is assumed to be Normally distributed with mean 0 and variance σ^2. L is the sib of Y, having parents J and K; X and Y are the parents of T, and V the nephews of L.

Appropriate recursions for peeling upwards (finally to J and K) are listed below:

(i) $(\cdot; P, Z) \rightarrow (X, Y; A, C) \cup (L; C^*)$ ($\cdot$ denotes T or V)

$$R'((X, Y; A, C) \cup (L; C^*)) = R((X, Y; A, C) \cup (L; C^*)) \int \int R(\cdot; P, Z)$$

$$\phi\left(\frac{P - A}{\sigma_P}\right) \phi\left(\frac{Z - P - C - C^*}{\sigma_E}\right) \delta.(Z - W) dPdE$$

since now for V or T, $Z - P - C - C^* = E$ is $N(0, \sigma_E^2)$.

(ii) $(X, Y; A, C) \cup (L; C^*) \rightarrow (X, Y; A) \cup (L; C^*)$

$$R'((X, Y; A) \cup (L; C^*)) = R((X, Y; A) \cup (L; C^*))$$

$$\int R((X, Y; A, C) \cup (L; C^*)) \phi\left(\frac{C}{\sigma_C}\right) dC$$

(iii) $(X, Y; A) \cup (L; C^*) \rightarrow (X, Y; A) \cup (J, K; A, C)$

$$R'((X, Y; A) \cup (J, K; A, C)) = R((X, Y; A) \cup (J, K; A, C)) R(L; P, Z)$$

$$\int \int \int R((X, Y; A) \cup (L; C^*)) \phi\left(\frac{P - A}{\sigma_P}\right) \phi\left(\frac{C^*}{\sigma_C}\right) \phi\left(\frac{Z - P - C - C^*}{\sigma_E}\right)$$

$$\delta_L (Z - W) dP dC^* dE$$

It should be noted here that one cannot peel $(X, Y; A) \cup (L, C^*)$ to $(X, Y; A) \cup (L; Z - C^*)$, that is, just integrating out the uncle–nephew common environment. If this were done (that is, if C^* were removed), the expression in the rectangular box becomes $(L; Z - C^*)$, and one cannot then peel $(L; W)$ onto that node, because the arc function is $\mathrm{OBS}(W, Z)$, and Z is no longer defined at the "box." In general, as discussed in Section 1, one cannot remove any linear component until the Z value has been used for all other arcs incident to the "box."

We have then

(iv) $(X, Y; A) \cup (J, K; A, C) \rightarrow (X, Y; P, Z) \cup (J, K; A, C)$

$$R'((X, Y; P, Z) \cup (J, K; A, C)) = R((X, Y; P, Z) \cup (J, K; A, C))$$

$$R(X, Y; A = \alpha(Y; P) + (1 - \alpha)(X; P))$$

(v) $(X, Y; P, Z) \cup (J, K; A, C) \rightarrow (Y; P, Z) \cup (J, K; A, C)$

$$R'((Y; P, Z) \cup (J, K; A, C)) = R((Y; P, Z) \cup (J, K; A, C)) \int \int \mathrm{ASSORT}(X, Y; Z)$$

$$R((X, Y; P, Z) \cup (J, K; A, C)) \mathrm{INIT}(X; P, Z) \delta_X (Z - W) dP dZ$$

(vi) $(Y; P, Z) \cup (J, K; A, C) \to (J, K; A, C)$

$$R'((J, K; A, C)) = R((J, K; A, C)) \int \int R((Y; P, Z) \cup (J, K; A, C))$$

$$\phi \left(\frac{P - A}{\sigma_P} \right) \phi \left(\frac{Z - P - C}{\sigma_E} \right) \delta_Y (Z - W) \, dP dE$$

We may on the other hand wish to work down to either of T or V, or possibly across onto L. Similar recursions apply, and in each case our final function will be on $(\cdot; P, Z)$ where "$\cdot$" denotes the final individual. As before, the key intervening split-sets will be, in some order, $(X, Y; Z, P)$, $(X, Y; A)$; $(J, K; A, C)$, $(X, Y; A, C)$; $(J, K; A, C)$, $(L, T, V; C^*)$; and $(J, K; A, C)$.

5.7. Analytic Recursions

Our derivation of recursions for R functions has not indicated how these are to be implemented. Where the attributes indexing the functions are discrete, there is no problem, since we have always functions over a finite set of discrete combinations of these attributes. For the major-gene model of Section 5.1, for example, only R functions over genotypes are required. A continuous phenotype creates no problem in this case. However, in models incorporating the direct transmission of a phenotype, or in some cases of assortative mating, as well as in the more complex cases of polygenic transmission and common environmental components, an R function over a continuous variable may be required.

One way to circumvent the problem is by polychotomizing the continuous attributes (Lalouel, 1978). However, this is an approximation and may also result in rounding errors in the computation of functions on extensive pedigrees if too many classes are allowed in the polychotomy. A compromise must be found between the large number required for accurate representation of the functions and the limitations imposed by storage space and computational accuracy.

In some cases an alternative procedure is available. Where all genetic and environmental components of the phenotype have Normal distributions, and where transmission of these components is also Normal, the R function will be of a multivariate Normal form. Thus we may replace our recursions, by exact analytic recursions for the means, variances, and covariances. This fact was noted by Elston and Stewart (1971) for the simple case of upwards peeling of a polygenic component, but the principle applies far more generally. It applies to peeling in any direction and onto any number of individuals. The only difference is that in peeling in different directions, our functions are sometimes probabilities that include the distribution of the variables which are attributes of the likelihood, and sometimes "likelihoods" conditional upon them. R functions do not necessarily integrate to 1, and we require additional recursions for a parameter-dependent multiplying factor. Analytic recursions are also applicable to a far wider class of models. In particular, they may be used in the polygenic model with a common-sib environment and assortative mating of Section 5.3, provided the function, $ASSORT(Z_X, Z_Y)$, is also of the form $\exp\{-\frac{1}{2}Q(Z_X, Z_Y)\}$, where Q is a quadratic form. They may be applied to the same model in a looped pedigree (Section 5.5), or to a model with Normally distributed environmental contributions, common to more distant relatives (Section 5.6). The explicit forms of the recursions for the model of Section 5.3 have been derived; these, and others, will be presented elsewhere.

6. Practical Aspects and Miscellaneous Problems

6.1. Optimization of Algorithms

For the computation of likelihoods of increasingly complex models on increasingly complex pedigrees to remain feasible, greater computational efficiency is required. Several aspects of the problem of optimizing the algorithms must be considered. The first, already discussed to some extent by CTS (1978), is in the derivation of optimal peeling sequences. In constructing any sequence, there is a tradeoff between optimizing use of processor time and memory requirements. In the analysis of complex pedigrees, the major factors are the size of the maximal split-set on which an R function must be stored and the maximal number of individuals that can be involved in any peeling operation, the latter being the major determinant of "time" and the former of memory required. This problem has been discussed further by Thompson, Cannings, and Skolnick (1978a) with reference to the complex genealogy of the Tristan da Cunha population; a program that determines locally optimal sequences in accordance with the criteria just cited is in operation, but a global optimum is not guaranteed.

Even for a zero-loop pedigree, the problem of optimal peeling sequences becomes important when complex models are involved. A program for determining a peeling sequence for the zero-loop branches of any pedigree has been developed, and an algorithm that produces a peeling sequence, minimizing the maximum number of R functions to be stored at any one time, has also been programmed. However, the peeling sequence does not determine the complete sequence of operations, and optimal procedures within each peeling operation should also be applied. For example, where limitations on memory are the major restricting factor and where very large numbers of genotypes are involved, it may be more efficient to complete the operation separately for each pivotal parent genotype than to consider all parental combinations jointly.

With the additional model complexities introduced in this paper, an extra dimension is added to the peeling sequence. A split-set is no longer defined by a set of individuals, but by the set of attributes of those individuals on which the

R function is held. We have developed the polygenic and mixed model with R functions defined jointly on the genetic components [P (and G)] and phenotype (Z), with an intermediate function on the common-sib–environmental component (C), and the parental–polygenic contribution (A) being used in peeling each offspring. However, subject to the restriction previously discussed (Sections 1 and 5.6) in peeling contributions to a phenotype which is the sum of such contributions, any sequence of nodes constituting a split-set can be used as the attribute set of an R function. Although in the case of a standard model, such as that of Section 5.3, the optimal form of the recursions is clear; however, in Section 5.6, it is no longer so, and optimization with respect to this aspect is required also. Such optimization complicates the presentation of a single form for the analytic recursions discussed in Section 5.7.

Another situation where efficient procedures are essential is in the maximization of likelihood with regard to specific parameters. Although general maximization routines may be applicable, our likelihood functions have special features which may permit more problem-specific procedures to be used. An important example is in the computation of derivatives of the parameters of a model.

Our basic recursion equation of Section 3 is

$$R'(\mathbf{I}^*; \mathbf{A}^*) = \sum_{(\mathbf{I}; \mathbf{A}) - (\mathbf{I}^*; \mathbf{A}^*)} \{R(\mathbf{I}; \mathbf{A})R(\mathbf{I}^*; \mathbf{A}^*)f((\mathbf{I}; \mathbf{A}), (\mathbf{I}^*; \mathbf{A}^*))\}$$

and parameter values enter the R functions via the function f. Differentiating the recursion equation with respect to any parameter ν we have

$$\begin{aligned}
\frac{\partial R'}{\partial \nu}(\mathbf{I}^*; \mathbf{A}^*) = \sum_{(\mathbf{I}; \mathbf{A}) - (\mathbf{I}^*; \mathbf{A}^*)} \Bigg\{ &\frac{\partial}{\partial \nu}(\mathbf{I}; \mathbf{A})R(\mathbf{I}^*; \mathbf{A}^*)f((\mathbf{I}; \mathbf{A}), (\mathbf{I}^*; \mathbf{A}^*)) \\
&+ R(\mathbf{I}; \mathbf{A})\frac{\partial}{\partial \nu}R(\mathbf{I}^*; \mathbf{A}^*)f((\mathbf{I}; \mathbf{A}), (\mathbf{I}^*; \mathbf{A}^*)) \\
&+ R(\mathbf{I}; \mathbf{A})R(\mathbf{I}^*; \mathbf{A}^*)\frac{\partial f}{\partial \nu}((\mathbf{I}; \mathbf{A}), (\mathbf{I}^*; \mathbf{A}^*)) \Bigg\}
\end{aligned}$$

Of course not all the components of the recursion will necessarily be functions of ν. The function on the previous split-set, $R(\mathbf{I}; \mathbf{A})$, will normally be so, except in peeling peripheral nodes or in peeling sections of the pedigree not including arcs involving the particular parameter. The previous R function on $(\mathbf{I}^*; \mathbf{A}^*)$ is often 1 and, hence, does not involve ν, but may otherwise do so. The function f may or may not depend on ν, depending on the type of arc to which ν relates. Parameters of the penetrance function will enter only on PEN arcs; those of transmission (e.g., recombination fractions) on TRANS arcs. Parameters of assortment enter via the ASSORT arc, but an INIT arc function may also depend on parameters of ASSORT or TRANS. Allele frequencies are parameters of an INIT arc function, but may also enter on ASSORT arc functions.

The above equation is a recursion for the derivative of the R function with respect to ν. Provided that at every stage both the value of the R function and its derivative are computed and stored, we may evaluate simultaneously the overall value of the R function and the derivative on the whole pedigree. Derivatives for several parameters may be handled simultaneously; all may be evaluated with a single sequence of peeling recursions. Exact values of first-order derivatives may greatly accelerate the maximization procedures. Differentiating the recursion again, with respect to the same or a different parameter, we see that joint and second-order derivatives are also theoretically feasible. We must simply compute and store, in addition, the joint and second-order derivatives at each stage in the peeling process. In practice, memory limitations will limit feasibility, but second-order derivatives at the maximum and, hence, variance estimates for estimators are certainly possible. Second-order derivatives with regard to particular parameters of interest may also be feasible in the course of the maximization procedure, and further speed that maximization.

6.2. Pedigree Structure and Sampling Procedures

In addition to optimality in the algorithms for the computation and maximization of likelihoods, we also require statistical efficiency. Different pedigree structures will have different levels of power to distinguish alternative modes of inheritance and different levels of information with regard to the estimation of different parameters (Thompson, Kravitz, Hill, and Skolnick, 1978). In addition to the structure of the pedigree, some phenotypic distributions will be far more informative than others. Pedigrees with a substantial number of affected individuals must provide more information about the inheritance of the disease than one which, perhaps simply because there are fewer relatives, contains very few affected individuals. However, concentration on pedigrees of "interest" creates ascertainment problems. In comparing alternative modes of inheritance, one should make the ascertainment correction appropriate to the sampling criteria which determined the selection of pedigrees for analysis. Although solutions in the context of an infinite population can be provided, given that the phenotypic event provoking analysis of the pedigree is known (Thompson and Cannings, 1979), the general problem of ascertainment corrections in pedigrees is complex and requires knowledge of the demographic structure of the population from which the pedigrees are taken (Cannings and Thompson, in preparation).

If pedigrees are studied by sequentially sampling members, the complexities of ascertainment bias are avoided and the efficiency of sampling is increased. Cannings and Thompson (1978) have shown that a sampling procedure dependent on phenotypic observations to date does not invalidate likelihood computations in that, within the context of a single pedigree, no further ascertainment correction is imposed by the sampling procedure. Even with a sibship, different sampling schemes may give substantially different amounts of information per individual sampled (Thompson, 1980), and on extensive pedigrees the effects may be large.

The question of the information content of a data set is also related to the alternative modes of inheritance to be compared in the analysis. However, even where (on a particular data set) complex models cannot be distinguished, the feasibility of computing likelihoods for such models is important. Only by comparing general models and by simulating the distribution of likelihood values given by such models on pedigrees can the statistical feasibility of model estimation be investigated. A general simulation package for use with pedigrees has been developed (Bishop and Cannings, 1979).

6.3. Comparison of Models Through Likelihood Analysis

A subject related to the distribution of likelihood values and the expected log-likelihood function is the question of comparing alternative models. Standard asymptotic likelihood theory predicts a chi-squared distribution for $-2 \log \Lambda$, where Λ is the likelihood ratio of a restricted model against a more general one. The degrees of freedom are the difference in dimensionality of the general and the restricted hypothesis; the noncentrality of the chi-squared is the minimum distance of the true hypothesis from the space of the restricted one in the metric of the information matrix. The above result holds, subject to a variety of regularity conditions on the joint distribution, when the data consist of independent observations and the location of the true parameter value is within an open set of full dimension with the parameter space of the unrestricted model (e.g., Berk, 1972). However, for the data of pedigree analysis a number of problems remain: (1) we do not have independent observations; (2) the models we wish to compare are often not submodels of each other and (3) the natural parameter space is restricted, with the possibility that true values may often be boundary points of the parameter space.

The first problem may be avoided if a sufficient number of disjoint pedigrees are available for analysis, for then each may be regarded as an independent observation, albeit not identically distributed since the pedigrees will usually be of different structures. The asymptotic distribution of maximum-likelihood estimates on a single large pedigree remains to be fully investigated. The second problem may be circumvented by comparing each model of interest to a general model which comprises them all (Elston and Stewart, 1971; Morton and MacLean, 1974). However, the composite model may have no genetic reality, and computation of its likelihood may not always be feasible. Moreover this approach does not enable direct comparisons of submodels to be made because the difference of the nonindependent chi-squareds is not chi-squared. The third problem is also relevant as many reasonable genetic models will have parameter values on the boundary of the composite space. In addition to the problem of the comparison of models, there may also be difficulty in determining the goodness of "fit." An approach has been given by Elston, Namboodiri, and Kaplan (1978), but the properties of their proposed statistics remain to be investigated.

Thus, in the absence of an appropriate theory or of extensive empirical studies, likelihood analysis should be regarded as an investigative tool in the construction and comparison of models. We are interested in more than the relative values of the likelihoods of different classes of models, at their respective maxima; additional information may be obtained from the shape of the likelihood surfaces with respect to the different classes of parameters. Many likelihood surfaces will have several local maxima (Kravitz *et al.*, 1978, 1979; Anderson, Bonné-Tamir, Carmelli, and Thompson, 1979), and the implication of this for inferences must be considered.

The absolute values of likelihoods computed on pedigrees are often very small, but this need not affect the strength of our conclusions. Inferences are based on relative values and the form of the surface. While models involving large numbers of polychotomized genotypes, or penetrance functions varying by many orders of magnitude over the range of normal variability, may result in additional computational complexities, there is no reason to suppose likelihood values are distorted by rounding error. Because smooth likelihood surfaces are obtained, and equal likelihood values given by very different peeling sequences (Thompson, 1977), it is clear that rounding errors are not operative. In considering likelihoods on pedigrees, we must note that we have an ordered observation on a large number of individuals. Viewed in this light, the likelihoods are not small; indeed they can be shown to be of exactly the order of magnitude expected.

6.4. Miscellaneous Problems

(a) Twins. Incorporating twin studies into the analysis is within the scope of the present method. In a small pedigree it is probably appropriate to ignore the possibility that the predisposition to produce fraternal twins is itself hereditary. If sufficient data on genetic markers and phenotypic traits are available, the zygosity of the twins can often be resolved. Identical twins can then be treated as a single genetic entity, with possibly disparate phenotypes, fraternal twins as ordinary sibs, although in each case additional common environmental components might be added. If no additional data are available, then we shall have to use the appropriate population frequencies for twin zygosities, and these will enter the peeling recursions. If, however, there is more than one pair of twins in the pedigree, then some incorporation of a model for the inheritance of twinning might be used and analyzed simultaneously with the characters of interest. It is unlikely, except in unusual circumstances, that this will produce very different results from the case where this possible inheritance is ignored. Fig. 8 illustrates a model structure diagram for MZ twins, incorporating common

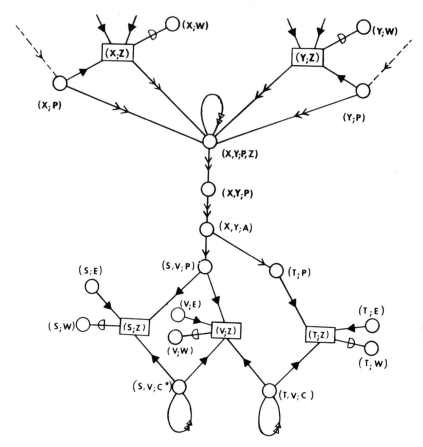

FIGURE 8. Model structure diagram for MZ twins (S, V) with common fetal environment. The twins are reared apart; one of the twins (V) shares common environment with his full sib (Z).

fetal environment, separate social environment, and common-sib environment between one twin and his full sib.

(b) Sequential Phenomena. We have assumed in all the models treated so far that the interdependence of the phenotypes of the sibs is caused by their common parentage or common environment, or both. Accordingly, the phenotypes of sibs were identically distributed and, given the parental genotypes and the common environmental contribution, independent. However, there are many other possible interactions between sibs which do not fall into this category. One of the commonest of these is that caused by parity. Variation in phenotypic expression with parity has been suggested for I.Q., for example, and due allowance for this possibility would need to be made in any analysis. We focus here, very briefly, on the type of phenomenon typified by Rh incompatability, in

which within certain matings the phenotype of the earlier offspring affect the survival of later ones. In this type of situation it is important to use as much information regarding mortalities as is available.

Suppose we consider a nuclear family where information about abortions, stillbirths, or other mortalities is available. Suppose further that there is not a simple phenotype–genotype correspondence, and that we must peel down from the parents to a specific offspring. It will then be necessary to proceed from the parents to the parents jointly with their first offspring (whether still alive or not), and from this group to the parents and the first two offspring and so on, until the whole family is involved in an R function. One can then peel the parents and the sibs to the one required. This process may, on occasion, be simplified if an adequate summary statistic can be found that can synthesize all the information regarding previous siblings; in some cases the total number of previous sibs of a certain phenotype may suffice; in others, the number of years since a particular phenotype was born will be sufficient. Some effort towards finding such a statistic would probably be necessary in such cases if a pedigree of any size is to be dealt with, as the number of individuals who can be jointly considered is limited in practice.

7. Summary

In this paper we have presented an algorithm for the calculation of likelihoods on a general set of genetic models. Our primary concern has been to demonstrate the very wide variety of models that can be analyzed within the framework of pedigree analysis. The computation of likelihoods for models that involve assortative mating, common environments, and linear components has been shown to be theoretically and computationally feasible. This feasibility, however, raises two classes of problem. The first is that the appropriate specification of models be consistent with population genetic theory. For this reason we have considered in detail a variety of models for transmission, penetrance, and assortative mating, with special emphasis on the effect of these factors on population equilibria. Second, we have considered the questions of optimization, of computational algorithms, and the statistical aspects of comparison of alternative models. These have been discussed briefly, and many questions in this area remain to be investigated.

Glossary of Notation

Individuals

X, Y	Parents of S, T and V
S, T, V	Offspring of X and Y
J, K, L	Others
$\mathbf{I}$	A set of individuals

Attributes

W	Observation
Z	Phenotype
P	Polygenic component
G	Major-genotype component
M	Major-genotype contribution to phenotype
C	Common-sib environment
C^*	Uncle–nephew common environment
E	Environment (individual)
$\mathbf{A}$	A set of attributes

Random Variables

$(\mathbf{I}; \mathbf{A})$	$\begin{cases} \text{All pairs of individuals in } \mathbf{I} \\ \text{and an attribute in } \mathbf{A} \end{cases}$
$(\mathbf{I}; \mathbf{A}) \cup (\mathbf{I}^*; \mathbf{A}^*)$	$\{$All random variables in $(\mathbf{I}; \mathbf{A})$ or in $(\mathbf{I}^*; \mathbf{A}^*)\}$

Population Parameters

p, q	Gene frequencies (diallelic locus)
q	(Gene) frequencies (with subscripts)
u, v, w	Genotype frequencies (diallelic locus)
Δ	Linkage disequilibrium
r	Recombination fraction
ϵ	Random noise
g	Density function of random noise
α, β, γ	Assortative mating parameters
χ	Assortative mating preference function
ϕ	Phenotypic density function
μ	Mean
σ^2	Variance
ρ	Parental correlation

Subscripts (other than defined above)

f	Female
m	Male

Functions

PROB, PEN, TRANS, OBS, INIT, ASSORT, SPLIT, JOIN, COND, LINCOMP (as defined in Table 1)

δ	Dirac delta-function

ACKNOWLEDGMENTS

We wish to thank Drs. Carmelli, Karlin, Elston, and Dadone for valuable comments and, in particular, Dr. Carmelli for discussion on Section 4.4.

References

Anderson, M. W., Bonné–Tamir, B., Carmelli, D., and Thompson, E. A. (1979), Linkage analysis and the inheritance of arches in a Habbanite isolate, *Am. J. Hum. Genet.* 31:620–629.

Berk, R. (1972), Consistency and asymptotic normality of MLE's for exponential families, *Ann. Math. Stat.* 43:193–204.

Binet, F. E., Sawyer, R. J., and Watson, G. S. (1958), Heredity counselling for sex-linked recessive deficiency diseases, *Ann. Hum. Genet. (London)* 22:144–152.

Bishop, D. T., and Cannings C. (1979), SIM: A simulation program for studying gene flow through a pedigree, Department of Medical Biophysics and Computing, University of Utah, Technical Report No. 11.

Boyle, C. R., and Elston, R. C. (1979), Multifactorial genetic models for quantitative traits in humans, *Biometrics* 35:55–68.

Bulmer, N. G. (1977), Assortative mating, *Nature* 266:195.

Cannings, C., and Thompson, E. A. (1978), Ascertainment in the sequential sampling of pedigrees, *Clin. Genet.* 12:208–212.

Cannings, C., Thompson, E. A., and Skolnick, M. H. (1976), The recursive derivation of likelihood on complex pedigrees, *Adv. Appl. Probab.* 8:622–625.

Cannings, C., Thompson, E. A., and Skolnick M. H. (1978), Probability functions on complex pedigrees, *Adv. Appl. Probab.* 10:26–61.

Cannings, C., Thompson, E. A., and Skolnick, M. (1979), Extension of pedigree analysis to include assortative mating and linear models, in *Genetic Analysis of Common Diseases: Applications to Predictive Factors in Coronary Disease* (C. F. Sing and M. Skolnick, eds.), Alan F. Liss, Inc., New York.

Cannings, C., Skolnick, M. H., de Nevers, K., and Sridharan, R. (1976), Calculation of risk factors and likelihoods for familial diseases, *Comp. Biomed. Res.* 9:393–407.

Cavalli-Sforza, L. L., and Feldman, M. W. (1973a), Cultural versus biological inheritance, *Am. J. Hum. Genet.* 25:618–637.

Cavalli-Sforza, L. L., and Feldman, M. (1973b), Models for cultural inheritance. I. Group mean and within group variation, *Theor. Popul. Biol.* 4:42–55.

Chakraborty, R., Shaw, M., and Schull, W. J. (1974), Exclusion of paternity: The current state of the art, *Am. J. Hum Genet.* 26:477–488.

Chase, G. A., Murphy, E. A., and Bolling, D. R. (1971), The ENSU scoring system. A strategy for solving a class of single-locus genetic counselling problems, *Clin. Genet.* 2:141–148.

Elston, R. C., and Stewart, J. (1971), A general model for the genetic analysis of pedigree data, *Hum. Hered.* 21:523–542.

Elston, R. C., and Yelverton, K. S. (1975), General models for segregation analysis, *Am. J. Hum. Genet.* 27:31–45.

Elston, R. C., Namboodiri, K. K., Glueck, C. J., Fallat, R., Tsang, R., and Leuba, V. (1975), Study of the genetic transmission of hypercholesterolemia and hypertriglyceridemia in a 195 member kindred, *Ann. Hum. Genet. (London)* 39:67–87.

Elston, R. C., and Rao, D. C. (1978), Statistical modeling and analysis in human genetics, *Ann. Rev. Biophys. Bioeng.* 7:253–286.

Elston, R. C., Namboodiri, K. K., and Kaplan, E. B. (1978), Resolution of major loci for quantitative traits, paper prepared for the Proceedings of the Conference on Genetic Epidemiology, Hawaii, October 1977, in *Genetic Epidemiology* (N. E. Morton and C. S. Chung, eds.), pp. 223–235, Academic Press, New York.

Falconer, D. S. (1965), The inheritance of liability to certain diseases, estimated from the incidence among relatives, *Ann. Hum. Genet.* 29:51–76.

Feldman, M. W., and Cavalli-Sforza, L. L. (1976), Cultural and biological evolutionary processes; selection for a trait under complex transmission, *Theor. Popul. Biol.* 9:238–259.

Fisher, R. A. (1918), The correlation between relatives on the supposition of Mendelian inheritance, *Trans. R. Soc. Edinburgh* 52:399–433.

Heuch, I., and Li, F. H. F. (1972), PEDIG – A computer program for calculation of genotype probabilities using phenotype information, *Clin. Genet.* 3:501–504.

Hilden, J. (1970), An algebraic approach to pedigree probability calculus, *Clin. Genet.* 1:319–348.

Johnson, F. H., Eyring, H., and Stover, B. J. (1974), *The Theory of Rate Processes in Biology and Medicine*, John Wiley, New York.

Karlin, S., and Scudo, F. M. (1969), Assortative mating based on phenotype – II. Two autosomal alleles without dominance, *Genetics* 63:499–510.

Karlin, S. (1979), Models of multifactorial inheritance. I. Formulation and basic convergence results, *Theor. Popul. Biol.* 15:308–355.

Kidd, K. K., and Records, M. A. (1979), Genetic methodologies for the study of speech, in *Neurogenetics: Genetic Approaches to the Nervous System* (X. O. Breakfield, ed.), Elsevier, New York.

Kidd, K. K., and Spence, M. A. (1976), Genetic analyses of pyloric stenosis suggesting a specific maternal effect, *J. Med. Genet.* 13:290–294.

Knudson, A. G. (1973), Mutation and human cancer, *Adv. Cancer Res.* 17:317–352.

Kravitz, K., Skolnick, M., Edwards, C., Cartwright, G., Cannings, C., Amos, B., Carmelli, D., and Baty, B. (1978), Pedigree analysis of the linkage between HLA and hemochromatosis, paper prepared for the Proceedings of the Conference on Genetic Epidemiology, Hawaii, October 1977, in *Genetic Epidemiology* (N. E. Morton and C. S. Chung, eds.), pp. 241–246, Academic Press, New York.

Kravitz, K., Skolnick, M., Cannings, C., Carmelli, D., Baty, B., Amos, B., Johnson, A., Mendell, N., Edwards, C., and Cartwright, G. (1979), Genetic linkage between hereditary hemochromatosis and HLA, *Am. J. Hum. Genet.* 31:601–619.

Lalouel, J.-M. (1978), Recurrence risks as an outcome of segregation analysis, in *Genetic Epidemiology* (N. E. Morton and C. S. Chung, eds.), Academic Press, New York.

Lange, M., and Elston, R. C. (1975), Extensions to pedigree analysis. I. Likelihood calculations for simple and complex pedigrees, *Hum. Hered.* 25:95–105.

Li, C. C. (1955), *Population Genetics*, University of Chicago Press, Chicago.

Morton, N. E. (1974), Analysis of family resemblance. I. Introduction, *Am. J. Hum. Genet.* 26:318–330.

Morton, N. E., and MacLean, C. F. (1974), Analysis of family resemblance. III. Complex segregation of quantitative traits, *Am. J. Hum. Genet.* 26:489–503.

Morton, N. E., and Rao, D. C. (1978), Quantitative inheritance in man, *Yearb. Phys. Anthropol.* 21:72–141.

Murphy, E. A. (1970), The ENSU scoring system in genetic counselling, *Ann. Hum. Genet.* 34:73–78.

O'Donald, P. (1960), Assortative mating in a population in which two alleles are segregating, *Heredity* 15:389–396.

Penrose, L. S. (1933), A study in the inheritance of intelligence, *Brit. J. Psychol.* 24:1–19.

Rao, D. C., Morton, N. E., and Yee, S. (1974), Analysis of family resemblance. II. A linear model for familial correlation, *Am. J. Hum. Genet.* 26:331–359.

Rao, D. C., Morton, N. E., and Yee, S. (1976), Resolution of cultural and biological inheritance by path analysis, *Am. J. Hum. Genet.* 28:228–242.

Roberts, D. G. (1968), Genetic effects of population size reduction, *Nature (London)* 220:1084–1088.

Smith, C. A. B. (1976), The use of matrices in calculating Mendelian probabilities, *Ann. Hum. Genet. (London)* 40:37–54.

Stanton, R. G. (1946), Filial and fraternal correlations in successive generations, *Ann. Eugen.* 13:18–24.

Stark, A. E. (1977), Comments on the Penrose–Stanton model of assortative mating, *Ann. Hum. Genet. (London)* 41:117–121.

Thompson, E. A. (1976a), Inference of genealogical structure, *Soc. Sci. Inform.* 15:477–526.

Thompson, E. A. (1976b), Peeling programs for zero-loop pedigree, Department of Medical Biophysics and Computing, University of Utah, Technical Report No. 5.

Thompson, E. A. (1977), Peeling programs for pedigrees of arbitrary complexity, Department of Medical Biophysics and Computing, University of Utah, Technical Report No. 6.

Thompson, E. A. (1978), Ancestral inference. II: The founders of Tristan da Cunha, *Ann. Hum. Genet. (London)* 42:239–253.

Thompson, E. A. (1980), Sequential sampling schemes for sibships, *Adv. Appl. Probab.*, in press.

Thompson, E. A., and Skolnick, M. H. (1977), Likelihoods on complex pedigrees for quantitative traits, Proceedings of the International Conference on Quantitative Traits, Iowa State University Press, Ames, Iowa.

Thompson, E. A., Cannings, C., and Skolnick, M. H. (1978), Ancestral inference. I. The problem and the method, *Ann. Hum. Genet. (London)* 42:95–100.

Thompson, E. A., Kravitz, K., Hill, J., and Skolnick, M. H. (1978), Linkage and the power of a pedigree structure, paper prepared for the Proceedings of the Conference on Genetic Epidemiology, Hawaii, October 1977, in *Genetic Epidemiology* (N. E. Morton and C. S. Chung, eds.), pp. 247–253, Academic Press, New York.

Thompson, E. A., and Cannings, C. (1979), Sampling schemes and ascertainment, in *Genetic Analysis of Common Diseases: Applications to Predictive Factors in Coronary Disease* (C. F. Sing and M. Skolnick, eds.), Alan F. Liss, New York.

Vetta, A. (1977a), Assortative mating, *Nature* **266**:195.

Vetta, A. (1977b), Reply to Bulmer, *Nature* **266**:195–196.

Vetta, A., and Smith, C. A. B. (1974), Comments on Fisher's theory of assortative mating, *Ann. Hum. Genet.* **38**:243–248.

Wagener, D. K. (1976), Preferential mating. Nonrandom mating of a continuous phenotype, *Theor. Popul. Biol.* **10**:185–204.

Watterson, G. A. (1959), Nonrandom mating, and its effect on the rate of approach to homozygosity, *Ann. Hum. Genet.* **23**:204–220.

Wilson, S. R. (1973), The correlation between relatives under the multifactorial model with assortative mating. I. The multifactorial model with assortative mating, *Ann. Hum. Genet. (London)* **37**:189–204.

Wright, S. (1921), Correlation and causation, *J. Agric. Res.* **20**:557–585.

10

Current Directions in Genetic Epidemiology

THEODORE REICH, BRIAN SUAREZ, JOHN RICE, and
C. ROBERT CLONINGER

1. Introduction

Genetic epidemiology is a new and burgeoning field of genetics which studies the familial and population distribution of non-Mendelian phenotypes in naturalistic settings (Morton and Chung, 1978). Since most of these traits show a variable age of onset, variation in severity, assortative mating, and are sex specific, failure to give simple Mendelian ratios is expected. Even when attempts have been made to control extraneous sources of variation, these phenotypes still do not fall into Mendelian categories.

The common familial diseases such as hypertension, arteriosclerotic heart disease, schizophrenia, and diabetes are perhaps the most important of these non-Mendelian phenotypes. In spite of this, they have received relatively little attention from geneticists because simple Mendelian subvarieties could not easily be defined. With respect to the common familial diseases, current thinking is that they are each caused by several possibly independent mechanisms and that both genes and nongenetic environmental effects are involved. The situation is quite complex because some of the environmental effects may be transmitted in the same families as the genetic factors.

THEODORE REICH, BRIAN SUAREZ, JOHN RICE, AND C. ROBERT CLONINGER • Department of Psychiatry, Washington University, School of Medicine and the Jewish Hospital of St. Louis, 216 South Kingshighway, St. Louis, Missouri 63110.   This work was supported in part by USPHS Grants MH-31302, AA-03539, MH-00048, MH-25430, and MH-14677.

Several examples of genotype—environment interaction are available to us and can serve as simple models for the more complex situations referred to above. Patients with phenylketonuria develop moderate to severe levels of mental retardation in a phenylalanine-rich environment, and the syndrome can be modified to a great degree if a diet free of phenylalanine is provided (Cavalli-Sforza and Bodmer, 1971). Similarly, individuals with alpha-1-antitrypsin deficiency often develop a severe, rapidly progressing form of emphysema if they are exposed to cigarette smoke or industrial pollutants (Pierce, Eisen, and Dhingra, 1969). Again, reduction of the environmental agents greatly reduces the severity and incidence of the disease.

2. The Heterogeneity Problem

The first and perhaps most important step in understanding the etiologic mechanisms responsible for the common familial diseases is their subdivision into increasingly homogeneous subforms. As an example, Goldstein, Schrott, Hazzard, Bierman, and Motulsky (1973) studied patients who had survived a myocardial infarction. Examining the families of these individuals, a form of hypercholesterolemia was detected which followed simple Mendelian ratios, and an important underlying genetic cause for myocardial disease was established.

The subdivision of a complex phenotypic entity, however, does not always lead to clear homogeneous mechanisms. The observation that juvenile onset, insulin-requiring diabetes is in linkage disequilibrium with the *HLA* locus, whereas adult onset diabetes is not, clearly separates diabetes into two groups (Rotter and Rimoin, 1978). However, the mode of transmission of each of these groups still remains a complex mystery.

One approach for dealing with the heterogeneity problem involves the examination of single large extended pedigrees (Elston, Namboodiri, Glueck, Fallat, Tsang, and Leuba, 1975). The logic of this method requires the assumption that the mode of transmission of the phenotype throughout the entire pedigree is unitary. That is, if a complex entity consists of more than one abnormality and if each abnormality is relatively rare, then a single abnormality should be found when examining a single kindred. The phenotype may be either quantitative or qualitative. Under these assumptions, genetic parameters relevant to the transmission of a major gene can be measured and predictions can be made about the presence or absence of the disorder in subsequent members of the family.

The extended pedigree method suggested by Elston is used to detect the presence of major loci when there are both major and minor loci. Detection of the major locus is also favoured by the observation of bimodality of the relevant phenotype in the general population. An example of the use of extended pedigrees to help define the mode of transmission of a complex phenotype is described in a paper by Moll, Powsner, and Sing (1979). In this endeavor both the presence of single major locus and relevant background genetic variation could be discerned.

Reich and co-workers (Reich, Rice, Wette, and James, 1979; Reich, Rice, Cloninger, and Lewis, 1980) have proposed that for polygenic or multifactorial traits the correlational architecture of nuclear families or extended pedigrees could be used to define independently transmissible subforms of a disorder. Using nuclear families they demonstrated that subforms of a single disorder or indeed two related disorders might be different degrees of the same process, environmental variants of the same process, or truly independently transmissible syndromes. In this latter case the extent to which the transmissible factors might be common between the two subforms is quantified. The goal of this phenotypic analysis is to categorize clinically observable heterogeneities and to use them to discover unitary pathological syndromes. By observing the correlational architecture in nuclear families of two disorders, or alternately a subdivided disorder, some insight might be gained into the extent to which unitary factors are operating. For example, Cloninger, Reich, and Guze (1975) were able to show that hysteria (Briquet's syndrome) and antisocial personality appeared to be different degrees of the same process implying a unitary etiology. By contrast the transmission of alchoholism from male and female probands indicated that non-familial environmental factors were more important in the etiology of alcoholism in females. This suggested that alcoholism in males and females was essentially a measure of the same underlying phenotypic process except that environmental nonfamilial factors were more important in determining the presence or absence of alcoholism in females (Reich et al., 1975). Finally, Cloninger and co-workers (Cloninger, Reich, and Wetzel, 1979; Cloninger, Rice, and Reich, 1979a, b) showed that the transmission of antisocial personality in the families of individuals with alcoholism and depression represented an independently transmissible entity. Since it is expected that independently transmissible entities are more likely to have either a unitary etiology or at least one distinct from the group from which they are split off, these clarifications of phenotypic classification using familial principles should be useful in ultimately determining the genetic and nongenetic mechanisms which lead to the manifestation of a phenotype.

3. Some Common Mechanisms

The most sought after mode of transmission by genetic epidemiologists is the single major locus mechanism. In this formulation genetic variation is due to two or more alleles at a single locus. The individual's phenotype depends only on his genotype and random nonfamilial environmental factors, as shown in Fig. 1.

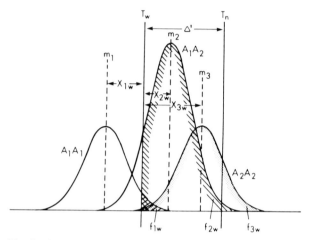

FIGURE 1. Distribution of phenotypes in genotypes A_1A_1, A_1A_2, A_2A_2. Each genotype truncated by two thresholds. $q = 0.5$, $m_1 - m_2 = 3$ S.D., $m_2 - m_3 = 1.5$ S.D.; m_1, mean of genotype A_1A_1; m_2, mean of genotype A_1A_2; m_3, mean of genotype A_2A_2; T, threshold; f_1, proportion of A_2A_2 affected by disease; X_1, X_2, X_3, normal deviates corresponding to f_1, f_2, f_3. Subscripts w and n refer to wide (more common) and narrow (less common) forms of the disease and are omitted when one threshold is considered. Δt, distance between thresholds in S.D. units.

In this figure, a single locus with two alleles is displayed. If the trait were quantitative, then m_1, m_2, and m_3 would be the mean value of each genotype. Variation about each genotypic mean is due to random nonfamilial factors. When dichotomous traits are considered, a threshold T may be present and individuals whose phenotype is greater than the threshold have the disease. In Fig. 1 two thresholds are displayed, as would be the case if there were a more and less common form of the disease. The discovery of this type of mechanism is important since it may be due to a relatively simple, biological process (Reich, James, and Morris, 1972).

A more complex formulation is the multifactorial model of disease transmission. In this model many genes of small effect and environmental factors are summed into a single variable termed the "liability," which is transmitted between parent and offspring. The effect of each variable is small in relation to the total variation and the liability score of an individual is the sum of genetic and environmental events which are relevant. If a dichotomous phenotype is being studied, then a threshold is used to define affected individuals whose phenotypic liability score is greater than the threshold. If a second threshold is present, perhaps due to variable severity or a sex effect, it may also be represented as in Fig. 2. A similar model may be used for quantitative phenotypes, where the phenotypic score is generally scaled so that it is normally distributed.

In Fig. 2, a single doubly truncated liability distribution is displayed along with the liability distributions of the relatives of individuals with two forms of

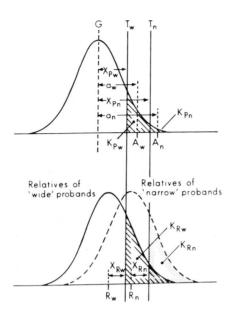

FIGURE 2. Three distributions representing the general population (above) and relatives of affected individuals (below) at two thresholds. T, threshold; G, mean liability of general population; A, mean liability of affected individuals; K_P, prevalence of disease in population; K_R, prevalence of disease in relatives or probands; X_P, deviation of threshold of probands from population mean, the normal deviation; X_R, deviation of threshold of relatives of probands from relative mean, the normal deviate; a, mean deviation of probands from population mean; w, more common form of disease (includes n); n, less common form of disease.

the disease. Using a model such as this, the correlation in liability between relatives for different forms of the disease can be computed.

This model is especially useful when behavioral traits are considered because it does not require that all transmission be genetic. Information may also be transmitted from parent to offspring by cultural mechanisms.

The most advanced models for the transmission of the common familial illnesses combine both single major loci and multifactorial mechanisms. Both major and minor genes may each contribute to the presence or absence of a phenotype or a phenotypic score. The model is most complex when major genes, minor genes, and cultural factors are all responsible for intergenerational transmission.

In order to apply these models to a data set, the genetic epidemiologist relies on the segregation distribution of the trait or quantitative scores within a nuclear or extended family. A number of computer programs are available which use maximum-likelihood techniques to estimate a set of parameters which most clearly resemble those of the data set. A statistical test can then be made for the presence or absence of the major gene or alternately of a multifactorial background. The principle of parsimony requires that an attempt be made to reduce the number of parameters to an acceptable minimum. The goal of these analyses is not only to fit an entire complex model to a set of data but to provide a vehicle for further hypotheses testing and critical experiments.

4. Detecting Major Loci

More than a century ago Mendel, by studying seven "constantly differentiating characters" of *Pisum*, conclusively demonstrated that allelic variation at a single major locus could explain the phenotypic variation he observed. He deliberately chose characters which could be accurately classified into one of the two dichotomous groups (e.g., long vs. short stems; smooth vs. wrinkled seeds) and neglected the residual variation which occurred within classes. Mendel was the first to identify a single major locus (SML) and since the rediscovery of his work, the search for major loci has steadily increased. Indeed, Elston and Stewart (1971) have asserted that perhaps the single most important question concerning the inheritance of any character is whether " . . . most of the genetic variation (is) due to one locus, or are many loci necessarily involved?"

The two major techniques that can be used to detect the presence of a major locus are segregation analysis and linkage analysis. Below is a brief review of the history of these techniques.

4.1. Segregation Analysis

Much of Mendel's success can be attributed to the characters he chose to study, that is, characters which presented two mutually exclusive (and exhaustive) phenotypic classes. Mendel hypothesized that a plant's phenotype was a simple function of its genotype at a SML, and by performing the appropriate crosses he was able to "test" his hypothesis by evaluating the proportion of offspring the model predicted to fall in each class against the observed proportion for any particular mating combination. This approach — testing observed proportions of offspring against those predicted from a SML model — is the essence of segregation analysis. The methodology has undergone a number of refinements which take into account such factors as method of ascertainment (Weinberg, 1912; Lenz, 1929; Hogben, 1931; Bailey, 1951c, d; Smith, 1959; Li and Mantel, 1968) and the presence of sporadics or, as they are sometimes called, phenocopies (Morton, 1959). Haldane (1932, 1949) and Fisher (1934) improved the efficiency of segregation analysis by introducing the principles of maximum-likelihood estimation, which was later extended by Bailey (1951c, d) and Smith (1956).

For the most part these techniques are appropriate for characters which can be sorted into mutually exclusive classes where each group is taken to

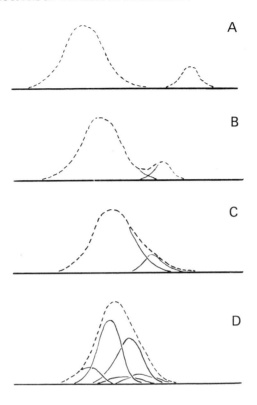

FIGURE 3. Possible phenotypic distributions resulting from the action of a single major locus. (A) The two distributions do not overlap so that the variation within each distribution can be neglected without loss of power. (B) The two distributions overlap slightly giving rise to an antimode. Classification based on the antimode will result in the misclassification of some individuals. (C) The genotypic distributions overlap to such an extent that a continuous, albeit skewed, phenotypic distribution results. (D) Distribution of enzymatic activity for the three allele red cell acid phosphatase locus. The sum of the individual genotypic distributions (solid curves) gives rise to a continuous and almost normal activity distribution (dashed curve). (After Harris, 1966)

reflect one or more genotypes such that, given the genotype, the phenotype is completely determined although the reverse may not be the case as, for example, when dominance is present. This situation is shown in part A of Fig. 3. In the simplest case one of the two distributions would contain one homozygote and only that homozygote, while the other distribution would contain the other homozygote and heterozygotes. When the distributions do not overlap, the variation within each can be ignored. But what if the classes determined by the SML are not discrete? The situation shown in part B of Fig. 3 is by no means atypical. Here the two distributions overlap. When their region of overlap is not too great and when the smaller distribution is not too small, an antimode can be discerned. The presence of an antimode does not guarantee the presence of a

SML (Murphy, 1964), although many such distributions are in fact known to result from a SML (see, for instance, Penrose, 1952; Perry, Hensen, Tischler, and Bunting, 1967; Weidman, Suarez, Falko, Witzum, Kolar, Raber, and Schonfeld, 1979). The greater the overlap between the distributions, the more difficult it becomes to detect the presence of a SML. This can be seen in Fig. 3C, where the observed population distribution contains no antimode but instead is significantly skewed. Like bimodality, skewness certainly does not guarantee the presence of a SML, but again examples are known where skewness is, in fact, the result of such a locus. Part D of Fig. 3 shows the activity distribution of red-cell acid-phosphatase (Harris, 1966). Even though this enzyme is known on electro-phoretic grounds to be determined by three alleles at a SML, if just the enzymatic-activity phenotype is studied, the population distribution is so close to normal that the major locus could easily be missed even though the SML accounts for about 60% of the phenotypic variability in activity (Eze, Tweedie, Bullen, Wren, and Evans, 1974).

If the distributions shown in Fig. 3D are liability distributions and if an individual's value exceeded a particular threshold, then the SML could give rise to a continuously distributed liability distribution which could, in turn, give rise to two phenotypes such as "affected" (those above the threshold) and "unaffected" (those below the threshold). In this case there is no powerful way to determine the transformation between genotype and phenotype (James, 1971; Suarez, Reich, and Trost, 1976; Suarez, Fishman, and Reich, 1977). When, however, the phenotype is determined by multiple thresholds giving rise to three or more classes, a unique transformation can be found (Reich, James, and Morris, 1972). Of course, it is also possible that a phenotypic discontinuity can result from a polygenic mechanism when a threshold is imposed. This situation was first modeled by Wright (1934) and refined by, among others, Edwards (1960), Falconer (1965), Smith (1971), Morton, Yee, and Lew (1971), and Reich, James, and Morris (1972).

Since it has become clear that a SML could give rise to a discrete distri-bution of phenotypes or a continuous distribution and, likewise, that a multi-factorial mechanism (with no SML) could also give rise to both a discrete and continuous distribution of phenotypes, it was only natural that these two basic models — multifactorial and SML — would be combined into a single model. These models, generally known as mixed models because they combined both types of transmission, actually are surprisingly old, having first been proposed by Mittman (1938). More recent and sophisticated formulations have been given by Morton and MacLean (1974), Elston and Yelverton (1975), and, for pedigrees of limited size, by Ott (1979). Recent reviews can be found in Elston and Rao (1978) and Morton and Rao (1978). These mixed models are designed to detect a SML in the presence of a multifactorial background. Among other things, the background tends to "smooth out" the effect of the major locus such that, at the population level at least, only a skewed phenotypic distribution may be evident. It is, of course, always possible to find a monotonic transformation that normalizes the distribution. To the extent that the transformation fails to normalize the phenotypic distribution in relatives from an enriched sample (i.e., one ascertained through one or more deviant probands), the major locus can be detected using currently available methods (MacLean, Morton, and Lew, 1975). In principle, segregation analysis can be extended to large pedigrees although ascertainment is difficult to deal with, cultural transmission can be confused with a SML, and present day computer technology is still too slow and costly.

Regardless of whether small nuclear families or large extended families are studied, segregation analysis is more sensitive to distribution assumptions than is path analysis. Especially troublesome is skewness, which can simulate a SML when none exists (MacLean, Morton, Elston, and Yee, 1976). Its elimination via an appropriate transformation, however, will weaken the evidence of the presence of a SML.

4.2. Linkage Analysis

Apart from identification of a specific biochemical gene product the *sine qua non* for detection of a SML is mapping it to a linkage group. Whereas the roots of segregation analysis can clearly be traced to Mendel and his pea experiments, linkage analysis is comparatively a new methodology. Indeed, the phenomenon of linkage constitutes a violation of Mendel's second "law," i.e., independent assortment.[†] For all together nongenetic reasons, it is quite possible for traits to segregate in families with patterns that simulate a SML. A classic example is the trait "attending medical school," which behaves much like a Mendelian recessive with a gene frequency of about 6% (Lilienfeld, 1959). It is much more difficult, however, for environmental factors to simulate linkage.

Linkage analysis can be traced to the early work of Bateson, Saunders, and Punnett (1905), Morgan (1910), and Sturtevant (1913). Human linkage studies date back to the 1920's, although it was not until the 1930's that real progress in methodology was made. Prior to 1930 no autosomal linkages had been found, although at least 15 X-linked loci were known. The usual method for detecting linkage prior to about 1930 was by simple inspection of pedigrees. Thus, Levine (1926) found no evidence for linkage between atopic hypersensitivity and the ABO blood groups. Likewise, Snyder (1929, 1931) was unable to demonstrate linkage between polydactylism or telangiectasis with the ABO locus.

The first serious attempt at devising a linkage methodology suitable for human autosomal data was made by Bernstein (1931). Bernstein's paper, like so much of his work, constitutes a landmark in human genetics as it laid out the theoretical possibility of constructing a map of the human genome. Moreover,

---

[†] The loci determining two of the seven traits Mendel studied are, in fact, linked with a recombination fraction of about 12cM (Blixt, 1975). Possible reasons why Mendel failed to detect the linkage have been given by Douglas and Novitski (1977).

he was the first to show that linkage could be both detected and the recombination fraction estimated using data involving only two generations. The following year Wiener (1932) devised an alternative but similar method.

Hogben (1934a) extended Bernstein's method to include cases where both linked loci show complete dominance and where one linked locus shows dominance while the other exhibits codominance (Hogben, 1934b).

Haldane (1934) further extended Bernstein's methods to include loci with three alleles. Especially noteworthy was a section of Haldane's (1934) paper that attempted to come to grips with the problems of incomplete penetrance and variable age of onset. These two problems, however, were treated as one and the same, and no general approach was developed. Nevertheless, some insight into incomplete penetrance for rare dominant genotypes was gained.

The scoring method of Bernstein was significantly improved by Fisher (1935a,b, 1936), who developed a maximum-likelihood scoring procedure that essentially made Bernstein's approach, as amended by Hogben and Haldane, obsolete. In the first of a series of three papers, Fisher (1935a) introduced his u statistics, which not only were more efficient than Bernstein's (and fully efficient in the limit for loose linkage), but also allowed for the combination of information provided by families of differing size. The first paper treated dominant abnormalities and the second paper extended the methodology to recessive abnormalities (Fisher, 1935b). In the third paper, Fisher (1936) extended the u score method to "partial" sex linkage and, moreover, showed how ancillary information provided by the number of affected children per family could be used to appropriately treat pedigrees collected with unknown ascertainment biases.

Fisher's pioneering work was later extended by Finney (1940, 1941a,b, 1942) to include various types of families. He tabulated his results in a manner that facilitated the combination of information contained in various mating types so that the units of the score divisor, the sampling variance, and the amount of information are all identical. Although he only considered two-allele loci, he demonstrated that information could be recovered from those families where the parents were of uncertain genotypes (families that had earlier been rejected by Fisher as useless). Finney also showed that for recessive traits, maximum recovery of information was possible for families where the ascertainment procedure is unknown. Finney's improvement on Fisher's method requires a considerable amount of algebraic manipulation when many different mating types are involved, and consequently his approach is not only time consuming but also greatly increases the chance of making arithmetic errors. Because of these considerations, Bailey (1951a, b) developed a general method of deriving u statistics (and their corresponding amounts of information) which allows a variety of special cases to be readily obtained from a few general equations.

The development of Fisher's u score approach represented a significant improvement over the methods of the early 1930's. Nevertheless, the method does have its disadvantages, as pointed out by Smith (1935) and Morton (1955). For instance, although u scores are easy to use when parental genotypes are completely specified (except, of course, for linkage phase), the calculation of the variance may be intractable when parental genotypes are unknown (although this criticism has largely been overcome with the advent of computers and efficient numerical optimization techniques). Moreover, as pointed out above, u scores are only fully efficient in the limit for loose linkage which generally cannot be detected anyway. The assumption of normality for the total score distribution may be far from true (Haldane, 1946, provided a normalizing transformation for such cases). Finally, information about linkage can be greatly increased by using families involving more than two generations because, among other reasons, linkage phase can often be deduced. Use of u scores is restricted to two generational nuclear families.

Haldane and Smith (1947) used the probability ratio test to extract information from nuclear families (and larger kindred). Their approach depends on the theorem that the expected value of the probability ratio is unity on the null hypothesis regardless of alternative hypotheses. Moreover, the ratio of the probability of the two hypotheses need not be normally distributed. From family data, maximum-likelihood estimates of the parameters can be obtained under the hypothesis that the recombination fraction is some value ($\leqslant 1/2$) and under the hypothesis that the recombination fraction is exactly $1/2$ (i.e., no linkage). The maximum of the likelihood curve with respect to the recombination fraction is then determined. Actually, the log of the likelihood is maximized (hence the name "lod," from: *l*ogarithm of the *od*ds). Each pedigree provides a lod score and these in turn can be summed to obtain an estimate of the recombination fraction and then confidence intervals can be constructed.‡

The lod score method underwent significant improvement when Morton (1955, 1956, 1957) applied the technique of Wald's (1947) sequential analysis. Morton showed that for double backcross sib pairs, sequential analysis requires about 33% as many observations (for a given significant level) as the u score method and about 20% as many observations as the Haldane–Smith nonsequential probability ratio test.

Further extensions of the sequential approach were accomplished when Morton (1956) used lod scores to obtain likelihood ratio tests of homogeneity and maximum-likelihood estimates of the recombination distance for multiple generational pedigrees. Shortly thereafter, the method was extended to include multiple alleles at the "test" locus (Steinberg and Morton, 1956), and the "trait" locus (Morton, 1957). It is noteworthy that the first clear-cut heterogeneity for what had been considered a "simple" autosomal trait (elliptocytosis) was found through linkage analysis.

‡ If the individual lod scores were computed as logarithms to the base 10, the correction factor 2.303 ($= \log_e 10$) is necessary in constructing the confidence interval since the theory is valid only for natural logarithms (Cavalli-Sforza and Bodmer, 1971).

The linkage techniques which we have briefly reviewed were designed to be applied to traits known in advance to be due to a SML with complete penetrance. When the mode of transmission is unknown, or when linkage analysis is being used to detect the presence of a SML, different techniques need to be employed. Perhaps the first such technique to be developed was Penrose's (1935) sib pair method. Sib pairs are arrayed in a 2×2 contingency table by determining if the pair is alike or unlike for the traits being investigated. If linkage is present, there will be an excess of pairs in the alike—alike and unlike—unlike cells over those expected on the basis of the marginal distributions (i.e., under the assumption of independence). The excess may be tested by use of chi-square test (or if the total number of pairs is small by Fisher's exact test) when there is only a single sib pair per family used. In general, however, it is better to use efficient scores (Penrose, 1946, 1950) especially since, in the presence of linkage, the direction of nonindependence is known *a priori* (Li, 1961).

Smith (1953) has provided a large-sample correction for Penrose's method. However, as Morton (1955) notes, its use destroys the principal advantage of the method, that of arithmetical simplicity. Another drawback of the sib pair method is its sensitivity to heterogeneity in gene frequencies when different populations are pooled (Finney, 1941a; Woolf in Smith, 1953). Bailey (1961) suggests that when the mode of transmission is unknown, Penrose's method has some advantages over the Fisherian approach in helping to *detect* linkage, but Morton (1955), for instance, finds the term "linkage" scarcely appropriate when the mode of transmission is not known with certainty. It is certainly clear that Penrose's sib pair method is highly sensitive to both incomplete penetrance and variable age of onset.

More recent and powerful approaches to the detection of SML using sib pairs have been developed (Day and Simons, 1976; Suarez, 1978; Suarez, Rice, and Reich, 1978; Fishman, Suarez, Hodge, and Reich, 1978). These sib pair methods are especially powerful when both sibs are affected and when the linked marker locus is highly polymorphic as with, for instance, the *HLA* polymorphism (Suarez and Hodge, 1979; Suarez, Hodge, and Reich, 1979).

Similar to the development of segregation analysis for continuously distributed traits, an effort has been made to detect SML via linkage analysis (Haseman and Elston, 1972; Hill, 1975; Smith, 1975). While these approaches are still in their infancy, we can expect that further developments will make them a powerful tool in the future for the detection of SML in humans.

5. Resolution of Polygenic and Cultural Inheritance

Whereas segregation and linkage analysis are useful for detecting major loci, path analysis is the most flexible and powerful method for resolving the multifactorial variation present in most common diseases into polygenic and environmental components (Morton, 1976). Rather than sterile preoccupation with heritability estimates, path models of combined polygenic–cultural inheritance permit specification of relevant cultural factors in addition to quantifying their transmission probabilities and heritabilities. After a prolonged period of quiescence, there have recently been rapid advances so that now appropriate methods for data analysis have been developed both for data on intact nuclear families and in the presence of variable family structure in extended pedigrees. The history of these developments will first be sketched and then models for analyzing intact families or separation data will be described. Finally, the direction of current and future work in this area will be briefly discussed.

5.1. History of the Path Analytic Models

Path analysis was introduced by Wright (1921) as a technique to explain the interrelationships among variables by analyzing their correlational structure. The relationships among the variables of a model are depicted by a path diagram as in Fig. 4, where each variable is assumed to have mean zero and variance one. Single-headed arrows indicate the direct influence of one (independent) variable on another (the dependent variable) and curved double-headed arrows indicate correlations between independent variables which are otherwise unexplained in the diagram. Path coefficients (standardized partial regression coefficients) are associated with each single-headed arrow and measure the change in the dependent variable when a unit change is made in that independent variable with all other independent variables held constant. The correlation between any two variables in the diagram may be obtained by tracing all paths connecting

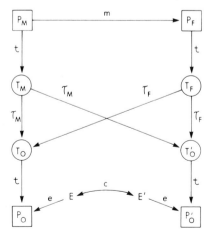

FIGURE 4. Path diagram of the transmission of complex (genetic and nongenetic) factors from parents to offspring when a sex-dimorphism is present.

them with the use of a simple set of rules (Li, 1975). Path analysis provides a comprehensive framework for modeling the familial transmission of complex traits.

The transmission of many complex traits appears to be influenced both by genic and by sociocultural factors. Until recently, except for an application by Wright (1931), direct parent-to-offspring transmission of environmental factors (cultural transmission) was precluded in models of familial resemblance. As a result, parent–offspring resemblance could only be interpreted as evidence for a genetic mechanism. Current path analytic models of familial resemblance simultaneously allow for cultural transmission, genetic transmission, assortative mating and common environment.

Morton (1974) and Rao, Morton, and Yee (1974, 1976) have described a general linear model of familial resemblance which incorporates cultural transmission, social homogamy, and a common environment of rearing. In addition, they incorporate an index of home environment and use the correlations between the phenotype and index as a source of additional information. Loehlin (1978) compares their model and the model of Jencks (1972) and the Birmingham model of Jinks, Eaves, and Fulker. More recently, Rao, Morton, and Cloninger (1979) have generalized their model to include mixed homogamy, i.e., assortative mating based on both social homogamy and phenotypic homogamy.

Cavalli-Sforza and Feldman have described several models of complex environment transmission (Cavalli-Sforza and Feldman, 1973, 1978; Feldman and Cavalli-Sforza, 1977) which also include selection and mutation. In their F-inheritance model there is a direct path from a parent's phenotype to an offspring's, while in their E-inheritance model genes and environmental factors are transmitted separately, and then combine to produce the offspring's phenotype. They allow for both types of transmission to occur simultaneously in their general model.

Rice, Cloninger, and Reich (1978) and Cloninger, Rice, and Reich (1979a, b) have developed two models of multifactorial inheritance which incorporate cultural transmission, assortative mating, and common environment. These models, termed the TAU and BETA models, are described in detail below.

5.2. The TAU Model

When data consist of observations on individuals reared in intact nuclear families without separation data or indices of environmental factors, it is not feasible to partition transmissible factors into discrete polygenic and cultural components. However, it may nevertheless be possible to detect cultural inheritance by allowing the probability for factors that are transmitted from parent to child to differ from the value of 1/2, which is expected for purely polygenic traits under the assumption of diploid autosomal inheritance. Such data may be treated rigorously using the TAU model (Rice, Cloninger, and Reich, 1978).

In the TAU model (Rice, Cloninger, and Reich, 1978), a continuous phenotype P is assumed to be partitioned as $P = T + E$, where T denotes both genic and cultural factors which are transmissible from parent to offspring and E denotes all other effects with the covariance between T and E equal to zero. To obtain the corresponding path equation, the variables P, T, and E must be standardized. Letting μ_X and σ_X denote the mean and standard deviation of a variable X, the equation above may be rewritten in the following manner:

$$P = T + E \tag{5.1}$$

$$P - \mu_P = (T - \mu_T) + (E - \mu_E) \tag{5.2}$$

$$\frac{P - \mu_P}{\sigma_P} = \frac{\sigma_T}{\sigma_P}\left(\frac{T - \mu_T}{\sigma_T}\right) + \frac{\sigma_E}{\sigma_P}\left(\frac{E - \mu_E}{\sigma_E}\right) \tag{5.3}$$

$$P = tT + eE \tag{5.4}$$

Equation (5.2) follows from Eq. (5.1) since the mean of the sum of two variables is always the sum of their means ($\mu_P = \mu_T + \mu_E$), and Eq. (5.3) follows from (5.2) using simple arithmetic. Recalling that a variable is standardized by subtracting its mean and dividing by its standard deviation, we can rewrite Eq. (5.3) as Eq. (5.4), where the symbols P, T, and E now represent the standardized variables. The coefficients $t = \sigma_T/\sigma_P$ and $e = \sigma_E/\sigma_P$ are path coefficients and Eq. (5.4) is a path equation.

Transmission from parent to offspring is given by the path equation

$$T_O = \tau_F T_F + \tau_M T_M + r_1 R_1 \tag{5.5}$$

where M, F, and O denote mother, father, and offspring, respectively, and R_1 is a residual variable which represents the nonfamilial factors which determine the T of an offspring. The path coefficients τ_F and τ_M measure the effectiveness of a parent in transmitting factors to his or her offspring. In the case of polygenic inheritance, $\tau_M = \tau_F = 1/2$ and R_1 is segregation from midparent genotype. For cultural inheritance, τ_M and τ_F need not be equal since either parent may contribute disproportionately as the result of sex-dependent roles in the rearing of children.

A correlation m between the phenotypes of mates which is based on phenotypic assortative mating (rather than based on resemblance for a component of the phenotype as in inbreeding or social homogamy) can be represented by the following path equation (Cloninger, Rice, and Reich, 1979a; Rice, Cloninger, and Reich, 1980a):

$$P_F = mP_M + r_2 R_2 \tag{5.6}$$

Other types of assortative mating can easily be included in the model (Cloninger, Rice, and Reich, 1979a; Rao, Morton, and Cloninger, 1979).

Although the nontransmissible environmental components (E) of parent and child are uncorrelated by definition, we allow for a correlation c between the E's of full siblings. Equations (5.4)–(5.6) are depicted in Fig. 4, which shows the relation among parents and two siblings reared together. Using the rules of path analysis, the father–offspring, mother–offspring, and sibling correlations are given by

$$r_{FO} = \tau_F(1 + m)t^2 \tag{5.7}$$

$$r_{MO} = \tau_M(1 + m)t^2 \tag{5.8}$$

$$r_{OO} = (\tau_F^2 + \tau_M^2 + 2\tau_F\tau_M mt^2)t^2 + ce^2 \tag{5.9}$$

General formulas for any vertical or collateral relatives reared in intact families are given by Rice, Cloninger, and Reich (1978).

All these correlations are determined once m, τ_F, τ_M, t^2 and c are known. These five numbers are called the parameters of the model and all correlations between relatives reared in intact homes may be expressed in terms of these parameters. In particular, a polygenic mechanism can predict the same correlations as a cultural mechanism with $\tau_M = \tau_F = 1/2$, so that the two could not be distinguished without separation data, no matter how many classes of relatives are observed.

The parameters themselves are in general not known and must be estimated from a set of observed correlations. This procedure is described mathematically below, but the idea is simple — choose parameter values which predict correlations as close as possible to the observed ones. If there are more correlations than parameters, then the goodness-of-fit of the model to the data may also be evaluated.

The TAU model has been extended to include a sex effect (Rice, Cloninger, and Reich, 1980b) where males and females may have different transmissible factors and where transmission from parent to offspring may depend on both the sex of the parent and the sex of the offspring. Reich *et al.* (1980) have applied the TAU model and segregation analysis with sex effect to a study of alcoholism using a threshold model. In a threshold model, a qualitative phenotype is assumed to reflect an underlying continuous liability scale with a threshold for which an individual is "affected" if his liability score is above the threshold, and "unaffected" otherwise.[†]

5.3. The BETA Model

When there is separation data or data about relevant environmental indices, it is feasible to partition polygenic and cultural factors using the BETA model (Cloninger, Rice, and Reich, 1979a, b). It is usually assumed that individuals are reared either in intact nuclear biological families or in intact nuclear adoptive families consisting of mother, father, and two children, but the BETA model

[†] Documented computer programs written in FORTRAN are available upon request which implement these models (Rice, 1979).

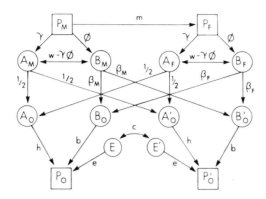

FIGURE 5. Path diagram depicting the causes of phenotypic resemblance between full sibs (P_O and P_O') in intact nuclear families (residuals omitted).

has been extended to allow for variable family structure (Cloninger, Rice, and Reich, 1979b). In this section we will consider the special case of intact nuclear families and comment on the general case later. The model of intact nuclear families is depicted in Fig. 5.

In the BETA model (Cloninger, Rice, and Reich, 1979a), the transmissible elements T are further partitioned as $T = A + B$, where A denotes additive genetic factors and B denotes heritable cultural factors. The determination of the phenotype P is given by

$$P = hA + bB + eE \qquad (5.10)$$

where h^2 is the polygenic heritability of the trait and b^2 is the proportion of heritable cultural factors.

Transmission from parent to offspring is given by the two equations

$$A_O = \tfrac{1}{2}A_F + \tfrac{1}{2}A_M + sS \qquad (5.11)$$

$$B_O = \beta_F B_F + \beta_M B_M + r_3 R_3 \qquad (5.12)$$

where S is segregation from midparent genic value and R_3 is fluctuation from midparent cultural value. The path coefficients β_F and β_M measure the effectiveness of a parent in transmitting cultural factors to his or her offspring.

As in the TAU model above, phenotypic assortative mating is represented by the path equation

$$P_F = mP_M + r_4 R_4 \qquad (5.13)$$

Even if A and B are uncorrelated in a random mating population, a correlation w between them will result from phenotypic assortative mating (Cloninger, Rice, and Reich, 1979a). In Fig. 5, the natural causal ordering for the determination of the parental phenotypes has been reversed. The correlation between the A's and B's of mates are $r_{AA} = m\gamma^2$ and $r_{BB} = m\phi^2$, where $\gamma = h + wb$ and $\phi = b + wh$.

The father–offspring, mother–offspring, and sibling correlations are given by

$$r_{FO} = \tfrac{1}{2}(1 + m)h\gamma + (\beta_F + m\beta_M)b\phi \tag{5.14}$$

$$r_{MO} = \tfrac{1}{2}(1 + m)h\gamma + (\beta_M + m\beta_F)b\phi \tag{5.15}$$

$$r_{OO} = \tfrac{1}{2}h^2(1 + r_{AA}) + (\beta_M^2 + \beta_F^2 + 2\beta_M\beta_F r_{BB})b^2 + 2whb + ce^2 \tag{5.16}$$

The correlations between relatives reared in intact families as well as between individuals reared in a wide spectrum of separated and extended situations can be found in Cloninger, Rice, and Reich (1979a,b).

The BETA model has been applied to IQ (Cloninger, Rice, and Reich, 1979a) and to an analysis of IQ and SES (Rice, Cloninger, and Reich, 1980a), where it was found that both b^2 and h^2 were significant.‡

5.4. Statistical Estimation and Hypothesis Testing

Let θ denote the set of parameters of a given model which must be estimated. For the TAU model, $\theta = \{m, \tau_M, \tau_F, t^2, c\}$ and for the BETA model $\theta = \{m, \beta_M, \beta_F, b, h, c, c_{DZ}, c_{MZ}\}$. Given a set of k observed correlations $\bar{r}_1, \ldots, \bar{r}_k$ with sample sizes $N_1, \ldots, N_k$, the parameters θ must be estimated. This is done by maximizing the log likelihood function L plus a constant, with

$$L = -\tfrac{1}{2} \sum_{i=1}^{k} \{f(\bar{r}_i) - f(r_i(\theta))\}^2 (N_i - 3) \tag{5.17}$$

where $r_i(\theta)$ is the correlation predicted from the model and f is Fisher's Z transformation. At the point of best fit, $-2L$ is approximately a value from the chi-square distribution with ν degrees of freedom, where ν equals k minus the number of parameters which are estimated.

Tests of linear constraints placed upon the parameters may be performed using the likelihood ratio test (Kendall and Stuart, 1973). Here, the model is fitted to the data twice, one with and once without the constraint. Twice the difference of the log likelihoods is asymptotically a value from a chi-square distribution whose degrees of freedom are equal to the number of linear constraints.

Using models described above analyses have been done on data sets which include alcoholism (Reich et al., 1980), spatial visualizing ability (Rice et al., 1980b), IQ (Rice, Cloninger, and Reich, 1980a), and height (Rice, Cloninger, and Reich, 1978).

5.5. Variable Family Structure

The high rates of separation and divorce in the U.S.A. and elsewhere combine with increased risk for early parental death to disrupt family structure

‡ A documented program for the BETA model is available upon request (Rice and Cloninger, 1979).

Table 1. Marital History Measures for Women Born between 1930 and 1941, United States, June 1971[a]

Measure	White	Black
Number of times married (%)	100.0	100.0
never married	3.8	8.4
married once	82.7	74.5
married twice	11.8	15.0
married 3+ times	1.7	1.9
% ever married	96.2	91.6
% currently divorced	4.8	11.2
% first marriage ending in divorce	15.3	24.1
% known to have been divorced	15.4	24.3
Median age at first marriage	20.2	20.4
Median age at divorce after first marriage	27.6	28.3
Median age at remarriage after first marriage ended in divorce	29.8	30.1
Median age at redivorce after second marriage	38.3	37.5

[a] Adapted from U.S. Bureau of the Census, *Current Population Reports*, Series P-20, No. 239, "Marriage, Divorce, and Remarriage by Year of Birth: June 1971," Tables A, C, D, E, R, G, and 1.

Table 2. Structure of the Families of 50 Alchoholic Patients (Mean Age = 41 years)

			Number of parents of rearing			
		1		2		3+
At age 10	mother	8%	mother–father	58%		
	other	6%	other	16%		
	total	14%	total	74%	total	12%
At age 15	mother	12%	mother–father	48%		
	other	16%	other	12%		
	total	28%	total	60%	total	12%
From 0–15			mother–father	40%		
			other	18%		
	total	0	total	58%	total	42%

for many diseases (Cloninger, Rice, and Reich, 1979b; Reich, Cloninger, Lewis, and Rice, 1978). Variation in family structure includes not only broken homes but also extensions in which grandparents, maiden aunts, stepparents, and others participate in child rearing. Family structure data from the 1971 census of the United States are shown in Table 1. Even higher roles of nonnuclear family structure (i.e., other than two-parent families) are associated with some diseases like alcoholism, as shown in Table 2.

In the presence of cultural inheritance, it is essential to describe the unit of cultural transmission accurately in order to obtain meaningful results. Variable family structure can have a marked influence on familial resemblance as shown by computer simulation elsewhere (Cloninger, Rice, and Reich, 1979b). Accordingly, the BETA model has been extended to allow for variable family structure and differences in parental influence due to separation, age, or stage of development of the child, birth order, or type of relationship.

5.6. Future Directions of Research

Available path models have been fully recursive linear models, but models allowing for reciprocal phenotype–environment interaction are currently being implemented by us. Models of assortative mating which allow for admixture of social and phenotypic homogamy are also being implemented (Rao, Morton, and Cloninger, 1979). The possibility of analyzing multiple correlated traits simultaneously appears feasible with available computer facilities and optimization routines but has not been fully implemented. Path and segregation analysis have been combined simultaneously only for the TAU model in nuclear families (Reich *et al.*, 1980), but there is no theoretical obstacle to implementation of the BETA model in extended pedigree structures.

The most important goal of current research is evaluation of methods for deriving environmental indices (Cloninger, Rice, and Reich, 1979a; Rice, Cloninger, and Reich, 1978). Early models required the dubious assumption that genetic factors did not influence a putative index, but recently this has been relaxed to permit tests of the magnitude of genetic influences. That is, an indexed trait may itself have complex inheritance. Further experience will be required to assess the robustness of alternative models in clinical applications (Loehlin, 1978).

6. Discussion

Early workers in the field attempted to use the analysis of variance or covariance to quantify the components of variation of a complex phenotype. Unfortunately, these workers very often used data collected at different centers, such as IQ scores. Their approach was heavily criticized as being an analysis only of a local situation, of being static and unable to predict future directions, and of requiring assumptions which were unrealistic. Furthermore, it was pointed out that the measurement of variance components, such as heritability, dominance deviation, and common environment, led to no further productive scientific investigation (Feldman and Lewontin, 1975).

At least in part as a response to these criticisms, the field of genetic epidemiology has been developing new dynamic models which do predict future changes in family distributions and in population structure. Furthermore, the important goal of genetic epidemiologists in specifying environmental factors, either nonfamilial or familial which may be responsible for the development of a disease, may well lead to modification of life styles, thereby decreasing the frequency of common diseases. Although it is probably true that a heritability estimate by itself has very little use, the specification of an environmental precursor to a major disease may well prevent the disease.

Massive shifts are taking place in the stability of the nuclear family. Biological and psychosocial environments of rearing are frequently not being offered by the same individuals and even on a theoretical level the consequences of this phenomenon is poorly understood. Only by understanding the impact of certain environmental factors on existing genetic substrates can some predictions be made.

Genetic epidemiology is controversial in another context. Sociobiologists frequently use naive generalizations of selection theory and suggest that complex human institutions are maintained by natural selection (Wilson, 1978). Unfortunately, these sweeping pronouncements have not incorporated the careful, logical analyses of population geneticists. Conclusions are drawn and social programs may be recommended on the basis of fragmentary evidence. To these scientists, the pace of genetic epidemiology may be far too slow since it requires careful measurement, controlled study, and replication. We fervently hope, however, that the lessons acquired in genetic epidemiology can be applied in a sensible fashion to general populations so that meaningful progress can be made.

It seems likely that the genetic makeup of an individual and the environment to which that individual is exposed can be combined into a statistical prediction that the individual will develop a common disorder. It is the goal of genetic epidemiology to demonstrate that by interfering with the cultural and environmental concomitants of the disorder it may be prevented or postponed. Our goal then is to optimize the duration and quality of life of the individual.

References

Bailey, N. T. J. (1951a), On simplifying the use of Fisher's u-statistics in the detection of linkage in man, *Ann. Eugen. (London)* **16**:26–32.

Bailey, N. T. J. (1951b), The detection of partially manifesting rare "dominant" and recessive abnormalities in man, *Ann. Eugen. (London)* **16**:33–44.

Bailey, N. T. J. (1951c), The estimation of the frequencies of recessiveness with incomplete multiple selection, *Ann. Eugen. (London)* **16**:215–222.

Bailey, N. T. J. (1951d), A classification of methods of ascertainment and analysis in estimating the frequencies of recessives in man, *Ann. Eugen. (London)* **16**:223–225.

Bailey, N. T. J. (1961), *Introduction to the Mathematical Theory of Genetic Linkage*, Clarendon Press, Oxford.

Bateson, W., Saunders, E. R., and Punnett, R. C. (1905), Experimental studies in the physiology of heredity, Reports to the Evolution Committee of the Royal Society, No. 2.

Bernstein, F. (1931), Zur Grundlegung der Chromosomenteorie der Vererbung beim Menschen mit besondere Berücksichtung der Blutgruppen, *A. Indukt. Abstamm. Vererbungsl.* 57:113–138.

Blixt, S. (1975), Why didn't Gregor Mendel find linkage?, *Nature* 256:206.

Cavalli-Sforza, L. L., and Bodmer, W. F. (1971), *The Genetics of Human Populations*, Freeman, San Francisco.

Cavalli-Sforza, L. L., and Feldman, M. W. (1973), Models of cultural inheritance. I. Group mean and within group variation, *Theor. Popul. Biol.* 4:47–55.

Cavalli-Sforza, L. L., and Feldman, M. W. (1978), The evolution of continuous variations. III. Joint transmission of genotype, phenotype and environment, *Genetics* 90: 391–425.

Cloninger, C. R., Reich, T., and Guze, S. B. (1975), The multifactorial model of disease transmission: III. Familial relationship between sociopathy and hysteria (Briquet's Syndrome), *Br. J. Psychiatry* 127:23–32.

Cloninger, C. R., Reich, T., and Wetzel, R. D. (1979), Alcoholism and affective disorders: Familial associations and genetic models, in *Alcoholism and the Affective Disorders* (D. Goodwin and C. Erickson, eds.), pp. 57–86, Spectrum, New York.

Cloninger, C. R., Rice, J., and Reich, T. (1979a), Multifactorial inheritance and cultural transmission and assortative mating. II. A general model of combined polygenic and cultural inheritance, *Am. J. Hum. Genet.* 31:176–198.

Cloninger, C. R., Rice, J., and Reich, T. (1979b), Multifactorial inheritance with cultural transmission and assortative mating. III. Family structure and the analysis of separation experiments, *Am. J. Hum. Genet.* 31:366–388.

Day, N. E., and Simons, M. J. (1976), Disease susceptibility genes – their identification by multiple case family studies, *Tissue Antigens* 8:109–119.

Douglas, L., and Novitski, E. (1977), What chance did Mendel's experiments give him of noticing linkage?, *Heredity* 38:253–257.

Edwards, J. H. (1960), The simulation of Mendelism, *Acta Genet. Stat. Med.* 10:63–70.

Elston, R. C., Namboodiri, K. K., Glueck, C. J., Fallat, R., Tsang, R., and Leuba, V. (1975), Study of the genetic transmission of hypercholesterolemia and hypertriglyceridemia in a 195 member kindred, *Ann. Hum. Genet., London* 39:67–87.

Elston, R. C., and Rao, D. C. (1978), Statistical modeling and analysis in human genetics, *Annu. Rev. Biophys. Bioeng.* 1:253–286.

Elston, R. C., and Stewart, J. (1971), A general model for the genetic analysis of pedigree data, *Hum. Hered.* 21:523–542.

Elston, R. C., and Yelverton, K. C. (1975), General models for segregation analysis, *Am. J. Hum. Genet.* 27:31–45.

Eze, L. C., Tweedie, M. C. K., Bullen, M. F., Wren, P. J. J., and Evans, D. A. P. (1974), Quantitative genetics of human red cell acid phosphatase, *Ann. Hum. Genet.* 37: 333–340.

Falconer, D. S. (1965), The inheritance of liability of certain diseases, estimated from the incidence among relatives, *Ann. Hum. Genet.* 29:51–76.

Feldman, M. W., and Cavalli-Sforza, L. L. (1977), The evolution of continuous variation. II. Complex transmission and assortative mating, *Theor. Popul. Biol.* 11:161–181.

Feldman, M. W., and Lewontin, R. C. (1975), The heritability hangup: The role of variance analysis in human genetics, *Science* 190:1163–1168.

Finney, D. (1940), The detection of linkage, *Ann. Eugen. (London)* 10:171–214.

Finney, D. (1941a), The detection of linkage II: Further mating types; scoring of Boyd's data, *Ann. Eugen. (London)* 11:10–30.

Finney, D. (1941b), The detection of linkage III: Incomplete parental testing, *Ann. Eugen. (London)* 11:115–135.

Finney, D. (1942), The detection of linkage IV: The loss of information from incompleteness of parental testing, *Ann. Eugen. (London)* 11:233–242.

Fisher, R. A. (1934), The effect of methods of ascertainment upon the estimation of frequencies, *Ann. Eugen. (London)* 6:13–25.

Fisher, R. A. (1935a), The detection of linkage with "dominant" abnormalities, *Ann. Eugen. (London)* 6:187–201.

Fisher, R. A. (1935b), The detection of linkage with recessive abnormalities, *Ann. Eugen. (London)* 6:339–351.

Fisher, R. A. (1936), Tests of significance applied to Haldane's data on partial sex linkage, *Ann. Eugen. (London)* 7:87–104.

Fishman, P. M., Suarez, B. K., Hodge, S. E., and Reich, T. (1978), A robust method for the detection of linkage in familial diseases, *Am. J. Hum. Genet.* 30:308–321.

Goldstein, J. L., Schrott, H., Hazzard, W., Bierman, E., and Motulsky, A. (1973), Hyperlipidemia in coronary heart disease. II. Genetic analysis of lipid levels in 176 families and delineation of a new inherited disorder, combined hyperlipidemia, *J. Clin. Invest.* 52:1544–1568.

Haldane, J. B. S. (1932), A method for investigating recessive characters in man, *J. Genet.* 25:251–255.

Haldane, J. B. S. (1934), Methods for the detection of autosomal linkage in man, *Ann. Genet. (London)* 6:26–65.

Haldane, J. B. S. (1946), The cumulants of the distribution of Fisher's "u_{11}" and "u_{31}" scores used in the detection and estimation of linkage in man, *Ann. Eugen. (London)* 13:122–134.

Haldane, J. B. S. (1949), A test for homogeneity of records of familial abnormalities, *Ann. Eugen. (London)* 14:339–341.

Haldane, J. B. S., and Smith, C. A. B. (1947), A new estimate of the linkage between the genes for colour-blindness and haemophilia in man, *Ann. Eugen. (London)* 14:10–31.

Harris, H. (1966), Enzyme polymorphisms in man, *Proc. R. Soc. London Ser. B.* 164:298–310.

Haseman, J. K., and Elston, R. C. (1972), The investigation of linkage between a quantitative trait and a marker locus, *Behav. Genet.* 2:3–19.

Hill, A. P. (1975), Quantitative linkage: A statistical procedure for its detection and estimation, *Ann. Hum. Genet.* 38:439–449.

Hogben, L. (1931), The genetic analysis of familial traits. I. Single gene substitution, *J. Genet.* 25:97–112.

Hogben, L. (1934a), The detection of linkage in human families. I. Both heterozygous genotypes indeterminate, *Proc. R. Soc. London Ser. B.* 114:340–352.

Hogben, L. (1934b), The detection of linkage in human families. II. One heterozygous genotype indeterminate, *Proc. R. Soc. London Ser. B.* 114:353–363.

James, J. W. (1971), Frequency in relatives for an all-or-none trait, *Ann. Hum. Genet.* 35:47–49.

Jencks, C. (1972), *Inequality: A Reassessment of the Affect of Family and Schooling in America*, Basic Books, New York.

Kendall, M. G., and Stuart, A. (1973), *The Advanced Theory of Statistics, Vol. 2, Inference and Relationship*, (3rd ed.), Hafner, New York.

Lenz, F. (1929), Methoden der menschlicken Erblichkeitsforschung, *Handbuch hygn. Untersuch. Jena*, Vol. III.

Levine, P. (1926), Atopic hypersensitiveness, *J. Immunol.* 11:283–297.

Li, C. C. (1961), *Human Genetics: Principles and Methods*, McGraw-Hill, New York.

Li, C. C. (1975), *Path Analysis – A Primer*, The Boxwood Press, Pacific Grove, California.

Li, C. C., and Mantel, N. (1968), A simple method of estimating the segregation ratio under complete ascertainment, *Am. J. Hum. Genet.* 20:61–81.

Lilienfeld, A. M., (1959), A methodological problem in testing a recessive genetic hypothesis in human disease, *Am. J. Public Health* **49**:199–204.

Loehlin, J. (1978), Heredity–environment analyses of Jenck's IQ correlations, *Behav. Genet.* **8**:415–435.

MacLean, C. J., Morton, N. E., and Lew, R. (1975), Analysis of family resemblance. IV. Operational characteristics of segregation analysis, *Am. J. Hum. Genet.* **27**:365–384.

MacLean, C. J., Morton, N. E., Elston, R. C., and Yee, S. (1976), Skewness in commingled distributions, *Biometrics* **32**:695–699.

Mittman, O. (1938), Vererbung durch ein Genpaar und Mitwirkung des Restgenotypes im statistischen Nachweis, *Z. Indukt. Abstamm. Vererbungsl.* **75**:191–232.

Moll, P. P., Powsner, R., and Sing, C. F. (1979), Analysis of genetic and environmental sources of variation in serum cholesterol in Tecumseh, Michigan: V. Variance components estimated from pedigrees, *Ann. Hum. Genet.* **42**:343–354.

Morgan, T. H. (1910), Sex limited inheritance in drosophila, *Science* **32**:120–122.

Morton, N. E. (1955), Sequential tests for the detection of linkage, *Am. J. Hum. Genet.* **7**:277–318.

Morton, N. E. (1956), The detection and estimation of linkage between genes for elliptocytosis and the Rh blood type, *Am. J. Hum. Genet.* **8**:80–96.

Morton, N. E. (1957), Further scoring types in sequential linkage tests, with a critical review of autosomal and partial sex linkage in man, *Am. J. Hum. Genet.* **9**:55–75.

Morton, N. E. (1959), Genetic test under incomplete ascertainment, *Am. J. Hum. Genet.* **11**:1–16.

Morton, N. E. (1974), Analysis of family resemblance. I. Introduction, *Am. J. Hum. Genet.* **26**:318–330.

Morton, N. E. (1976), Resolution of cultural inheritance, polygenes and major loci, in Excerpta Medica International Congress Series No. 397, Fifth International Congress of Human Genetics, Armendares, S., and Lisker, R. (eds.), Excerpta Medica, Amsterdam.

Morton, N. E., and Chung, C. S. (eds.), (1978), *Genetic Epidemiology*, Academic Press, New York.

Morton, N. E., and MacLean, C. J. (1974), Analysis of family resemblance. III. Complex segregation of quantitative traits, *Am. J. Hum. Genet.* **26**:489–503.

Morton, N. E., and Rao, D. C. (1978), Quantitative inheritance in man, *Yearb. Phys. Anthropol.* **21**:12–41.

Morton, N. E., Yee, S., and Lew, E. (1971), Complex segregation analysis, *Am. J. Hum. Genet.* **23**:602–611.

Murphy, E. A. (1964), One cause? Many causes? The argument from the bimodal distribution, *J. Chronic Dis.* **17**:301–324.

Ott, J. (1979), Maximum likelihood estimation by counting methods under polygenic and mixed models in human pedigrees, *Am. J. Hum. Genet.* **31**:161–175.

Penrose, L. S. (1935), The detection of autosomal linkage in data which consists of pairs of brothers and sisters of unspecified parentage, *Ann. Eugen. (London)* **6**:133–138.

Penrose, L. S. (1946), A further note on the sib-pair linkage method, *Ann. Eugen. (London)* **13**:25–29.

Penrose, L. S. (1950), Data for the study of linkage in man: Red hair and the ABO locus, *Ann. Eugen. (London)* **15**:243–247.

Penrose, L. S. (1952), Measuring the pleiotropic effects in phenylketonuria, *Ann. Eugen. (London)* **16**:134–141.

Perry, T. L., Hansen, S., Tischler, B., and Bunting, R. (1967), Determination of heterozygosity for phenylketonuria on the amino acid analyzer, *Clin. Chem. Acta.* **18**:51–56.

Pierce, J., Eisen, A., and Dhingra, H. (1969), Relationship of antitrypsin deficiency to the pathogenesis of emphysema, *Trans. Assoc. Am. Physicians* **82**:87.

Rao, D. C., Morton, N. E., and Yee, S. (1974), Analysis of family resemblance. III. A linear model for familial correlation, *Am. J. Hum. Genet.* **26**:331–359.

Rao, D. C., Morton, N. E., and Yee, S. (1976), Resolution of cultural and biological inheritance by path analysis, *Am. J. Hum. Genet.* **28**:228–242.

Rao, D. C., Morton, N. E., and Cloninger, C. R. (1979), Path analysis under generalized assortative mating. I. Theory, *Genet. Res.* **33**:175–188.

Reich, T., James, J. W., and Morris, C. A. (1972), The use of multiple thresholds in determining the mode of transmission of semi-continuous traits, *Ann. Hum. Genet.* **36**:163–184.

Reich, T., Mullaney, J., and Winokur, G. (1975), The transmission of alcoholism, in *Genetic Research in Psychiatry* (R. Fieve, D. Rosenthal and H. Brill, eds.), The John Hopkins University Press, Baltimore.

Reich, T., Cloninger, C. R., Lewis, C., and Rice, J. (1978), Familial structures in models of cultural inheritance, in *Genetic Epidemiology* (N. E. Morton and C. S. Chung, eds.), pp. 183–191, Academic Press, New York.

Reich, T., Rice, J., Wette, R., and James, J. (1979), The use of multiple thresholds and segregation analysis in analyzing the phenotypic heterogeneity of multifactorial traits, *Ann. Hum. Genet.* **42**:371–390.

Reich, T., Rice, J., Cloninger, C. R., and Lewis, C. (1980), The contribution of affected parents to the pool of affected individuals: Path analysis of the segregation distribution for alcoholism, in *The Social Consequences of Psychiatric Illness*, (L. N. Robins, P. Clayton, and J. Wing, eds.), Brunner/Mazel, New York.

Rice, J. (1979), GENLIB: A library of computer programs for the genetic analysis of family data. Available upon request.

Rice, J., Cloninger, C. R., and Reich T. (1978), Multifactorial inheritance with cultural transmission and assortative mating. I. Description and basic properties of the unitary models, *Am. J. Hum. Genet.* **30**:618–643.

Rice, J., Cloninger, C. R., and Reich, T. (1980a), The analysis of behavioral traits in the presence of cultural transmission and assortative mating: Applications to IQ and SES, *Behav. Genet.*, in press.

Rice, J., Cloninger, C. R., and Reich, T. (1980b), General causal models for sex differences in the familial transmission of multifactorial traits: An application to human spatial visualizing ability, *Social Biology*, in press.

Rotter, J. I., and Rimoin, D. L. (1978), Heterogeneity in diabetes mellitus – update 1978 – Evidence for further genetic heterogeneity within juvenile onset insulin dependent diabetes mellitus, *Diabetes* **27**:599.

Smith, C. (1971), Recurrence risks for multifactorial inheritance, *Am. J. Hum. Genet.* **23**:578–588.

Smith, C. A. B. (1953), The detection of linkage in human genetics, *J. R. Statist. Soc. B.* **15**:153–192.

Smith, C. A. B. (1956), A test for segregation ratios in family data, *Ann. Hum. Genet.* **20**:257–265.

Smith, C. A. B. (1959), A note on the effects of method of ascertainment on segregation ratios, *Ann. Hum. Genet.* **23**:311–323.

Smith, C. A. B. (1975), A non-parametric test for linkage with a quantitative character, *Ann. Hum. Genet.* **38**:451–460.

Snyder, L. (1929), *Blood Grouping and Its Relation to Clinical and Legal Medicine*, Williams and Wilkins, Baltimore.

Snyder, L. (1931), Linkage in man, *Eugenical News* **16**:177–179.

Steinberg, A. G., and Morton, N. E. (1956), Sequential test for linkage between cystic fibrosis of the pancreas and the MNS locus, *Am. J. Hum. Genet.* 8:177–189.

Sturtevant, A. H. (1913), The linear arrangement of six sex-linked factors in *Drosophila* as shown by their mode of association, *J. Exp. Zool.* 14:43–59.

Suarez, B. K. (1978), The affected sib pair IBD distribution for *HLA* linked susceptibility genes, *Tissue Antigens* 12:87–93.

Suarez, B. K., and Hodge, S. E. (1979), A simple method to detect linkage for rare recessive diseases: An application to juvenile diabetes, *Clin. Genet.* 15:126–136.

Suarez, B. K., Reich, T., and Trost, J. (1976), Limits of the general two-allele single locus model with incomplete penetrance, *Ann. Hum. Genet.* 40:231–244.

Suarez, B. K., Fishman, P. M., and Reich, T. (1977), Estimating the parameters of the uncompletely penetrant single locus model using multiple populations, *Hum. Hered.* 27:336–351.

Suarez, B. K., Rice, J., and Reich, T. (1978), The generalized sib pair IBD distribution: Its use in the detection of linkage, *Ann. Hum. Genet.* 42:87–94.

Suarez, B. K., Hodge, S. E., and Reich, T. (1979), Is juvenile diabetes determined by a single gene closely linked to *HLA*?, *Diabetes* 28:527–532.

Wald, A. (1947), *Sequential Analysis*, Wiley, New York.

Weidman, S. W., Suarez, B., Falko, J. M., Witztum, J. L., Kolar, J., Raben, M., and Schonfeld, G. (1979), Type III hyperlipoprotememia: development of a VLDL ApoE gel iso-electric focusing technique and application in family studies, *J. Lab. Clin. Med.* 93: 549–569.

Weinberg, W. (1912), Methode und Fehlerquellen der Untersuchung auf Mendelsche Zahlen beim Menschen, *Arch. Rass. Ges. Biol.* 9:165–174.

Wiener, A. S. (1932), Method of measuring linkage in human genetics, with special reference to blood groups, *Genetics* 17:335–350.

Wilson, E. O. (1978), *On Human Nature*, Harvard University Press, Cambridge.

Wright, S. (1921), Correlation and causation, *J. Agric. Res.* 20:557–585.

Wright, S. (1931), Statistical methods in biology, *Proc. Am. Stat. Assoc.* 26:155–163.

Wright, S. (1934), An analysis of variability in numbers of digits in an inbred strain of guinea pigs, *Genetics* 19:506–536.

Wright, S. (1978), *Evolution and the Genetics of Populations, Vol. 4, Variability Within and Among Natural Populations*, The University of Chicago Press, Chicago.

PART IV

ANALYTICAL THEORY: ILLUSTRATED BY EXAMPLE

11

Segregation Analysis

R. C. Elston

1. Introduction

The statistical detection of Mendelian ratios in human sibships has long been known as segregation analysis. More generally, we can define segregation analysis as the statistical methodology used to determine from family data the mode of inheritance of a particular phenotype, especially with a view to elucidating single-gene effects; it is thus a basic tool in human genetics. There have been many reviews of the early literature on this topic (see, e.g., Smith, 1956, 1959; Steinberg, 1959; Morton, 1962, 1964, 1969; Elandt-Johnson, 1974), and this will not be repeated here; rather the present chapter will concentrate on the developments in this area over the last decade.

The fast development of the subject in recent years can be largely attributed to the increasing availability of electronic computers, allowing the use of sophisticated analyses that would otherwise be impossible. Therefore, on the assumption that appropriate computer programs will soon be widely available, this chapter will pay more attention to the statistical principles involved, and less to methods of computation. In Section 2 the various models are defined mathematically, so as to give precision to the assumptions that are made. The general-likelihood method of hypothesis testing and parameter estimation is taken up in Section 3, and its application to recent examples of segregation analysis is illustrated in Section 4.

R. C. ELSTON • Department of Biometry, Louisiana State University, Medical Center, New Orleans, Louisiana 70112. This work was supported in part by a Public Health Service Research Scientist Award (MH31732) and research grant (MH26721) from the National Institute of Mental Health, and by a research grant (GM16697) from the National Institute of General Medical Sciences. This is a modified version of a longer article by the same title appearing in Volume II of *Advances in Human Genetics* (Harris, H. and Hirschorn, K., eds.), Plenum, New York (to be published).

2. Mathematical Formulation of Genetic Models

Segregation analysis is based on a mathematical model that has four major components. The first two components describe the genetic basis for the phenotypic variability of a trait in a population, the third describes how that variability is passed on from one generation to the next, while the last component describes the way in which a sample of individuals is selected from the population for study. Each of these components will be discussed in turn: the joint genotypic distribution of mating individuals, the relationship between phenotype and genotype, the mode of inheritance, and the sampling of data. In this way it will be possible to build up a general model for segregation analysis, following the papers by Elston and Stewart (1971) and Elston and Yelverton (1975).

2.1. Joint Genotypic Distribution of Mating Individuals

When there is random mating, the joint genotypic distribution of mating individuals is simply the product of the genotypic distributions for males and females in the parental population. If furthermore there is no selection or mutation, and the population has reached equilibrium, these genotypic distributions depend only on the gene frequencies at the various loci.

In general we can let ψ_t be the probability that an individual in the parental population has genotype t. For two alleles at an autosomal locus, A and a, say, with gene frequencies q and $1 - q$, respectively, the genotypic distribution under random mating is given by the Hardy–Weinberg proportions $\psi_{AA} = q^2$, $\psi_{Aa} = 2q(1 - q)$, and $\psi_{aa} = (1 - q)^2$. If we consider in addition two alleles at a second autosomal locus, the genotypic distribution at equilibrium is obtained by multiplying together the probabilities for the genotypes at the individual loci.

This procedure can be extended to obtain the equilibrium genotypic distribution for any number of autosomal loci, but the number of genotypes, and hence the number of different probabilities that need to be considered, soon becomes prohibitively large. If, however, we replace the genotype by the total number of "capital letters" it contains, the total being over all loci, for a large number of loci this number will tend to be normally distributed in the population. This is illustrated in Fig. 1, where the distribution of this number for two alleles at each of three autosomal loci, all gene frequencies being equal to a half, is depicted. This gives the basis for the usual additive polygenic model in which it is assumed that there is an underlying polygenic genotype, which I shall call the "polygenotype" of an individual, that is normally distributed in the population. Without loss of generality the polygenotype can be assumed to have a mean of zero, and its variance will be denoted σ_G^2. Thus, using the notation

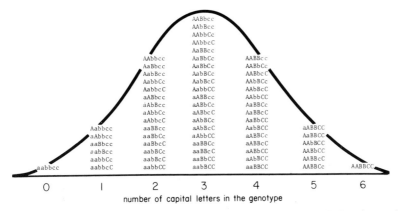

FIGURE 1. Population genotypic distribution when the genotype is classified by the number of "capital letters" it contains. The histogram gives the distribution for two alleles at each of three independent loci; the smooth curve gives the distribution in the limit as the number of loci tends to infinity. [Adapted from Roberts (1977)]

$$\phi(x, \sigma^2) = \frac{1}{(2\pi)^{1/2}\sigma} \exp\left[-\frac{1}{2}\left(\frac{x}{\sigma}\right)^2\right] \tag{2.1}$$

and letting G denote polygenotype, the distribution of polygenotype in the population is given by $\psi_G = \phi(G, \sigma_G^2)$.

Thus, using the symbols s and t to denote genotypes at one or a few loci ("monogenotype" or "oligogenotype"), the distribution of the mating type $s \times t$ under random mating is $\psi_s\psi_t$, and this is easily expressible in terms of gene frequencies; using the symbols F and G to denote polygenotypes, the distribution of the mating type $F \times G$ is $\psi_F\psi_G = \phi(F, \sigma_G^2)\phi(G, \sigma_G^2)$; and if the total genotype contains both components, oligogenotype and polygenotype, the distribution of the mating type $sF \times tG$ is $\psi_s\phi(F, \sigma_G^2)\psi_t\phi(G, \sigma_G^2)$.

2.2. Relationship between Phenotype and Genotype

Once we know the genotypic distribution, the relationship between phenotype and genotype can be completely described by specifying, separately for each genotype, the phenotypic distribution. Let the phenotype that is being investigated be z, assumed to be a single observation on each individual, and denote the distribution of z conditional on genotype t $g_t(z)$. If the genotype is polygenic, G, we write the conditional distribution $g_G(z)$; and if both monogenotype and polygenotype are involved we have $g_{tG}(z)$. Classical segregation analysis was limited to qualitative phenotypes — dichotomies such as presence or absence of a disease, or polychotomies such as the patterns of agglutination possible with a set of standard antisera. Recently, however, segregation analysis has been extended to allow for quantitative traits such as the concentration of a particular component in serum. We now discuss how the distributions $g_t(z)$, $g_G(z)$, and

$g_{tG}(z)$ may be mathematically specified to build up a segregation analysis model. In each case one or more of the various parameters may be sex specific, but this point will not be belabored.

2.2.1 Dichotomous Phenotype

The simplest genetic model for a dichotomy, affected $(z = 1)$ vs. unaffected $(z = 0)$, is that of two alleles at one autosomal locus. The phenotypic distributions are then completely specified by the three "penetrances" $g_{AA}(1), g_{Aa}(1)$, and $g_{aa}(1)$, since $g_{AA}(0) = 1 - g_{AA}(1)$, $g_{Aa}(0) = 1 - g_{Aa}(1)$, and $g_{aa}(0) = 1 - g_{aa}(1)$. If the allele A is dominant to a we have $g_{AA}(1) = g_{Aa}(1)$; a dominant disorder with complete penetrance is equivalent to these quantities being unity, with the absence of sporadic cases corresponding to $g_{aa}(1) = 0$. Similarly if the allele a causes a completely penetrant recessive disorder we have $g_{aa}(1) = 1$, with absence of sporadic cases corresponding to $g_{AA}(1) = g_{Aa}(1) = 0$.

When we turn to a normally distributed polygenotype, the usual model is to assume that the penetrance is an increasing function of G. In particular, this function is taken to be of the form

$$g_G(1) = \Phi[(G - \theta)/\sigma_E] \qquad (2.2)$$

where Φ is the cumulative normal function defined by

$$\Phi[(G - \theta)/\sigma] = \int_{-\infty}^{(G-\theta)/\sigma} \frac{1}{(2\pi)^{1/2}\sigma} \exp\left(-\frac{1}{2}u^2\right) du$$

$$= \int_{-\infty}^{G} \frac{1}{(2\pi)^{1/2}\sigma} \exp\left[-\frac{1}{2}\left(\frac{x - \theta}{\sigma}\right)^2\right] dx \qquad (2.3)$$

This function, which is often called a risk funtion, is illustrated in Fig. 2 for two different values of θ: θ_1 and θ_2; the other parameter, σ_E, determines how steeply the risk rises as a function of G.

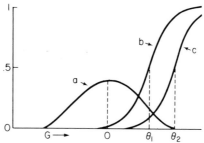

FIGURE 2. Pictorial representation of two cumulative normal risk functions in relation to an underlying normally distributed polygenotype, G. (a) Distribution of G, $\psi_G = \phi(G, \sigma_G^2)$. (b) Risk function $\Phi[(G - \theta_1)/\sigma_E]$. (c) Risk function $\Phi[(G - \theta_2)/\sigma_E]$. The risk function is the probability that an individual with polygenotype G is affected; this probability may depend upon the genotype at a major locus or upon the severity of the disorder. [From Elston and Rao (1978)]

It must be understood that the form of this risk function is arbitrary, and has no biological justification. It does, however, correspond to the usual threshold model for the polygenic inheritance of a dichotomous trait. Assume the existence of a normally distributed random variable L, called liability; it is made up of two uncorrelated components: the polygenotype G, normally distributed with variance σ_G^2, and an environmental component E, also assumed to be normally distributed but with variance σ_E^2. Let an individual be affected if and only if his liability is greater than θ, a parameter called the threshold. This model is illustrated in Fig. 3; the two models illustrated in Figs. 2 and 3, although seemingly different, are mathematically identical.

Since the trait we are considering is merely a dichtomous classification, and not a quantitative measure, it is impossible to give unique values separately to σ_G^2 and σ_E^2; it is only their *relative* magnitudes that is relevant. Thus without loss of generality some authors take $\sigma_G^2 = 1$ (e.g., Curnow, 1974), while others take $\sigma_G^2 + \sigma_E^2 = 1$ (e.g., Falconer, 1965); in the latter case σ_G^2 is the heritability of the liability to the disorder (Elston, 1973).

Morton and MacLean (1974) extended the threshold model to allow for a genotype that has both monogenic and polygenic components. Denoting the genotype tG, the "penetrance" becomes

$$g_{tG}(1) = \Phi[(G - \theta_t)/\sigma_E] \qquad (2.4)$$

analogous to Eq. (2.2). In this model differences at the major genotype locus are reflected as shifts of the risk function (Fig. 2) or the threshold (Fig. 3) to the right or left. For two alleles at an autosomal locus there are three thresholds, θ_{AA}, θ_{Aa}, and θ_{aa}, two of which are identical if dominance is assumed.

2.2.2. Polychotomous Phenotype

It is a simple matter to generalize the above phenotypic distributions to allow for a polychotomy, and this will be demonstrated with particular reference to a trichotomy. As before we can let $z = 0$ for unaffected individuals, but now we have $z = 1$ or 2 for affected individuals, representing two different forms of the disorder; in particular we can let $z = 1$ represent the less severe or "intermediate" form, while $z = 2$ represents the fully affected form.

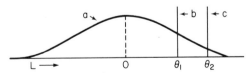

FIGURE 3. Pictorial representation of the threshold approach to the polygenic model for a qualitative trait. (a) Distribution of liability L, $\phi(L, \sigma_G^2 + \sigma_E^2)$. (b) Threshold θ_1. (c) Threshold θ_2. Individuals whose total liability is greater than the threshold are affected; the threshold may depend upon the genotype at a major locus or upon the severity of the disorder. [From Elston and Rao (1978)]

For two alleles at one autosomal locus the distributions are completely specified by the six penetrances $g_t(j)$, $t = AA$, Aa, or aa, and $j = 1$ or 2. By an appropriate choice of six constants θ_{jt} we can equate

$$g_t(2) = \Phi(-\theta_{2t})$$

and

$$g_t(1) = \Phi(-\theta_{1t}) - \Phi(-\theta_{2t}) \tag{2.5}$$

This, together with the assumption that there exist five constants μ_{AA}, μ_{Aa}, μ_{aa}, θ_1, and θ_2 such that

$$\theta_{jt} = \theta_j - \mu_t \tag{2.6}$$

forms the basis of the monogenic trichotomy model proposed by Reich, James, and Morris (1972). This assumption can be rationalized by supposing the existence of three normal liability distributions, one for each genotype: in each case the variability around the mean is environmentally caused, and the liability distribution for genotype t has mean μ_t. Furthermore two thresholds are assumed, θ_1 and θ_2, such that individuals with liabilities above θ_2 are affected, while individuals with liabilities between θ_1 and θ_2 are intermediate. This model is illustrated in Fig. 4, and leads to penetrances satisfying (2.5) and (2.6). [It can be noted in passing that the goodness-of-fit test for a monogenic hypothesis proposed by Reich, James, and Morris (1972) is as much a test of whether Eq. (2.6) is true as it is of a monogenic mechanism.]

For a pure polygenic model we generalize Eq. (2.2) to obtain the phenotypic distribution

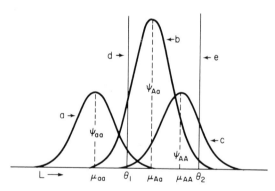

FIGURE 4. Pictorial representation of a monogenic trichotomy model. There are three component liability distributions: (a) $\phi(L - \mu_{aa}, \sigma_E^2)$, for aa individuals, (b) $\phi(L - \mu_{Aa}, \sigma_E^2)$, for Aa individuals, (c) $\phi(L - \mu_{AA}, \sigma_E^2)$, for AA individuals; (d) threshold θ_1, below which individuals are unaffected; (e) threshold θ_2, above which individuals are fully affected. Individuals whose liabilities fall between θ_1 and θ_2 have an intermediate form of the disorder. [Adapted from Reich et al. (1972)]

$$g_G(2) = \Phi[(G - \theta_2)/\sigma_E]$$

$$g_G(1) = \Phi[(G - \theta_1)/\sigma_E] - \Phi[(G - \theta_2)/\sigma_E] \qquad (2.7)$$

$$g_G(0) = 1 - \Phi[(G - \theta_1)/\sigma_E]$$

as illustrated in Figs. 2 and 3. This can be further generalized into the mixed model with both monogenic and polygenic components by making θ_1 and θ_2 monogenotype specific, i.e., by substituting θ_{1t} and θ_{2t} for them, respectively, as follows:

$$g_{tG}(2) = \Phi[(G - \theta_{2t})/\sigma_E]$$

$$g_{tG}(1) = \Phi[(G - \theta_{1t})/\sigma_E] - \Phi[(G - \theta_{2t})/\sigma_E] \qquad (2.8)$$

$$g_{tG}(0) = 1 - \Phi[(G - \theta_{1t})/\sigma_E]$$

If we assume in addition that Eq. (2.6) holds, we arrive at the mixed-model phenotypic distributions proposed by Morton and MacLean (1974) for a trichotomous trait.

2.2.3 Quantitative Phenotype

For a quantitative trait it is usual to assume that the distribution of z conditional on genotype is normal. Both the mean and variance of this normal distribution could in principle depend on genotype, but in order not to have too many unknown parameters, in practice the variance is taken to be the same, σ_E^2, for all genotypes. Thus for a monogenotype we take $g_t(z) = \phi(\mu_t - z, \sigma_E^2)$, and the resulting distribution of z in the population is

$$\sum_t \psi_t \phi(\mu_t - z, \sigma_E^2) \qquad (2.9)$$

as depicted in Fig. 5 for the special case of two alleles at an autosomal locus. For

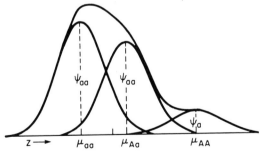

FIGURE 5. Population distribution of a quantitative trait dependent on the segregation of two alleles at an autosomal locus, assuming a normal distribution for each monogenotype. The variance within each component distribution is σ_E^2 for the monogenic model, and $\sigma_G^2 + \sigma_E^2$ for the mixed monogenic and polygenic model. [Adapted from Morton and MacLean (1974)]

a polygenotype we take $g_G(z) = \phi(G + \mu - z, \sigma_E^2)$, so that analogous to (2.9) the distribution of z in the population is (recalling $\psi_G = \phi(G, \sigma_G^2)$ and replacing summation by integration)

$$\int_{-\infty}^{\infty} \phi(G, \sigma_G^2)\phi(G + \mu - z, \sigma_E^2)dG = \phi(\mu - z, \sigma_G^2 + \sigma_E^2) \qquad (2.10)$$

i.e., normal with mean μ and variance $\sigma_G^2 + \sigma_E^2$. In this situation, however, unlike the case of qualitative phenotypes, both σ_G^2 and σ_E^2 are separately estimable. The extension to the case of mixed monogenotype and polygenotype is, as proposed by Elston and Stewart (1971), $g_{tG}(z) = \phi(G + \mu_t - z, \sigma_E^2)$; the population distribution is then again a mixture of normal distributions, such as is shown in Fig. 5, but now the variance within each distribution is $\sigma_G^2 + \sigma_E^2$ rather than just σ_E^2.

All the parameters in these distributions can be made to depend on the effects of age, sex, or other measurable factors such as may be environmentally determined, but usually the effects on the means μ and μ_t are more important than the effects on the variance. If one is willing to assume that these effects are independent of genotype, approximate allowance can often be made for them by subjecting the data to initial analyses to find appropriate overall adjustments. The original phenotypes are then adjusted to a "common" age, sex, and environment prior to undergoing segregation analysis.

2.3. Mode of Inheritance

The mode of inheritance from one generation to the next can be summarized mathematically by the genotypic distributions of the offspring conditional on the two parental genotypes. Let p_{stu} be the probability that an individual has genotype u given that his parents' genotypes are s and t. These conditional probabilities p_{stu} can be viewed as the elements of a three-dimensional stochastic matrix called the genetic transition matrix. Alternatively, the genetic transition matrix can be considered a two-dimensional matrix whose elements are probability distributions. This will now be explained for the hereditary mechanisms usually considered in segregation analysis. The extensions to other hereditary mechanisms are given by Elston and Stewart (1971).

2.3.1. Monogenic Inheritance

Table 1 gives the genetic transition matrix for segregation of two alleles at one autosomal locus. We order the genotypes $1 = AA$, $2 = Aa$, and $3 = aa$, so that the sth row corresponds to genotype s for one of the parents and the tth column corresponds to genotype t for the other parent. The (s, t)th entry in the matrix is the vector $[p_{st1}\ p_{st2}\ p_{st3}]$, i.e. the genotypic distribution of offspring from the mating $s \times t$. Now define the transmission probability τ_{tA} as the probability that an individual with genotype t transmits A to his offspring, so that $1 - \tau_{tA}$ is the

Table 1. Genetic Transition Matrix for Two Alleles at One
Autosomal Locus. Each Entry is a Genotypic Distribution
$[p_{st1} p_{st2} p_{st3}]$. [From Elston and Stewart (1971)]

		t	
s	$1 = AA$	$2 = Aa$	$3 = aa$
$1 = AA$	$[1\ 0\ 0]$	$[\frac{1}{2}\ \frac{1}{2}\ 0]$	$[0\ 1\ 0]$
$2 = Aa$	$[\frac{1}{2}\ \frac{1}{2}\ 0]$	$[\frac{1}{4}\ \frac{1}{2}\ \frac{1}{4}]$	$[0\ \frac{1}{2}\ \frac{1}{2}]$
$3 = aa$	$[0\ 1\ 0]$	$[0\ \frac{1}{2}\ \frac{1}{2}]$	$[0\ 0\ 1]$

probability that he transmits a. Then the entries in Table 1 can be generated
quite simply from

$$[p_{st1}\ p_{st2}\ p_{st3}] = [\tau_s \tau_t\ \ \tau_s(1 - \tau_t) + \tau_t(1 - \tau_s)\ \ (1 - \tau_s)(1 - \tau_t)] \quad (2.11)$$

substituting $\tau_{AA} = 1$, $\tau_{Aa} = \frac{1}{2}$, and $\tau_{aa} = 0$, which are the appropriate Mendelian
values if there is no mutation or meiotic drive.

2.3.2. Polygenic and Mixed Inheritance

In the usual additive polygenic model an individual's polygenotype is the
sum of the gametic values he inherits, one from each parent. The population of
gametic values transmitted by any polygenotype, G, is normally distributed with
mean $G/2$ and variance $\sigma_G^2/2$, and any two such gametic values produced by G
have correlation $\frac{1}{2}$. It follows that under random mating the offspring genotypic
distribution conditional on the parental polygenotypes F and G is normally
distributed with mean $(F + G)/2$ and variance $\sigma_G^2/2$; i.e., letting H be the offspring polygenotype, we have

$$p_{FGH} = \phi[H - (F + G)/2, \sigma_G^2/2] \quad (2.12)$$

The distribution for a mixed model containing both monogenic and polygenic components is obtained by multiplying together the two corresponding
distributions, i.e., we can write

$$p_{sF\ tG\ uH} = p_{stu} p_{FGH} \quad (2.13)$$

2.4. Sampling Scheme

2.4.1. Random Sampling

Random sampling implies the existence of a well-defined population of
distinct sampling units, each of which has equal probability of being sampled.
When the sampling unit is a sibship this kind of sampling is, in principle at least,
feasible. All the persons living in a specified geographic area define a population
of distinct sibships (including sibships of single individuals). The fact that some
individuals in this population may have sibs residing outside the specified

geographic area is not critical, as we can define our population of sibships as being comprised of individuals living within the specified area only. We can also define sibships such that half sibs are automatically reckoned as being in different sibships. The important point is that we can define our sampling unit in such a way that every individual in the population belongs to exactly one sampling unit. When this is so, standard sampling methodology can be used to obtain a random sample of sampling units.

But suppose we try to make our sampling unit a larger structure, for example, the nuclear family (parents and offspring). We immediately run into the difficulty that many individuals belong to two such units, since they have both offspring and parents. In order to have a population of distinct nuclear families, and hence make random sampling possible, it becomes necessary to exclude from consideration many of the individuals living in the specified area. There will also be some individuals who have neither offspring nor parents, and so belong to "degenerate" nuclear families. These difficulties become further magnified when an attempt is made to have even larger (pedigree) structures as the sampling unit.

Fortunately, however, it is not necessary to have random sampling in the strict sense in order to make valid statistical inferences, so long as certain conditions hold. Suppose we take a random sample of individuals from the population and call these individuals "random probands." We then augment the sample of random probands by including also some of their relatives. Whether or not some of the original random probands are related to each other, we can sort the final sample out into unrelated family structures. It is then possible to treat this sample of unrelated family structures as though it is a random sample from the population, and this will lead to valid results provided the decision to include the extra relatives, and the number of such extra relatives included for each random proband, are independent of the proband's phenotype. The simplest way to ensure that these conditions hold is to decide beforehand just what types of relatives (e.g., all first-degree relatives, all first- and second-degree relatives) will be included in the sample, provided they exist in the population. If this is done the only possible sources of bias are (i) the existence of certain types of relatives in the population may depend on the random proband's phenotype and (ii) the willingness of individuals to be sampled, whether probands or relatives, may depend on their phenotypes. We shall use the term "random sampling" to denote those situations in which the probands are a random sample from the population and these potential biases do not exist; and assume as a model for the actual sampling scheme random sampling of family units from a large population of similar discrete unrelated family units.

2.4.2. Nonrandom Sampling

Random sampling is not a very efficient way to study the genetics of rare conditions, since it leads to a sample that is largely devoid of individuals with the

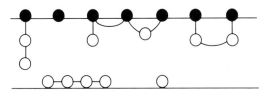

FIGURE 6. Model for ascertainment of families via affected probands. Black circles represent affected individuals; white circles represent unaffected individuals. Only the floating black circles are visible to the sampler; when a black circle is sampled, so also are all the other circles linked to it. [From Batschelet (1963)]

condition and hence largely uninformative. Typically families are selected for study because at least one member of the family has the condition, but the actual sampling scheme used is often poorly defined. Here we shall present a model that has been suggested to describe the kind of nonrandom sampling, or ascertainment via affected probands, that commonly occurs.

Ascertainment was originally considered in terms of a dichotomous trait segregating in sibships (e.g., by Fisher, 1934; Bailey, 1951; Morton 1959), using the model illustrated in Fig. 6. In this model black circles floating on the water represent affected individuals, while white circles that sink down in the water represent unaffected individuals; individuals in the same sibships are linked together. The white circles are invisible to the sampler, who picks black circles (probands) at random, each with equal probability π; and when a black circle is picked, all the circles linked to it are also drawn into the sample. This sampling procedure can be described mathematically by defining a function $\pi(z)$ which specifies the sampling probability that an individual with phenotype z in the population becomes a proband, i.e.,

$$\pi(z) = \begin{cases} \pi & \text{if } z = 1 \\ 0 & \text{if } z = 0 \end{cases} \tag{2.14}$$

In the limit as π tends to 0, the probability that a sibship enters the sample is proportional to the number of affected members it contains; this will be called single ascertainment. When π equals 1, the probability that a sibship enters the sample is independent of the number of affected members it contains, provided it contains at least one affected member; this is called complete ascertainment. The situation where π takes on any other value between 0 and 1 is called multiple ascertainment. The function $\pi(z)$ has been generalized by Elston and Yelverton (1975) to quantitative traits.

In theory this same ascertainment model could be used for sampling larger pedigree structures. We could imagine Fig. 6 to include all the individuals living in a well-defined geographic area, with all related individuals linked together. However, this implies that once a proband is drawn, *all* his relatives living in the specified area, however remote the relationship, are included in the sample;

otherwise (for example, if we take his first- and second-degree relatives only) we have the same problem as before, namely, that the population is not made up of discrete sampling units. Since it is usually impractical to sample all of a proband's relatives — and, furthermore, this would tend to defeat the original purpose of nonrandom sampling — Elston and Sobel (1979) have used the same principle as suggested above for random sampling: the family structures finally sampled for study are assumed to be taken from a similar conceptual population of discrete unrelated family units. However, it is necessary to note that the final sample will often contain individuals who, whatever their phenotype, could never be probands. For example, these could be individuals who live outside the specified geographic area, or who, when probands are chosen from the records of a particular hospital, would go to a different hospital for treatment, if affected; or a sampling scheme may be used whereby only individuals of a certain age or sex could be probands. Elston and Sobel's (1979) model assumes that each individual in the sample can be unequivocally classified as to whether he could or could not be a proband, and they discuss possible ways of achieving this. Other ascertainment models have been recently discussed (Stene, 1977; Cannings and Thompson, 1977; Thompson and Cannings, 1979) but, for those cases where these models would yield theoretically different results, it is not yet clear that they have any practical advantages.

3. The Likelihood Method

Given a mathematical basis for the four components of a segregation analysis model, an expression can be derived for the likelihood of a set of observed data: the probability (or, for continuous data, the density) of the actual observations being associated with the sample, under the assumed model. The likelihood can be thought of as summarizing the information the sample contains with respect to that model. In this section the appropriate likelihood is first derived for randomly sampled data, and then a modification is shown to be necessary when sampling is via probands of a particular phenotype. Since the likelihoods are derived in a general way, the same basic expressions can allow for all the genetic mechanisms that have been discussed so far. In the last part of this section the principles underlying the use of these likelihoods for segregation analysis are discussed.

3.1. Likelihood of Randomly Sampled Data

3.1.1. Nuclear Families and Sibships

First consider a nuclear family of two parents and n children, with k possible genotypes affecting the phenotype. Denote the phenotypes of the father and mother z_f and z_m, respectively, and those of their offspring $z_j (j = 1, 2, \ldots, n)$.

The likelihood that the jth offspring has phenotype z_j, conditional on his having genotype u, is $g_u(z_j)$; and the same likelihood, but conditional on his parents having genotypes s and t, is $\sum_{u=1}^{k} p_{stu} g_u(z_j)$. Now assume that, conditional on their own respective genotypes, the phenotypes of the offspring are independent of one another; then the likelihood for the whole sibship, given the parents' genotypes are s and t, is

$$\prod_{j=1}^{n} \sum_{u=1}^{k} p_{stu} g_u(z_j) \tag{3.1}$$

It is to be understood that the summation over u in this expression is performed separately for each offspring, and the sums are then multiplied together. From now on symbols such as Π_j and Σ_u will be written, since the limits will be clear.

Under random mating the likelihood for the two parents can be written as

$$\sum_s \psi_s g_s(z_f) \sum_t \psi_t g_t(z_m) \tag{3.2}$$

which is the sum of k^2 terms, each term corresponding to a particular mating type $s \times t$. Multiplying each term in this sum by the likelihood for the sibship conditional on s and t, i.e., expression (3.1), we arrive at the likelihood for the whole nuclear family:

$$\sum_s \psi_s g_s(z_f) \sum_t \psi_t g_t(z_m) \prod_j \sum_u p_{stu} g_u(z_j) \tag{3.3}$$

This expression assumes that, conditional on their genotypes, the phenotypes of all the family members are mutually independent; in other words it assumes that there are no environmentally caused correlations among the phenotypes.

The likelihood under a completely additive polygenic model is the same, except that ψ_s and ψ_t are replaced by ψ_F and ψ_G, p_{stu} is replaced by p_{FGH}, and integration replaces summations. Thus, using the results given earlier, expressions (3.2) and (3.3) become, respectively,

$$\int_{-\infty}^{\infty} \phi(F, \sigma_G^2) g_F(z_f) \int_{-\infty}^{\infty} \phi(G, \sigma_G^2) g_G(z_m) dG \, dF \tag{3.4}$$

and

$$\int_{-\infty}^{\infty} \phi(F, \sigma_G^2) g_F(z_f) \int_{-\infty}^{\infty} \phi(G, \sigma_G^2) g_G(z_m) \prod_j \int_{-\infty}^{\infty} \phi[H - (F + G)/2, \sigma_G^2/2] g_H(z_j) dH \, dG \, dF \tag{3.5}$$

In this expression there is a separate integration over H for each offspring, just as in expression (3.3) there is a separate summation over u for each offspring.

Similarly, if the model contains both monogenic and polygenic components, we can combine expressions (3.2) and (3.3) to obtain, for the two parents,

$$\sum_s \psi_s \int_{-\infty}^{\infty} \phi(F, \sigma_G^2) g_{sF}(z_f) \sum_t \psi_t \int_{-\infty}^{\infty} \phi(G, \sigma_G^2) g_{tG}(z_m) dG \, dF \tag{3.6}$$

and we can combine expressions (3.3) and (3.5) to obtain, for the whole nuclear family

$$\sum_s \psi_s \int_{-\infty}^{\infty} \phi(F, \sigma_G^2) g_{sF}(z_f) \sum_t \psi_t \int_{-\infty}^{\infty} \phi(G, \sigma_G^2) g_{tG}(z_m) \times$$

$$\prod_j \sum_u p_{stu} \int_{-\infty}^{\infty} \phi[H - (F + G)/2, \sigma_G^2/2] g_{uH}(z_j) dH \, dG \, dF \qquad (3.7)$$

All these likelihoods assume that, conditional on their genotypes, the phenotypes of the individuals in the family are mutually independent. Morton and MacLean (1974) introduced a model in which, in addition to both monogenic and polygenic inheritance, there is an environmental component, C, common to all members of the same sibships; furthermore, C is assumed to be normally distributed among sibships with mean 0 and variance σ_C^2. The likelihood for the parents under this model is still (3.6); but that for the whole nuclear family is slightly different from (3.7), the factor in the second line being modified:

$$\sum_s \psi_s \int_{-\infty}^{\infty} \phi(F, \sigma_G^2) g_{sF}(z_f) \sum_t \psi_t \int_{-\infty}^{\infty} \phi(G, \sigma_G^2) g_{tG}(z_m) \times$$

$$\int_{-\infty}^{\infty} \phi(C, \sigma_C^2) \prod_j \sum_u p_{stu} \int_{-\infty}^{\infty} \phi[H - (F + G)/2, \sigma_G^2/2] g_{uHC}(z_j) dH \, dC \, dG \, dF \qquad (3.8)$$

where $g_{uHC}(z_j)$ is the probability density function of z_j conditional on monogenotype u, polygenotype H, and common environment C. Under this model the total environmental variance σ_E^2 is partitioned into σ_C^2 and a residual σ_R^2. Thus if, for a dichotomous trait, $g_{tG}(1) = \Phi[(G - \theta_t)/\sigma_E]$ for a parent, then for an offspring

$$g_{uHC}(1) = \Phi[(C + H - \theta_u)/\sigma_R] \qquad (3.9)$$

Similarly for a quantitative trait, corresponding to $g_{tG}(z) = \phi(G + \mu_t - z, \sigma_E^2)$ for a parent, we have for an offspring

$$g_{uHC}(z) = \phi(C + H + \mu_u - z, \sigma_R^2) \qquad (3.10)$$

In all of the above cases, the likelihood of a set of independent nuclear families is simply the product of the likelihoods for each of the separate families. If, however, members of two different nuclear families are in any way related, these two families should be considered as part of a single pedigree structure, including if necessary linking individuals whose phenotypes are unknown: all such individuals must be included in the likelihood that will now be derived, with $g(z)$ for them being set equal to unity whenever they occur.

3.1.2. Pedigrees

So far an individual's phenotype has been denoted z. It will now be convenient, following Elston and Stewart (1971), to use two different symbols for phenotype, corresponding to the two different kinds of individuals who can

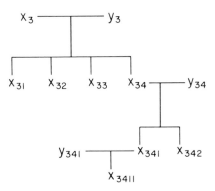

FIGURE 7. Illustration of the notation for the phenotypes of the members of a pedigree: this is the third pedigree ($i_o = 3$) in a set of pedigrees. [From Elston and Rao (1978)].

appear in a simple pedigree – a pedigree which contains no loops and starts with a single set of original parents. Persons who are related to someone in a previous generation of the pedigree will have their phenotype denoted x, and unrelated persons "marrying into" the pedigree will have their phenotypes denoted y. In the case of the original parents, however, one will be arbitrarily denoted x and the other y.

It is also convenient to use subscripts on subscripts to denote the generation, starting with o for the original generation. Let the phenotypes of the original parents of the i_oth pedigree be x_{i_o} and y_{i_o}; let the phenotype of their i_1th child be $x_{i_o i_1}$, and let his or her spouse's phenotype be $y_{i_o i_1}$; similarly let the phenotype of the i_2th child of this i_1th child be $x_{i_o i_1 i_2}$, and that of his or her spouse $y_{i_o i_1 i_2}$, and so on. This notation is illustrated in Fig. 7.

If we now rewrite expression (3.3) in this new notation for the i_oth set of parents, at the same time using subscripts s_o and t_o to indicate genotypes in the original generation, and s_1 (replacing u) for genotypes in the offspring generation, we obtain

$$\sum_{s_o} \psi_{s_o} g_{s_o}(x_{i_o}) \sum_{t_o} \psi_{t_o} g_{t_o}(y_{i_o}) \prod_{i_1} \sum_{s_1} p_{s_o t_o s_1} g_{s_1}(x_{i_o i_1}) \qquad (3.11)$$

Thus the joint likelihood of a set of independent nuclear families can be written as the product of this expression over i_o. Furthermore, if we define the operator

$$\Gamma_j = \prod_{ij} \sum_{s_j} p_{s_{j-1} t_{j-1} s_j} g_{s_j}(x_{i_o i_1 \ldots ij}) \sum_{t_j} \psi_{t_j} g_{t_j}(y_{i_o i_1 \ldots ij}) \qquad (3.12)$$

the likelihood for a set of simple pedigrees of any number of generations can be written as the sequence of operations $\Gamma_o(\Gamma_1(\Gamma_2(\Gamma_3 \ldots)))$, provided we define $p_{s_{j-1} t_{j-1} s_j} = \psi_{s_o}$ when $j = 0$.

In the same manner, we can define Γ_j for the polygenic model as

$$\prod_{ij} \int_{F_j} \phi[F_j - (F_{j-1} + G_{j-1})/2, \sigma_G^2/2] g_{F_j}(x_{i_o i_1} \ldots ij) \int_{G_j} \phi(G_j, \sigma_G^2) g_{G_j}(y_{i_1 i_2} \ldots ij)$$
$$(3.13)$$

where the symbol $\int_F$ indicates integration of everything following it with respect to F from minus infinity to plus infinity; then the likelihood of a pedigree under the polygenic model is similarly given by the sequence of operations Γ_j, provided we now replace $\phi[F_j - (F_{j-1} + G_{j-1})/2, \sigma_G^2/2]$ by $\phi(F_o, \sigma_G^2)$ when $j = 0$.

The likelihood under a model that contains both monogenic and polygenic components is obtained by defining Γ_j to be a combination of expressions (3.12) and (3.13), analogous to the way in which expression (3.7) is a combination of expressions (3.3) and (3.5); and the modification to allow for an environmental correlation within sibships can similarly be incorporated, analogous to expression (3.8).

The approach followed here to derive the likelihood of a simple pedigree can be extended to allow for twins and half sibships (Elston and Yelverton, 1975); it can also be extended, for an oligogenic model, to allow for arbitrary pedigree structures (Lange and Elston, 1975; Cannings, Thompson, and Skolnick 1978).

3.2. Likelihood when Sampling via Selected Probands

3.2.1. Conditioning on the Parental Phenotypes

If our sample consists of independent nuclear families, each of which is ascertained via one or more probands with a particular phenotypic condition, and if in every case the proband is a parent, there is a relatively simple way of constructing a likelihood that will yield valid results when using the general maximum-likelihood procedures that will be described later. All one need do is to take, instead of one of the likelihoods just derived, the likelihood for the phenotypes of the sibship conditional on the phenotypes of the two parents. For a single family this conditional likelihood is equal to expression (3.3) divided by expression (3.2) for a monogenic model; to expression (3.5) divided by expression (3.4) for a polygenic model; and to expressions (3.7) or (3.8) divided by expression (3.6) for mixed monogenic and polygenic models, according to whether a sibling environmental correlation is assumed absent or present. If, furthermore, the model is such that each parent can only have one genotype, then there is only one term in the numerator of each such quotient, and the denominator is a constant that can be factored out. This is the basis for many of the early segregation analyses of data on sibships ascertained through the parents, in which it is commonly assumed that the parental mating type is known.

3.2.2. Conditioning on the Sampling Model

Although there may be easier ways to obtain a likelihood that will give rise to valid results, the most informative likelihood will in general be the one that gives the probability (or density) of the sampled data conditional on the exact manner in which that sampling took place. This can be derived for any pedigree, if we can assume the sampling model proposed by Elston and Sobel (1979), as follows.

Let L(pedigree $|\geq 1$ proband) be the likelihood of the pedigree conditional on it containing at least one proband among those individuals in it who could be probands: this is thus the likelihood we need. Then we have

$$L(\text{pedigree} \,|\geq 1 \text{ proband}) = L(\text{pedigree}) \cdot \frac{L(\geq 1 \text{ proband} \,|\, \text{pedigree})}{L(\geq 1 \text{ proband})} \quad (3.14)$$

where L(pedigree) is the likelihood of the pedigree phenotypes assuming that the pedigree has been randomly sampled from a population of pedigrees of the same size and structure; $L(\geq 1$ proband $|$ pedigree) is the likelihood that the pedigree, given the phenotypes of the individuals who could be probands, contains at least one proband; and $L(\geq 1$ proband) is the likelihood that an arbitrary pedigree of the same size and structure contains at least one proband among those whose particular positions are occupied by individuals who could be probands. We have already derived expressions for L(pedigree) under various models, so we now consider the correction factor by which this is multiplied on the right side of Eq. (3.14).

Suppose there are n individuals in the pedigree who could be probands, with phenotypes denoted $z_i (i = 1, 2, \ldots, n)$, and m individuals who could not, with phenotypes denoted $z_j^* (j = 1, 2, \ldots, m)$. Let the proband status of the ith individual who could be a proband be b_i: $b_i = 1$ if that individual is a proband, $b_i = 0$ if not. Furthermore define an ascertainment function $\alpha(z, b)$ for each individual who could be a proband as follows: $\alpha(z, 0) = 1 - \pi(z), \alpha(z, 1) = \pi(z)$. Then (assuming independent ascertainments) the joint likelihood of all the proband statuses observed, conditional on the phenotypes in the pedigree, is

$$L(\text{proband statuses} \,|\, \text{pedigree}) = \prod_{i=1}^{n} \alpha(z_i, b_i) \quad (3.15)$$

and hence the numerator of the correction factor is

$$L(\geq 1 \text{ proband} \,|\, \text{pedigree}) = 1 - \prod_{i=1}^{n} \alpha(z_i, 0) = 1 - \prod_{i=1}^{n} [1 - \pi(z_i)] \quad (3.16)$$

The denominator is obtained by summing the whole numerator in Eq. (3.14) over all possible phenotypes for each individual, i.e.,

$$L(\geq 1 \text{ proband}) = \sum_{z_1} \cdots \sum_{z_n} \sum_{z_1^*} \cdots \sum_{z_m^*} L(\text{pedigree}) L(\geq 1 \text{ proband} \,|\, \text{pedigree}) \quad (3.17)$$

(If z is continuous, the summations are replaced by integrations.)

Substitution of expressions (3.16) and (3.17) into (3.14) yields basically the same likelihood as has been commonly used, for the simple case of sibships ascertained through affected children, when the parental mating type is assumed known. For the case where the parental mating type is not known, Elandt-Johnson (1971) and Morton and MacLean (1974) have proposed that the likelihood should be further conditioned on the parental phenotypes; but this can be expected to lead to a loss of information (Go, Elston, and Kaplan, 1978). Prior to Elston and Sobel (1979), however, it appears never to have been suggested that account should be taken of which individuals could, and which individuals could not, be probands.

3.3. Parameter Estimation and Testing Hypotheses

3.3.1. General Principles

There are different statistical methods of estimating parameters and testing hypotheses, but the method most commonly used in segregation analysis is that based on maximum likelihood. Maximum-likelihood estimates of parameters are those values of the parameters that make the likelihood a maximum. They may not be unique, nor may they even exist for permissable values of the parameters. A variance, for example, must be positive; but the likelihood may be maximized by a negative value of a variance.

Provided they occur at a mathematical maximum of the likelihood, all maximum-likelihood estimates enjoy the following properties asymptotically, i.e., as the size of the sample increases without bound. First, they are unbiased — the mean of many such estimates is equal to the true value of the parameter being estimated. Second, they are efficient — the variance of many such estimates is the smallest possible for any asymptotically unbiased estimate. Third, the estimates are normally distributed, and this fact can be used to obtain approximate confidence limits for the estimates.

To test a null hypothesis under a particular model we can use the likelihood ratio criterion, which is the ratio of the maximum value of the likelihood under the null hypothesis to the maximum value of the likelihood under the model. Each null hypothesis corresponds to one or more restrictions being placed on the model, and hence leads to a smaller maximum likelihood. The smaller the likelihood ratio, the less likely is the null hypothesis to be true; the test thus consists of rejecting the null hypothesis, at a specified significance level, if this ratio is smaller than a certain quantity. Asymptotically, if the null hypothesis is true, minus twice the natural logarithm of the likelihood ratio is distributed as a chi-square, the number of degrees of freedom being the difference in the number of independent parameters over which the likelihood is maximized in the denominator and numerator, respectively; i.e., the number of degrees of freedom is equal to the number of independent restrictions corresponding to the particular null hypothesis. The null hypothesis is rejected if this statistic is greater than the appropriate tabulated value of chi-square.

Maximizing the likelihood, with or without restrictions, is a computational problem that can be tackled numerically in various ways. It is important to note that the likelihood surface may have several local maxima, and there is no general way of knowing how many such maxima exist. In practice it is often necessary to search for more than one local maximum whenever a particular hypothesis is tested. When, after appropriate hypothesis testing, a decision is arrived at regarding the most appropriate genetic mechanism, the final parameter estimates quoted should be those obtained on assuming that particular mechanism as the underlying model.

The method of maximum likelihood has intuitive appeal, as well as theoretical justification asymptotically. All results based on it, however, are model dependent; they are only valid if the assumed model does in fact allow as a possibility, at least approximately, the actual mechanism underlying the variability in the data. If the model is wrong, the result of any test may be meaningless: the test may be either invalid or powerless. Furthermore there are inherent difficulties in interpreting analyses of nonexperimental data (Kempthorne, 1978). For these reasons caution is necessary in drawing conclusions from segregation analysis.

3.3.2. Testing Genetic Hypotheses

If we assume one of the general genetic models discussed above — monogenic, polygenic, or mixed monogenic and polygenic — we can use these principles and the corresponding likelihoods to test various relevant hypotheses. Under a monogenic model of two alleles at one autosomal locus, for example, the hypothesis of Hardy–Weinberg equilibrium proportions, i.e., the hypothesis that the genotypic distribution is given by $\psi_{AA} = q^2$, $\psi_{Aa} = 2q(1-q)$, and $\psi_{aa} = (1-q)^2$, corresponds to the restriction

$$\psi_{Aa} = 2(\psi_{AA}\,\psi_{aa})^{1/2} \tag{3.18}$$

which can be tested via a chi-square statistic with one degree of freedom. The hypothesis of dominance corresponds to one of the two restrictions

$$g_{Aa}(z) = g_{AA}(z), \qquad \text{or} \qquad g_{Aa}(z) = g_{aa}(z) \tag{3.19}$$

which can also be tested via a chi-square statistic with one degree of freedom if $g_{Aa}(z)$ differs from $g_{AA}(z)$ or $g_{aa}(z)$ with respect to only one parameter.

The mixed model of monogenic and polygenic inheritance is a particularly interesting one, since under it one can attempt to test "what is possibly the single most important question concerning the inheritance of any character: is most of the genetic variation due to one locus, or are many gene loci necessarily involved?" (Elston and Stewart, 1971). Thus, using the likelihood (3.7) and assuming just three major genotypes, absence of segregation at a major locus corresponds to either of the set of restrictions

$$g_{AA\ G}(z) = g_{Aa\ G}(z) = g_{aa\ G}(z), \qquad \text{or} \qquad \psi_{AA} = \psi_{Aa} = 0 \tag{3.20}$$

and absence of polygenic inheritance corresponds to the restriction

$$\sigma_G^2 = 0 \tag{3.21}$$

If, furthermore, a sibling environmental correlation is also incorporated into the model [using (3.8)], absence of such a correlation corresponds to the restriction

$$\sigma_C^2 = 0 \tag{3.22}$$

Unfortunately, the application of such a mixed model to large pedigrees is not yet computationally feasible. There is, however, a way of generalizing to pedigrees the classical tests for Mendelian segregation in sibships. The usual test for a rare autosomal dominant gene is to consider the segregation ratio in sibships where one parent is affected, assuming the parental mating type is $Aa \times aa$; thus the Mendelian null hypothesis that is tested is $p_{Aa\ aa\ aa} = p_{Aa\ aa\ Aa} = \frac{1}{2}$. Similarly for a rare autosomal recessive, assuming the parental mating type is $Aa \times Aa$, the null hypothesis that is tested is $p_{Aa\ Aa\ aa} = \frac{1}{4}$. In terms of transmission probabilities, both these null hypotheses correspond to the restriction $\tau_{Aa\ A} = \frac{1}{2}$. Thus Elston and Stewart (1971) suggest that the likelihood under a two-allele one-locus autosomal model be parametrized in terms of the three transmission probabilities, as given in Eq. (2.11), and Mendelian segregation be tested by the null hypothesis

$$\left.\begin{array}{rcl} \tau_{AA} & = & 1 \\[2mm] \tau_{Aa} & = & \frac{1}{2} \\[2mm] \tau_{aa} & = & 0 \end{array}\right\} \tag{3.23}$$

against the unrestricted model in which the transmission probabilities can take on any values between zero and unity. The advantage of this test lies in the fact that the model includes the possibility that the offspring phenotypes are distributed independently of their parents' phenotypes, a hypothesis that corresponds to the restrictions

$$\tau_{AA\ A} = \tau_{Aa\ A} = \tau_{aa\ A} \tag{3.24}$$

Under this general model it is always possible for there to be three types of individuals in the population, AA, Aa, and aa, and for these to have different phenotypic distributions: thus under the hypothesis (3.24) the individuals in a pedigree can come from a mixture of phenotypic distributions, even though there is no genetic transmission from one generation to the next. When segregation at a major locus is tested by the null hypothesis (3.20) under a mixed model, however, there is the critical assumption that, conditional on polygenotype G, $g_{tG}(z)$ accurately represents the phenotypic distribution of z. It follows that this test for monogenic segregation is very sensitive to nonnormality if it is used together with the assumption that $g_{tG}(z)$ is a normal distribution (MacLean, Morton, and Lew, 1975).

4. Examples of Segregation Analysis

In this section two recent examples of segregation analysis are described to illustrate the use of the segregation analysis models derived above. The first example concerns the inheritance of a quantitative trait, serum cholesterol level, in a single large pedigree; it shows how in this pedigree segregation analysis strongly suggested that much of the variability of this trait is due to monogenic inheritance, a finding that has more recently been confirmed by linkage analysis (Elston, Namboodiri, Go, Siervogel, and Glueck, 1976). The second example reexamines the inheritance of the ability to taste phenylthiocarbamide (PTC); it shows that a single-gene mode of inheritance is confirmed, with no evidence for residual polygenic variation or sibling environmental correlation.

4.1. Segregation of Hypercholesterolemia in a Large Pedigree

Elston, Namboodiri, Glueck, Fallat, Tsang, and Leuba (1975) investigated a 195-member pedigree, extending over five generations, for the transmission of hypercholesterolemia and hypertriglyceridemia; here we shall review the analysis they performed as it refers to elevated serum cholesterol levels. The pedigree was ascertained through four related probands, all of whom were separately referred and studied within a four-week period; two had elevated cholesterol levels, and two were referred for evaluation because of a strong family history of premature death from myocardial infarction, which is associated with elevated cholesterol levels. The 195 individuals whose cholesterol levels were analyzed included only one of these probands, who thus represented a very small fraction of 40 or so others with elevated cholesterol levels. For this reason, and to simplify the computations, the pedigree was analyzed as though it had been randomly sampled, ignoring the trivial bias in the segregation ratios that might be induced by the nonrandom sampling. It was recognized, however, that the estimate of gene frequency obtained is biased upward: it represents the gene frequency of the y individuals *in this pedigree*, rather than in the population from which the pedigree was sampled.

The first step in the analysis ignored the pedigree structure, assuming the data to come from a random sample of individuals. There was no significant sex effect, but there was a significant effect of age. Linear regression of log cholesterol on age was found to account for a larger fraction of the total variance than linear regression of cholesterol on age, and empirical cumulative plots indicated that a log-normal distribution fits the data better than a normal distribution. All further analyses were therefore conducted on the log cholesterol values. Figure 8 shows a cumulative plot of these values, adjusted to age 30, together with the best fitting single log-normal distribution and the best fitting

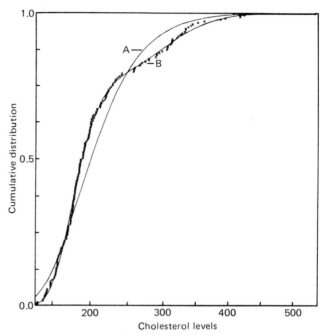

FIGURE 8. Empirical and theoretical cumulative plots of the kindred sample when one
normal (A) and a mixture of two normal distributions (B) are fitted to $\log_e$ cholesterol
values (after adjusting to age 30 by linear regression). The ordinate for the data points is
rank/196; the original scale of cholesterol values is used as abscissa. [From Elston et al.
1975)]

Table 2. Maximum Likelihood Estimates Obtained from 195 $\log_e$ Cholesterol
Values When (i) Assumed to be a Random Sample from a Mixture of Two
Distributions; (ii) Assumed to be Generated by Dominant Mendelian
Inheritance; and (iii) Assumed to Follow a Model with Arbitrary Transmission
Probabilities. All Mean Values Adjusted to Age 30. [Adapted from Elston et al.
(1975)]

	(i)	(ii)	(iii)
Mean of higher distribution (μ_{AA} and μ_{Aa})	5.748	5.755	5.754
Mean of lower distribution (μ_{aa})	5.151	5.161	5.159
Common standard deviation (σ_E)	0.170	0.167	0.167
Proportion in higher distribution ($\psi_{AA} + \psi_{Aa}$)	0.215	0.102	0.097
Proportion in lower distribution (ψ_{aa})	0.785	0.898	0.903
Linear regression coefficient on age (β)	0.005	0.005	0.005

mixture of two log-normal distributions. It is clear that a mixture of two distributions fits much better ($P < 0.001$), and the estimates of the parameters of this
mixture, together with the regression coefficient used for age adjustment, are
given in column (i) of Table 2.

The segregation analysis was based on a pedigree likelihood that utilized the operation (3.12) with the following parameter specification of the component functions:

(i) p_{stu} were functions of the three transmission probabilities, as indicated in Eq. (2.11).

(ii) ψ_t were the three parameters ψ_{AA}, ψ_{Aa}, ψ_{aa}; but since they must add to unity, these represent only two independent parameters.

(iii) $g_t(z)$ was taken to be $\phi(\mu_t + \beta a - z, \sigma_E^2)$, where a is age and z is log cholesterol; this function thus depended on five independent parameters: μ_{AA}, μ_{Aa}, μ_{aa}, σ_E^2, and β, the linear regression coefficient on age.

First the fit of Hardy–Weinberg equilibrium proportions to the data was tested, i.e., (3.18). Since there was no significant departure from this hypothesis, it was assumed when conducting the later tests. Then the hypothesis of dominance, (3.19), was tested. Two local maxima were found on the likelihood surface, one corresponding to the higher levels of cholesterol being dominant, the other corresponding to their being recessive. In neither case did the likelihood become significantly larger when μ_{Aa} was estimated as a separate parameter, but here again there were two corresponding maxima. However, the hypothesis that the distribution with higher mean is composed of two dominant genotypes gave a much larger likelihood (by a factor of 640), and so this was assumed in testing the hypothesis of Mendelian segregation, namely, (3.23). Twice the difference between the two log likelihoods for this test was found to be 1.05, which, when compared to the chi-square distribution with three degrees of freedom, is not significant. Finally the hypothesis of no genetic transmission from one generation to the next, i.e., (3.24), was tested: there was found to be a highly significant departure from this hypothesis ($P < 0.001$).

Columns (ii) and (iii) of Table 2 show the maximum-likelihood estimates obtained, assuming Hardy–Weinberg equilibrium and dominance, respectively when Mendelian transmission probabilities are assumed and when the transmission probabilities are estimated to maximize the likelihood. The estimates are seen to be remarkably similar to each other, as well as to the estimates obtained when pedigree structure is ignored [column (i)]. The greatest discrepancy is in the proportions, which in any case may be expected to differ: the values in the first column are estimates of the proportions among all 195 individuals, whereas those in the last two columns (which are very similar to each other) are estimates of the proportions among the y individuals only. The similarities in this table strongly support, but do not prove, that a single dominant gene accounts for much of the variability in cholesterol levels in this family. But, as pointed out by Elston et al. (1975), this analysis does not deny the possibility that there may be polygenic variation or environmentally caused correlations among relatives.

4.2. Segregation of Phenylthiocarbamide (PTC) Taste Sensitivity

Rao and Morton (1977) performed segregation analysis of PTC taste sensitivity among a total of 4335 individuals distributed in nuclear families – 2090 parents and 2245 children. The method of Morton and MacLean (1974) was used, i.e., the analysis was based on the likelihood of the children's phenotypes conditional on their parents' phenotypes, expression (3.8) divided by expression (3.6), with the following specifications:

   (i) p_{stu} were fixed at their Mendelian values for two alleles at one autosomal locus.

   (ii) ψ_t were functions of the gene frequency, Hardy–Weinberg equilibrium being assumed.

   (iii) $\bar{g}_{tG}(z)$ were taken to be as given in (2.8), together with the assumption (2.6); they thus involve six independent parameters: $\mu_{AA}, \mu_{Aa}, \mu_{aa}, \theta_1, \theta_2$, and σ_E. However, it was assumed with no loss of generality that the underlying liability has mean zero ($\psi_{AA}\mu_{AA} + \psi_{Aa}\mu_{Aa} + \psi_{aa}\mu_{aa} = 0$) and variance 1 ($\psi_{AA}\mu_{AA}^2 + \psi_{Aa}\mu_{Aa}^2 + \psi_{aa}\mu_{aa}^2 + \sigma_G^2 + \sigma_E^2 = 1$).

   (iv) $g_{uHC}(z)$ were taken to be as given in (3.9), but generalized to a trichotomy as in (2.6) and (2.8), i.e.,

$$g_{uHC}(2) = \Phi[(C + H + \mu_u - \theta_2)/\sigma_R]$$

$$g_{uHC}(1) = \Phi[(C + H + \mu_u - \theta_1)/\sigma_R] - \Phi[(C + H + \mu_u - \theta_2)/\sigma_R]$$

$$g_{uHC}(0) = 1 - \Phi[(C + H + \mu_u - \theta_1)/\sigma_R]$$

where $\sigma_R^2 = \sigma_E^2 - \sigma_C^2$.

Given these assumptions, there are seven independent unknown parameters in the model. However, by assuming that the population prevalences of the three phenotypes are known, there are only five independent unknown parameters; in other words the thresholds θ_1 and θ_2 that separate the nontaster, intermediate, and taster phenotypes are implicitly defined by the other parameters and the prevalences

$$\sum_t \psi_t \int_{-\infty}^{\infty} \phi(G, \sigma_G^2) g_{tG}(2) dG \qquad \text{for tasters}$$

and

$$\sum_t \psi_t \int_{-\infty}^{\infty} \phi(G, \sigma_G^2) g_{tG}(1) dG \qquad \text{for intermediates}$$

Table 3 gives the parametrization used by MacLean and Morton, together with the corresponding quantities in the notation developed here. It should be noted that Rao and Morton call B "sibling environmental correlation," a term that is better reserved for the quantity σ_C^2/σ_E^2.

When all five parameters are estimated simultaneously it is found that $\sigma_C^2 = 0$, and so this is assumed in the following tests. Absence of segregation at a

Table 3. Parameters and Notation Used by MacLean and Morton (1974), with Equivalent Notation Used Here; It Is Assumed That Liability Has Mean 0 and Variance 1

	Notation	
Parameter	MacLean and Morton	Here
Polygenic heritability	H	σ_G^2
Relative variance due to common environment	B	σ_C^2
Gene frequency at major locus	q	$\psi_{AA}^{1/2} = 1 - \psi_{aa}^{1/2}$
Displacement at major locus	t	$\mu_{AA} - \mu_{aa}$
Degree of dominance at major locus	d	$(\mu_{Aa} - \mu_{aa})/(\mu_{AA} - \mu_{aa})$

major locus is tested in the presence of polygenic inheritance by the hypothesis (3.20), i.e., $t = d = 0$ or $q = 0$, leading to a chi-square value of 33.6. It is not clear whether this should be compared to the tabulated chi-square with one or two degrees of freedom, but in any case it is highly significant, indicating that under this model we cannot assume absence of a major locus. On the other hand it is found that the hypotheses $H = d = 0$ and $H = B = d = 0$ both give rise to a chi-square value of 0.61, which is not significant whether compared to the tabulated chi-square with two or three degrees of freedom; this indicates that under this model there is no evidence for any polygenic inheritance or departure from complete dominance of the taster allele.

This study thus provides strong support for the monogenic hypothesis that has been previously based on the following classical evidence: bimodality of the taste threshold distribution in the population, rarity of taster children from two nontaster parents, and agreement with Snyder's ratio when the threshold distribution is dichotomized at its antimode. Rao and Morton note that such evidence is not beyond cavil, but conclude that their mixed model analysis "demonstrates that in this population skepticism about simple recessivity on the liability scale is unwarranted." However, although this analysis is far superior to any previous segregation analysis of taste sensitivity, it must be recognized that the results do depend on certain assumptions, in particular that conditional on genotype the phenotypic distributions are given by equations (2.8) and (2.6). It is conceivable, but highly unlikely, that this is a critical assumption; and one can never be absolutely certain that in a particular situation Mendelian segregation is not being simulated by an environmental mechanism.

5. Conclusion

Segregation analysis has seen many advances in the last decade, both in the generality of the statistical models used and in the complexity of the family structures to which it is applied. This review has been an attempt to bring these advances together into a coherent statement of the art at the present time.

Comparing current methods with the classical methods of segregation analysis, there have been three major changes: the phenotype that is studied no longer need be a dichotomy, the underlying statistical model need not be dependent on just one or two parameters, and the analysis need not be restricted to data on sibships. All these changes can be correlated with the availability of increasingly powerful methods of computation, in terms of both computer hardware and computer software. Computer technology is still advancing exponentially, and we can expect newer and better methods of segregation analysis to follow quickly. Two areas in which advances may be expected in the near future are the incorporation of more environmental correlations into segregation analysis models (Boyle and Elston, 1979; Cannings, Thompson, and Skolnick, this volume), and the use of multivariate phenotypes to define single-gene effects (Weiss, 1976; Goldin, Elston, Graham, and Miller, 1980). With these elaborations we can expect segregation analysis to be even more useful in the detection of major genes. It must always be remembered, however, that segregation analysis is but one tool at the geneticist's disposal, and that its use is limited unless complemented by other methodologies such as linkage and/or biochemical analysis.

References

Bailey, N. T. J. (1951), A classification of methods of ascertainment and analysis in estimating the frequencies of recessives in man, *Ann. Eug.* **16**:223–225.

Batschelet, E. (1963), Testing hypotheses and estimating parameters in human genetics if the age of onset is random, *Biometrika* **50**:265–279.

Boyle, C. R., and Elston, R. C. (1979), Multifactorial genetic models for quantitative traits in humans, *Biometrics* **35**:55–68.

Cannings, C., and Thompson, E. A. (1977), Ascertainment in the sequential sampling of pedigrees, *Clin. Genet.* **12**:208–212.

Cannings, C., Thompson, E. A., and Skolnick, M. H. (1978), Probability functions on complex pedigrees, *Adv. Appl. Probab.* **10**:26–61.

Curnow, R. N. (1974), The use of additional information in estimating disease risks from family histories, *Biometrics* **30**:655–665.

Elandt-Johnson, R. C. (1971), Complex segregation analysis. II. Multiple classification, *Am. J. Hum. Genet.* **23**:17–32.

Elandt-Johnson, R. C. (1974), Segregation analysis: An overview, in, *Proceedings of the 9th International Biometrics Conference, Constanta, Romania* (L. C. A. Corsten and T. Postelnicu, eds.), pp. 313–323. Academiei Republicii Socialiste Romania.

Elston, R. C. (1973), Discussion to symposium on schizophrenia: methodologies in human behavior genetics, *Soc. Biol.* **20**:276–279.

Elston, R. C., and Rao, D. C. (1978), Statistical modeling and analysis in human genetics, *Ann. Rev. Biophys. Bioeng.* **7**:253–286.

Elston, R. C., and Sobel, E. (1979), Sampling considerations in the gathering and analysis of pedigree data, *Am. J. Hum. Genet.* **31**:62–69.

Elston, R. C., and Stewart, J. (1971), A general model for the genetic analysis of pedigree data, *Hum. Hered.* **21**:523–542.

Elston, R. C., and Yelverton, K. C. (1975), General models for segregation analysis, *Am. J. Hum. Genet.* **27**:31–45.

Elston, R. C., Namboodiri, K. K., Glueck, C. J., Fallat, R., Tsang, R., and Leuba, V. (1975), Study of the genetic transmission of hypercholesterolemia and hypertriglyceridemia in a 195 member kindred, *Ann. Hum. Genet.* **39**:67–87.

Elston, R. C., Namboodiri, K. K., Go, R. C. P., Siervogel, R. M., and Glueck, C. J. (1976), Probable linkage between essential familial hypercholesterolemia and C3, in *Baltimore Conference (1975): Third International Workshop on Human Gene Mapping,* Vol. 12, pp. 294–297, Birth Defects: Original Article Series, 1976, The National Foundation, New York.

Falconer, D. C. (1965), The inheritance of liability to certain diseases, estimated from the incidence among relatives, *Ann. Hum. Genet.* **29**:51–76.

Fisher, R. A. (1934), The effect of methods of ascertainment upon the estimation of frequencies, *Ann. Eugen.* **6**:13–25.

Go, R. C. P., Elston, R. C., and Kaplan, E. B. (1978), Efficiency and robustness of pedigree segregation analysis, *Am. J. Hum. Genet.* **30**:28–37.

Goldin, L. R., Elston, R. C., Graham, J. B., and Miller, C. H. (1980), Genetic analysis of Von Willebrand's disease in two large pedigrees: a multivariate approach, *Am. J. Med. Genet.*, in press.

Kempthorne, O. (1978), Logical, epistemological and statistical aspects of nature-nurture data interpretation, *Biometrics* **34**:1–23.

Lange, K., and Elston, R. C. (1975), Extensions to pedigree analysis. I. Likelihood calculations for simple and complex pedigrees, *Hum. Hered.* **25**:95–105.

MacLean, C. J., Morton, N. E., and Lew, R. (1975), Analysis of family resemblance. IV. Operational characteristics of segregation analysis, *Am. J. Hum. Genet.* **27**:365–384.

Morton, N. E. (1959), Genetic tests under incomplete ascertainment, *Am. J. Hum. Genet.* **11**:1–16.

Morton, N. E. (1962), Segregation and linkage, in *Methodology in Human Genetics* (J. Burdette, ed.) pp. 17–52, Holden-Day, San Francisco.

Morton, N. E. (1964), Models and evidence in human population genetics, in, *Genetics Today (Proceedings of the XI International Congress of Genetics, The Hague, The Netherlands, 1963)* (S. J. Geerts, ed.), pp. 935–951, Pergamon Press, Oxford.

Morton, N. E. (1969), Segregation analysis, in, *Computer Applications in Genetics* (N. E. Morton, ed.), pp. 129–139, University of Hawaii Press, Honolulu.

Morton, N. E., and MacLean, C. J. (1974), Analysis of family resemblance III. Complex segregation analysis of quantitative traits, *Am. J. Hum. Genet.* **26**:489–503.

Rao, D. C., and Morton, N. E. (1977), Residual family resemblance for PTC taste sensitivity, *Hum. Genet.* **36**:317–320.

Reich, T., James, J. W., and Morris, C. A. (1972), The use of multiple thresholds in determining the mode of transmission of semi-continuous traits, *Ann. Hum. Genet.* **36**: 163–184.

Roberts, D. F. (1977), Methods and problems in physiological genetics, in, *Physiological Variation and its Genetic Basis (Symposia of the Society for the Study of Human Biology*, Vol. 17) (J. S. Weiner, ed.), pp. 23–41, Taylor and Francis, London.

Smith, C. A. B. (1956), A test for segregation ratios in family data, *Ann. Hum. Genet.* **20**: 257–265.

Smith, C. A. B. (1959), A note on the effects of method of ascertainment on segregation ratios, *Ann. Hum. Genet.* **23**:311–323.

Steinberg, A. G. (1959), Methodology in human genetics, *J. Med. Educ.* **34**:315–334.

Stene, J. (1977), Assumptions for different ascertainment models in human genetics, *Biometrics* **33**:523–527.

Thompson, E. A. and Cannings, C. (1979), Sampling schemes and ascertainment, in *The Genetic Analysis of Common Diseases: Applications to Predictive Factors in Coronary Heart Disease* (C. F. Sing, and M. Skolnick, eds.), Alan Liss, New York.

Weiss, V. (1976), Die Erkennung von Hauptgenen quantitativer morphologischer Merkmale mit Familienmaterial, Geschwister und Elter–Kind-Paaren am Beispiel der Kopflänge des Menschen, *Gegenbaurs Morph. Jahrb. Leipzig* **122**:875–881.

12

Path Analysis of Quantitative Inheritance

D. C. Rao and N. E. Morton

1. Introduction

Path analysis was developed by Sewall Wright (1921, 1968, 1978) to explain correlations between variables under a linear model. This powerful method remained untapped in human genetics for a few decades despite its invention by a pioneer population geneticist; an exception to this is Wright's own application to human IQ (1931). The human geneticists of the twenties and thirties were almost entirely confined to various aspects of *biometrical genetics* dependent on traditional methods of *analysis of variance*. As interests grew beyond biometrical methods, path analysis was introduced into human genetics during this decade (Jencks, 1972; Morton, 1974; Rao, Morton, and Yee, 1974), a few years after its rediscovery in social sciences (Duncan, 1966). Jencks in 1972 studied the consequences of phenotypic assortative mating on human IQ. It was in 1974 that a distribution theory was introduced giving tests of hypotheses in path analysis; emphasis on environmental indices greatly improved the power of resolution between biological and cultural causes of family resemblance (Morton, 1974; Rao, Morton, and Yee, 1974). Assortative mating was elaborated in two directions depending on whether the phenotypic marital correlation is considered secondary (called *social homogamy*: Rao and Morton, 1978; Morton and Rao, 1978) or primary (called *phenotypic homogamy*:

D. C. RAO AND N. E. MORTON ● Population Genetics Laboratory, University of Hawaii, Honolulu, Hawaii 96822. This work was partially supported by Grants GM24941, GM17-173, and HL16774 from the U.S. National Institutes of Health. PGL Paper No. 216.

Wright, 1978; Cloninger, Rice, and Reich, 1979). These two types have recently been combined into a general form called *mixed homogamy* (Morton and Rao, 1979; Rao, Morton, and Cloninger, 1979). In this chapter we shall present the underlying linear model, discuss the mechanics of assortative mating, present methods of analysis of quantitative data in nuclear families, and conclude with a few applications.

2. The Linear Model

Consider the linear model

$$P^* = G^* + C^* + R^* \qquad (2.1)$$

where P^* is the phenotype, G^* the relevant genotype (poygenic) assumed to be additive, C^* the relevant "family environment," consisting of all nonrandom nongenetic factors, and R^* is the residual, with

$$\text{var}(P^*) = \sigma_p^2, \qquad \text{var}(G^*) = \sigma_g^2, \qquad \text{var}(C^*) = \sigma_c^2, \qquad \text{var}(R^*) = \sigma_r^2$$

$$\text{cov}(G^*, C^*) = \sigma_{gc} \qquad \text{and} \qquad \text{cov}(G^*, R^*) = \text{cov}(C^*, R^*) = 0$$

Therefore the total phenotypic variance is, from (2.1),

$$\sigma_p^2 = \sigma_g^2 + \sigma_c^2 + \sigma_r^2 + 2\sigma_{gc} \cdots \qquad (2.2)$$

Dividing both sides of (2.1) by σ_p we get

$$\frac{P^*}{\sigma_p} = \frac{\sigma_g}{\sigma_p} \frac{G^*}{\sigma_g} + \frac{\sigma_c}{\sigma_p} \frac{C^*}{\sigma_c} + \frac{\sigma_r}{\sigma_p} \frac{R^*}{\sigma_r}$$

or,

$$P = hG + cC + rR \cdots \qquad (2.3)$$

where the standardized variables are denoted by P, G, C, and R, and

$$h = \sigma_g/\sigma_p$$
$$c = \sigma_c/\sigma_p \qquad (2.4)$$
$$r = \sigma_r/\sigma_p$$

Equations such as (2.3) are called *structural equations*, which are implicit in path diagrams. The coefficients h, c, r in Eq. (2.3) are called path coefficients. Taking variance on both sides of (2.3) yields

$$1 = h^2 + c^2 + 2hca + r^2 \cdots \qquad (2.5)$$

which is called the *equation for complete determination*, where $\text{cov}(G, C) = a = \sigma_{gc}/\sigma_g\sigma_c$.

The components of Eq. (2.2) are called *variance components*. In path analysis, variance components relative to the total phenotypic variance [components of (2.5)] are automatically obtained as functions of path coefficients. *Genetic heritability* is defined as the proportion of phenotypic variance due to genetic factors (σ_g^2/σ_p^2). In the presence of dominance (and epistasis) the genetic variance is split:

$$\sigma_g^2 = \sigma_a^2 + \sigma_n^2$$

where σ_a^2 is the additive genetic variance and σ_n^2 is the genetic variance due to gene—gene interactions.

Accordingly one defines two types of genetic heritability:

$$h_N^2 \text{ (narrow sense)} = \sigma_a^2/\sigma_p^2$$

$$h_B^2 \text{ (broad sense)} = \sigma_g^2/\sigma_p^2$$

When gene—gene interactions are absent, as we assume, $h^2 = h_N^2 = h_B^2$. For approximate treatment of gene—gene interactions see Wright (1978) and Rao, MacLean, Morton, and Yee (1975). Estimation of broad heritability is not credible in man, and heritability without specification means narrow heritability. Intergenerational differences are incorporated: Whereas the genetic heritability is h^2 for children, it is $h^2 z^2$ for adults. In the absence of such differences, $z = 1$. *Cultural heritability* is defined as the proportion of phenotypic variance due to family environment (σ_c^2/σ_p^2), which is c^2 for children and $c^2 y^2$ for adults. In the absence of intergenerational differences, $y = 1$.

Family environment consists of two components: partly transmitted from parents to children, and nontransmitted sibship environment (B). The total family environment (transmitted and nontransmitted) is denoted by C, and estimated by indices.

Covariance between genotype and family environment (*genotype—environment covariance*) measured by the parameter a, is assumed to be in equilibrium. The concept of genetic heritability was challenged in the presence of such covariance (Moran, 1973). However, as Holroyd (1975) pointed out, genetic heritability is simply defined as σ_g^2/σ_p^2 regardless of a.

Cultural inheritance determines family environment, which is sometimes called common environment or indexed environment. Specific maternal effects are incorporated through different effects of parental environments on the environment they provide to their children (f_F, f_M). Sibship environment which is not transmitted from parents to children is included.

Family environment is not directly observable, and so it is estimated by an *environmental index*. For behavioral traits like IQ we used the socioeconomic status (SES) as the index (Rao and Morton, 1978). In general when such data are available, we regress the phenotype on relevant environmental factors and define the discriminant as index. An index is not assumed to be a perfect estimator of the relevant family environment: a path coefficient (i for children, i_F for fathers, and i_M for mothers) measures the reliability of the index as an estimate of the environment. Since indices may be of unequal precision for parents and children, we consider separate indices for fathers, mothers, and children. Sibs are allowed to have separate environments and indices in recent models (Rao, Morton, and Cloninger, 1979).

Assortative mating is a system in which either like individuals (positive) or unlike individuals (negative) preferentially mate with each other. This preference may be based on two broad characteristics: social class including status, tastes, contacts, and other aspects of group membership, or phenotype. Assortative mating may accordingly be classified into two major types: *social homogamy* and *phenotypic homogamy*. A generalization incorporating phenotypic homogamy and social homogamy as two special cases is called *mixed homogamy* (Morton and Rao, 1979; Rao, Morton, and Cloninger, 1979). In the next three sections we shall briefly consider the consequences of these types of homogamy.

In depicting structural equations in terms of path diagrams, we shall follow the conventions of Rao, Morton, Elston, and Yee (1977) and show causes by ellipses and effects by rectangles. Only capital letters are used to denote causes or effects (including indices). Subscripts F, M, 1, and 2 are used to denote father, mother, and two children, respectively. Residual paths not contributing to familial correlations are not shown.

3. Social Homogamy

Under social homogamy mates choose each other on the basis of their group membership, which generates primary correlations between the genotypes and environments of spouses, and the phenotypic correlation between spouses becomes secondary. The group membership is in terms of a variable called social homogamy (H), which has a path coefficient $u^{1/2}$ to the environment and $m^{1/2}$ to the genotype of each spouse. This gives rise to the marital correlations: m, between genotypes of spouses; u, between environments of spouses; $(mu)^{1/2}$, between genotype and spouse's environment.

Inbreeding is included as the special case of social homogamy with $u = 0$. Similarly, assortment based on correlated environments alone is obtained for $m = 0$. Figure 1 presents the path diagram for a couple under social homogamy. All the path coefficients are defined in Table 1. Observe that in Fig. 1, the genotype—environment correlation for parents has two components: a direct path $[a - (mu)^{1/2}]$, and an indirect path $(mu)^{1/2}$ through H, preserving the total correlation a.

4. Phenotypic Homogamy

Under this system, mates choose one another strictly on the basis of their phenotypes. Phenotypic correlation between mates is therefore primary,

Table 1. Parameters of the Mixed Homogamy Model

Symbol	Parameter
h	effect of genotype on child's phenotype (square root of "heritability")
hz	effect of genotype on adult's phenotype
c	effect of child's indexed environment on the child's phenotype
cy	effect of adult's indexed environment on the adult's phenotype
p	primary correlation between parental phenotypes, not due to secondary resemblance through social homogamy (H)
m	correlation between parental genotypes through social homogamy (H)
u	correlation between parental indexed environments through social homogamy (H)
f_F	effect of father's indexed environment on child's indexed environment
f_M	effect of mother's indexed environment on child's indexed environment
b	effect of nontransmitted common sibship environment on child's indexed environment
bx	effect of nontransmitted common sibship environment on adult's indexed environment
i	effect of child's indexed environment on the child's index
i_F	effect of father's indexed environment on father's index
i_M	effect of mother's indexed environment on mother's index

Derived:

$\gamma = hz + cya$, correlation between the genotype and phenotype of an adult

$\phi = cy + hza$, correlation between the indexed environment and phenotype of an adult

$s = (mu)^{1/2}$, correlation between an adult's indexed environment and spouse's genotype under social homogamy

$a =$ correlation between genotype and indexed environment of an individual

$\psi = f_\text{F}^2 + f_\text{M}^2 + 2f_\text{F}f_\text{M}(u + p\phi^2)$, correlation between indexed environments of sibs derived from parental environments

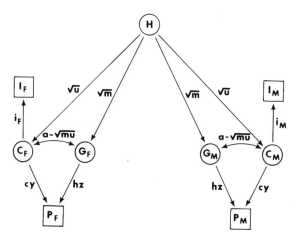

FIGURE 1. Path diagram for a couple under social homogamy. G, C, P, I, and H denote genotype, family environment, phenotype, environmental index, and homogamy, respectively. Subscripts F and M denote father and mother, respectively. See Table 1 for definition of the path coefficients.

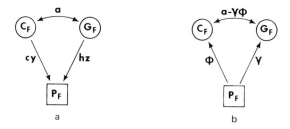

FIGURE 2. Path diagram showing the effect of reversing arrows. G, C, P denote genotype, family environment, and phenotype, respectively; subscript F denotes father. (a) G_F and C_F are shown as causes of P_F. Total correlation between G_F and C_F is a, shown by one correlational path. (b) Paths are reversed between G_F, C_F, and P_F conserving the total correlations between all pairs of variable $\gamma = hz + cya$ and $\phi = cy + hza$.

leading to derived correlations between genotypes and environments of mates.

Treatment of this system in path analysis is greatly simplified by reversing paths from effects to causes, and avoiding duplication of variables (Wright, 1978; Cloninger, Rice, and Reich, 1979). To explain the principles involved, consider Fig. 2. Figure 2a shows G and C as causes of an adult phenotype P. In Fig. 2b, the same variables are shown except that the paths from G and C to P are reversed. Whenever paths are reversed, new path coefficients should be assigned in a way consistent with the original causal system. For example, the total correlation between G and P should be the same whether derived from Fig. 2a

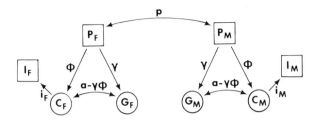

FIGURE 3. Path diagram for a couple under phenotype homogamy. G, C, P, I denote genotype, family environment, phenotype, and environmental index, respectively. Note that $\gamma = hz + cya$ and $\phi = cy + hza$ (see Fig. 2b).

or 2b: equating the two expressions we get

$$\gamma = hz + cya \tag{4.1}$$

Similarly, equating the correlations derived between C and P gives

$$\phi = cy + hza \tag{4.2}$$

Equating the correlations between G and C gives

$$a = (a - \gamma\phi) + \gamma\phi \tag{4.3}$$

Equations such as (4.1)–(4.3) specify the equivalences between Figs. 2a and 2b. In reversing paths, care must be taken to redefine the path coefficients.

Fig. 3 presents the path diagram for a couple under phenotypic homogamy, which is shown by the path p. Notice that the genotype–environment correlation for parents has two components: a direct path $(a - \gamma\phi)$, and an indirect one through the phenotype $(\gamma\phi)$ adding to a. All the parameters are defined in Table 1.

5. Mixed Homogamy

At this laboratory we have so far concentrated on social homogamy (Morton and Rao, 1978; Rao and Morton, 1978) with major interest in physiological traits such as lipoprotein concentrations (Rao, Morton, Gulbrandsen, Rhoads, Kagan, and Yee, 1979) and blood pressure (Morton, Gulbrandsen, Rao, Rhoads, and Kagan, 1979). Other investigators with primary interest in behavioral traits like I.Q. preferred phenotypic homogamy (Jencks, 1972; Wright, 1978; Cloninger, Rice, and Reich, 1979). Choice between these two models of assortative mating has so far been arbitrary. Generalization of assortative mating, called mixed homogamy, includes social homogamy and phenotypic homogamy as two special cases (Morton and Rao, 1979; Rao, Morton, and Cloninger, 1979).

Figure 4 displays the relationships between the variables (G, C, P) of a

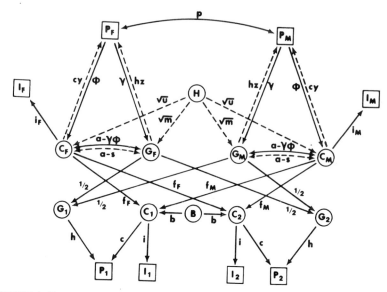

FIGURE 4. Treatment of mixed homogamy in nuclear families. P, G, C, I denote phenotype, genotype, indexed environment, and index, respectively. Subscripts F and M denote father and mother, 1 and 2 denote two children, respectively. B denotes nontransmitted common environment for a sibship. Table 1 defines the parameters of the model: $\gamma = hz + cya$, $\phi = cy + hza$, $s = (mu)^{1/2}$.

couple under mixed homogamy. Phenotypic homogamy, shown in Fig. 4 by a direct path (p), is represented by solid lines. The compound path coefficients γ and ϕ are already defined in (4.1) and (4.2). Let us now superimpose social homogamy (H), denoted by broken lines. This system of parallel paths (solid and broken lines) does not represent reciprocal causation (Wright, 1968). In this setup, the extent of premarital resemblance is measured by p, m, and part of u, and postmarital resemblance, if induced by cohabitation, by the remainder of u. Note that, in Fig. 4, $p = 0$ corresponds to social homogamy and $m = u = 0$ corresponds to phenotypic homogamy. In deriving expected correlations under mixed homogamy, two new rules have to be adhered to:

(i) Within an individual, either solid lines or broken lines are used but not both.

(ii) Between individuals, any given chain may contain either the solid paths or the broken paths between mates but not both; only those paths in a chain that connect two mates need to be either all solid or all broken.

6. Nuclear Families

Figure 5 displays the path diagram showing biological and cultural inheritance in nuclear families under mixed homogamy. The correlation between

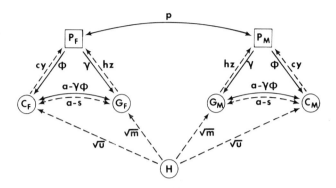

FIGURE 5. Path diagram for assortative mating under mixed homogamy. P, G, C, H denote phenotype, genotype, indexed environment, and social homogamy, respectively. Subscripts F and M denote father and mother. See Table 1 for definition of the parameters.

genotype and family environment of a child is derived from Fig. 5 as

$$[a + (mu)^{1/2} + \gamma p\phi](f_F + f_M)/2$$

which is a under equilibrium. The admissible root of

$$a^2 + a\beta + 1 + \frac{(mu)^{1/2}}{phzcy} = 0 \qquad (6.1)$$

gives a as a function of other parameters, where

$$\beta = \frac{\lambda p(h^2 z^2 + c^2 y^2) - 1}{\lambda phzcy}$$

and $\lambda = (f_F + f_M)/(2 - f_F - f_M)$.

Expected correlations derived from Fig. 5 are presented in Table 2. Expected correlations in nuclear families under social homogamy are obtainable from Table 2 by setting $p = 0$. Similarly, specialization of $m = u = 0$ in Table 2 gives expectations under phenotypic homogamy. Recently Cloninger (1979) incorporated phenotype–environment reciprocal interactions into mixed homogamy.

Notice that there are three nonlinear constraints on the parameters. Let us denote the total relative variances of child's phenotype, adult's phenotype, and child's family environment, respectively, by $\Sigma_{PC} + \sigma_{PC}^2$, $\Sigma_{PA} + \sigma_{PA}^2$, and $\Sigma_{CC} + \sigma_{CC}^2$, each of which equals 1, where the σ^2's are residual components and

$$\Sigma_{PC} = h^2 + c^2 + 2hca$$

$$\Sigma_{PA} = h^2 z^2 + c^2 y^2 + 2hzcya$$

$$\Sigma_{CC} = f_F^2 + f_M^2 + 2f_F f_M (u + p\phi^2)$$

Therefore, the three constraints are

$$\Sigma_{PC} \leqslant 1, \qquad \Sigma_{PA} \leqslant 1, \qquad \Sigma_{CC} \leqslant 1$$

7. Other Relatives

Correlations for various types of vertical, collateral, and other relatives were presented by Rao, Morton, and Cloninger (1979) under mixed homogamy. Some of these phenotypic correlations not covered in Table 2 are presented in Table 3.

8. Statistical Analysis

Consider a set of sample correlation coefficients $r_1, r_2, \ldots, r_m$ and their sample sizes $n_1, n_2, \ldots, n_m$. Since the large-sample distribution of r_i is normal with variance

$$\text{var}(r_i) = (1 - \rho_i^2)^2 / n_i$$

we consider

$$\chi^2 = \sum_{i=1}^{m} n_i (r_i - \rho_i)^2 / (1 - \rho_i^2)^2 \qquad (8.1)$$

and take the log likelihood as

$$\ln L = -\chi^2/2 + \text{constant} \qquad (8.2)$$

In (8.1) above, ρ is an expected correlation which is a function of path coefficients. Therefore, (8.1) and hence (8.2) is a function of the parameters. We can estimate some or all of the unknown parameters by minimizing (8.1), or equivalently, maximizing the log likelihood of (8.2). When k parameters are estimated, the residual χ^2 of (8.1) asymptotically follows a chi-square distribution with $m - k$ degrees of freedom, which provides a goodness-of-fit test. We can also use the residual χ^2 values to carry out likelihood ratio tests of null hypotheses. For example, let χ^2_{m-k-w} be the residual χ^2 after estimating $k + w$ parameters, and χ^2_{m-k} be another value after estimating only k of the $k + w$ parameters, the other w parameters being fixed under a null hypothesis. Then $\chi^2_w = \chi^2_{m-k} - \chi^2_{m-k-w}$ is asymptotically distributed as chi-square with w degrees of freedom (df) under the null hypothesis, and thus it provides the likelihood ratio test of the null hypothesis.

Table 2. Expected Correlations in Nuclear Families under Mixed Homogamy [See Fig. 5]

Relation	Variables	Expected correlation $(\rho)^a$
FMT (marital)	P_F, I_F	ϕi_F
	P_F, P_M	$p + (hz)^2 m + (cy)^2 u + 2hzcys$
	P_F, I_M	$(p\phi + hzs + cyu)i_M$
	I_F, P_M	$(p\phi + hzs + cyu)i_F$
	I_F, I_M	$(p\phi^2 + u)i_F i_M$
	P_M, I_M	ϕi_M
OPT (parent–offspring)	P_F, P_C	$\frac{1}{2}h[\gamma(1+p)+hzm+cys] + c\phi(f_F + pf_M) + cf_M(hzs + cyu)$
	P_F, I_C	$[\phi(f_F + pf_M) + f_M(hzs + cyu)]i$
	I_F, P_C	$[\frac{1}{2}h(a+s+\gamma p\phi) + cf_F + cf_M(u + \phi^2 p)]i_F$
	I_F, I_C	$[f_F + f_M(u + p\phi^2)]ii_F$
	P_M, P_C	$\frac{1}{2}h[\gamma(1+p)+hzm+cys] + c\phi(f_M + pf_F) + cf_F(hzs + cyu)$
	P_M, I_C	$[\phi(f_M + pf_F) + f_F(hzs + cyu)]i$
	I_M, P_C	$[\frac{1}{2}h(a+s+\gamma p\phi) + cf_M + cf_F(u + p\phi^2)]i_M$
	I_M, I_C	$[f_M + f_F(u + p\phi^2)]ii_M$
SST (filial)	(P_1, I_1) or (P_2, I_2)	$(c + ha)i$
	(P_1, I_2) or (P_2, I_1)	$[ha + c(b^2 + \psi)]i$
	I_1, I_2	$(b^2 + \psi)i^2$
	P_1, P_2	$\frac{1}{2}h^2(1 + m + p\gamma^2) + c^2(b^2 + \psi) + 2hca$

^{a} Note: $s = (mu)^{1/2}$, $\gamma = hz + cya$, $\phi = cy + hza$, $\psi = f_F^2 + f_M^2 + 2f_F f_M(u + p\phi^2)$.

Table 3. Expected Phenotypic Correlations under Mixed Homogamy for Some Relationships outside Regular Nuclear Families

Relation	Expected correlation between phenotypes (ρ)[a]
MZ twins reared together	$h^2 + c^2 + 2hca$
MZ twins reared apart, one by true parents	$(h^2 + hca)\theta$
DZ twins reared together (same as full sibs)	$h^2(1 + m + p\gamma^2)/2 + c^2 + 2hca$
DZ twins reared apart, one by true parents	$[h^2(1 + m + p\gamma^2)/2 + hca]\theta$
Foster sibs reared together	$c^2\theta^2(b + \psi)$
Offspring–parent living apart	$h\theta[\gamma(1 + p) + hzm + cys]/2$
Offspring–foster father[b]	$c\theta[\phi(f_F + pf_M) + (f_M + pf_F)(hzs + cyu)]$
Paternal half sibs reared together by parents of one[b]	$h^2(1 + 3m + 2\gamma^2p + \gamma^2p^2)/4 + c^2(b^2 + \psi) + hca + hc[a + f_M(\gamma p^2\phi + s - a)]/2$
Paternal half sibs reared separately by own parents[b]	$h^2(1 + 3m + 2\gamma^2p + \gamma^2p^2)/4 + c^2[b^2 + \psi - f_M^2(1 - u - \phi^2p^2)] + hc[a + f_M(\gamma p^2\phi + s - a)]$
Children of male MZ twins[b]	$K_2^2 + 2aK_2\Lambda_2 + (b^2x^2 + \psi)\Lambda_2^2$
Cross first cousins[b]	$K_2K_2'(1 + m + p\gamma^2)/2 + (b^2x^2 + \psi)\Lambda_2\Lambda_2' + a(K_2\Lambda_2' + \Lambda_2K_2')$
Uncle–niece[b]	$K_2'hz(1 + m + p\gamma^2)/2 + cy(b^2x^2 + \psi)\Lambda_2' + cyaK_2' + hza\Lambda_2'$

[a] Note: $\theta = 1/(1 - 2hca)^{1/2}$; $\psi = f_F^2 + f_M^2 + 2f_Ff_M(u + p\phi^2)$; $\gamma = hz + cyu$; $\phi = cy + hza$; $K_2 = h(1 + m^* + \gamma phz)/2 + cf_M(s^* + \phi phz)/2$; $m^* = (m - as)/(1 - a^2)$; $s^* = (mu)^{1/2}$; $\Lambda_2 = c[f_F + f_M(u^* + \phi pcy)] + h(t^* + \gamma pcy)/2$; $u^* = (u - as)/(1 - a^2)$; $t^* = (s - am)/(1 - a^2)$; K_2' and Λ_2' are obtained from K_2 and Λ_2 by reversing the subscripts F and M.

[b] When sex of the relevant parent is changed, expected correlations are obtained by reversing the subscripts F and M.

As an alternative to (8.1), we recommend using z transformations of correlations. We take

$$z_i = \frac{1}{2} \ln \frac{1 + r_i}{1 - r_i}$$

which is almost normally distributed with asymptotic mean

$$\bar{z}_i = \frac{1}{2} \ln \frac{1 + \rho_i}{1 - \rho_i}$$

and variance, $\text{var}(z_i) = 1/n_i$. Expression for χ^2 would then be

$$\chi^2 = \sum_{i=1}^{m} n_i(z_i - \bar{z}_i)^2 \tag{8.3}$$

instead of (8.1). Earlier we suggested small sample refinements (Rao, Morton, and Yee, 1974) which had negligible effects on the results (Goldberger, 1978). In large sample theory equations (8.1) and (8.3) are equivalent: good agreement lends credibility to use of large-sample theory.

9. Examples

In this section we shall consider a few applications of these methods to data on palmar ridge counts, skin color, periodontal disease, and human IQ. Except for IQ, other data sets were analyzed under social homogamy ($p = 0$). Equation (8.3) was used for the analyses.

9.1. Palmar Ridge Counts

Methods of social homogamy ($p = 0$) were employed to test hypotheses concerning the inheritance of $a - b$, $b - c$, and $c - d$ palmar ridge counts (Sciulli and Rao, 1975). Maternal effects were neglected. Both genetic and cultural heritabilities were found to be significant, which accounted for most of the variation at each of the three ridge count areas, where "cultural heritability" includes uterine environment. The genetic heritabilities ($\pm$ s.e.) are 0.613 ± 0.065, 0.929 ± 0.057, and 0.564 ± 0.066, respectively for $a - b$, $b - c$, and $c - d$; the corresponding cultural heritabilities are 0.258 ± 0.039, 0.119 ± 0.035, and 0.239 ± 0.040.

9.2. Skin Color

Post and Rao (1977) have analyzed skin reflectance measurements on a sample of 164 MZ and 181 DZ twin pairs to determine the effects of genetic and environmental factors under social homogamy ($p = 0$). Both genetic and environmental effects were found to be significant. The genetic and cultural heritabilities were estimated as 0.722 ± 0.034 and 0.224 ± 0.032, respectively.

9.3. Periodontal Health

The two data sets on palmar ridge counts and skin color are inadequate to demonstrate the full power of the methods of path analysis. For this purpose we shall here describe a study of periodontal health in nuclear families.

Chung, Kau, Chung, and Rao (1977) measured periodontal health by the first principal component of eight symptoms, adjusted for age and sex effects. Chung and Morton (1979) created environmental indices in terms of education, occupation, smoking history, and frequency of brushing, and generated 16 correlations in nuclear families (with only one index for all members of a sibship). These data were analyzed under the methods of social homogamy ($p = 0$) with the restriction that $\psi + b^2 = 1$ (see Table 1 for ψ), since only one index was allowed for each sibship. The general model with $m = 0$ gave an excellent fit ($\chi_6^2 = 7.13$). While cultural heritability (0.267 ± 0.047) was highly significant ($\chi_2^2 = 787.67$), genetic heritability (0.222 ± 0.143), maternal effects and inter-generational differences were not ($\chi_4^2 = 4.18$). High estimates of i, i_F, and i_M were obtained, indicating that the indices are good estimates of the environments. The most parsimonious hypothesis yields a cultural heritability of 0.338 ± 0.024, the same for children and adults, with zero genetic heritability. This example illustrates that (i) nuclear families can powerfully resolve biological and cultural inheritance, (ii) path analysis has no genetic bias, and (iii) family resemblance is attributed only to environmental factors when that is appropriate.

9.4. Human IQ

Rao and Morton (1978) have compiled a data set consisting of 65 estimates of correlations on human IQ covering 16 distinct relationships. Results of a preliminary analysis of this data set under mixed homogamy are presented in Table 4. Due to previous experience (Rao and Morton, 1978) we assume that $m = 0$ and $f_F = f_M = f$, say. The two interesting special cases $u = 0$ and $p = 0$ were tried in addition to mixed homogamy.

Total heterogeneity among multiple estimates of the same correlation due to differences in sampling and measurement was found to be highly significant ($\chi_{49}^2 = 142.46$). To offset this we have used $s^2 = 142.46/49 = 2.907$ as the error variance. Accordingly, tests of hypotheses are carried out in terms of F ratios. If χ_{m-k}^2 and χ_m^2 are the residual χ^2 values under the model and a specific null hypothesis, respectively, the F ratio on k and 49 df for testing the null hypothesis is calculated as

$$F = (\chi_m^2 - \chi_{m-k}^2)/ks^2$$

Goodness-of-fit of the model is tested by

$$F = \chi_{m-k}^2/(m - k)s^2$$

on $m - k$ and 49 df. Mixed homogamy gave a good fit (F ratio $= 2.01$ on 7, 49 df, $P > 0.05$). Unlike recent claims (Cloninger, Rice, and Reich, 1979; Rice, Cloninger, and Reich, 1979) phenotypic homogamy does not fit the data ($F = 22.90$ on 1, 49 df, $P < 0.001$), whereas social homogamy gives essentially identical results as those under mixed homogamy. It is interesting that the smallest adult genetic heritability was obtained under phenotypic homogamy. This is contrary to the suggestion that intergenerational differences were evident only under social homogamy (Loehlin, 1978, Rice, Cloninger, and Reich, 1979). It is surprising that even for a trait like IQ phenotypic homogamy is not even partially supported ($p = 0.000$).

10. Discussion

In recent years analyses of human IQ were excessively criticized mostly for ideological reasons (Kamin, 1974; Lewontin, 1975; Goldberger, 1977). What is overlooked is the impressive record of methodological developments that followed attempts to describe inheritance of IQ. Somewhat different results obtained for IQ under social homogamy and phenotypic homogamy (Loehlin,

Table 4. Analysis of Human IQ under Mixed Homogamy with $m = 0$ and $f_F = f_M = f$

Variable	Mixed homogamy $(\hat{p}, \hat{u})$	Phenotypic homogamy $(u = 0, \hat{p})$	Social homogamy $(p = 0, \hat{u})$
Residual χ^2	40.99^a	107.56^b	40.99^a
d.f.	7	8	8
F ratio	2.01	22.90	0.00
P	> 0.05	< 0.001	> 0.99
Genetic heritability:			
children (h^2)	0.689	0.626	0.690
adults ($h^2 z^2$)	0.310	0.015	0.311
Cultural heritability:			
children (c^2)	0.157	0.112	0.156
adult ($c^2 y^2$)	0.545	0.629	0.549
Marital correlations:			
p	0.000	0.532	0
u	0.951	0	0.939
Cultural inheritance:			
transmitted (f)	0.476	0.608	0.476
nontransmitted (b)	0.342	0	0.349
Gene–environment correlation (a)	0.000	0.177	0

[a] This solution was constrained to have $b = (1 - \psi)^{1/2}$, since $b^2 + \psi > 1$ when unconstrained (See Table 1 for ψ).

[b] This solution was constrained to have $\psi = 1$ (and hence $b = 0$), since $\psi > 1$ when unconstrained.

1978) encouraged generalization to mixed homogamy. Thus methods developed for IQ analyses helped to delineate the roles of genes and environment for other traits, most importantly the disease-related ones such as lipoprotein concentrations (Rao et al., 1979), blood pressure (Morton et al., 1979), and uric acid (Gulbrandsen, Morton, Rao, Rhoads, and Kagan, 1979).

Recent developments in path analysis have given rise to some questions: Why path analysis? Why not variance components? Why a linear model? What can path analysis do that regression analysis cannot? One category of questions is directed to path analysis almost exclusively (such as mentioned above). The second category includes ideological questions which apply to all methods of scientific inference. Some of the latter questions were adequately and effectively addressed by Dobzhansky (1976).

Path analysis and regression analysis are similar except in two respects. Firstly, they serve different purposes: given a set of variables, path analysis attempts to explain the interrelationships between the variables by erecting a causal scheme, whereas regression analysis maximizes the prediction of the dependent variable(s) from the independent variables with no causal implication. Secondly, path analysis is applicable even when the independent variables are unobserved or observed with error.

Investigators working with linear models do not pretend that nature always acts additively, but when the causes are not directly measured only linear models permit data analysis and have been shown to predict the essential features when applied to data generated under nonlinear models (Rao and Morton, 1974; Rao, Morton, and Yee, 1976). Before linearity is criticized excessively, a nonlinear model should be demonstrated to be determinate and give a better fit to the data.

Given a specific linear model, path analysis and variance components methods should yield essentially identical results, at least in large samples. To this extent, it is largely a matter of taste as to which method is used. Maximum-likelihood theories developed for the methods of variance components (Lange, Westlake, and Spence, 1976) and path analysis (Rao et al., 1979, appendix) reflect their close resemblance. In the former, absolute variance components are estimated from an appropriate likelihood function. Under the latter method, sample correlations are first estimated from the likelihood, and to these correlations path coefficients are fitted, giving as a byproduct relative variance components. If desired, the calculations could be made more similar. Even though these two methods are large sample equivalents for a given model, there are reasons for favoring path analysis. More elaborate models have been developed under path analysis and successfully applied to several data sets. Path analysis offers greater flexibility in model specification, such as the treatment of assortative mating. Many relationships are predictable functions of a few path coefficients, which generate a larger number of variance components. Maybe the day will come when advocates of variance components will develop better models, but we have to move a long way from present models specifying environmental effects which are either inconsistent (see Goldberger, 1977) or greatly over-simplified (Lange, Westlake, and Spence, 1976).

References

Chung, C. S., Kau, M. C. W., Chung, S. S. C., and Rao, D. C. (1977), A genetic and epidemi-ologic study of periodontal disease in Hawaii. II. Genetic and environmental influence, *Am. J. Hum. Genet.* **29**:76–82.

Cloninger, C. R. (1979), Resolution of polygenic and cultural inheritance from reciprocal phenotype–environment interaction. I. Introduction and description of the general dynamic model, submitted to *Genet. Res.*

Cloninger, C. R., Rice, J., and Reich, T. (1979), Multifactorial inheritance with cultural transmission and assortative mating. II. A general model of combined polygenic and cultural inheritance, *Am. J. Hum. Genet.* (in press).

Dobzhansky, T. H. (1976), The myths of genetic predestination and of tabula rasa, *Persp. Biol. Med.* **19**:156–170.

Duncan, O. D. (1966), Path analysis – sociological examples, *Am. J. Sociol.* **72**:1–6.

Goldberger, A. (1977), *Models and Methods in the IQ Debate: Part I*, SSRI workshop series, University of Wisconsin, Madison.

Goldberger, A. (1978), Pitfalls in the resolution of IQ inheritance, in *Genetic Epidemiology* (N. E. Morton and C. S. Chung, eds.); Academic Press, New York.

Gulbrandsen, C. L., Morton, N. E., Rao, D. C., Rhoads, G. G., and Kagan, A. (1979), Deter-minants of plasma uric acid, *Hum. Genet.* **50**:307–312.

Holroyd, R. G. (1975), On Moran's note on heritability, *Ann. Hum. Genet.* **38**:379.

Jencks, C. (1972), *Inequality*, Basic Books, New York.

Kamin, L. (1979), *The Science and Politics of IQ*, Eribaum Assoc., Potomac, Maryland.

Krieger, H., Morton, N. E., Rao, D. C., and Azevedo, E. (1979), Race and blood pressure in northeastern Brazil (in preparation).

Lange, K., Westlake, J., and Spence, M. A. (1976), Extensions to pedigree analysis. III. Variance components by the scoring method, *Ann. Hum. Genet.* **39**:485–491.

Lewontin, R. C. (1975), Genetic aspects of intelligence, *Ann. Rev. Genet.* **9**:387–405.

Loehlin, J. (1978), Heredity–environment analysis of Jenck's IQ correlations, *Behav. Genet.* **8**:415–435.

Moran, P. A. P. (1973), A note on heritability and the correlation between relatives, *Ann. Hum. Genet.* **37**:217.

Morton, N. E. (1974), Analysis of family resemblance. I. Introduction, *Am. J. Hum. Genet.* **26**:318–330.

Morton, N. E., and Rao, D. C. (1978), Quantitative inheritance, in *Yearb. Phys. Anthropol.* **21**:12–41.

Morton, N. E., and Rao, D. C. (1979), Causal analysis of family resemblance, in *The Genetic Analysis of Common Diseases: Application to Predictive Factors in Coronary Heart Disease* (C. F. Sing and M. Skolnick, eds.), Alan R. Liss Publishing, New York.

Morton, N. E., Gulbrandsen, C. L., Rao, D. C., Rhoads, G. G., and Kagan, A. (1979), Deter-minants of blood pressure in Japanese-American families, *Hum. Genet.* (in press).

Post, P. W., and Rao, D. C. (1977), Genetic and environmental determinants of skin color, *Am. J. Phys. Anthropol.* **47**:399–402.

Rao, D. C., and Morton, N. E. (1974), Path analysis of family resemblance in the presence of gene–environment interaction, *Am. J. Hum. Genet.* **26**:767–772.

Rao, D. C., and Morton, N. E. (1978), IQ as a paradigm in genetic epidemiology, in *Genetic Epidemiology* (N. E. Morton and C. S. Chung, eds.), Academic Press, New York.

Rao, D. C., Morton N. E., and Yee, S. (1974), Analysis of family resemblance. II. A linear model for familial correlation, *Am. J. Hum. Genet.* **26**:331–359.

Rao, D. C., MacLean, C. J., Morton, N. E., and Yee, S. (1974), Analysis of family resemblance. V. Height and weight in northeastern Brazil, *Am. J. Hum. Genet.* **27**:509–520.

Rao, D. C., Morton, N. E., and Yee, S. (1976), Resolution of cultural and biological inheritance by path analysis, *Am. J. Hum. Genet.* **28**:228–242.

Rao, D. C., Morton, N. E., Elston, R. C., and Yee, S. (1977), Causal analysis of academic performance, *Behav. Genet.* **7**:147–159.

Rao, D. C., Chung, C. S., and Morton, N. E. (1979), Genetic and environmental determinants of periodontal disease, *Am. J. Med. Genet.* **4**:39–45.

Rao, D. C., Morton, N. E., and Cloninger, C. R. (1979), Path analysis under generalized assortative mating. I. Theory, *Genet. Res.* **33**:175–188.

Rao, D. C., Morton, N. E., Gulbrandsen, C. L., Rhoads, G. G., Kagan, A., and Yee, S. (1979), Cultural and biological determinants of lipoprotein concentrations, *Ann. Hum. Genet.* **42**:467–477.

Rice, J., Cloninger, C. R., and Reich, T. (1979), The analysis of behavioral traits in the presence of cultural transmission and assortative mating: Application to IQ and SES, *Behav. Genet.* (in press).

Sciulli, P. W., and Rao, D. C. (1975), Path analysis of palmar ridge counts, *Am. J. Phys. Anthropol.* **43**:291–294.

Spence, M. A., Rao, D. C., Ritenbaugh, C. K., and Yee, S. (1979), Family resemblance for height and weight in Pima Indians, *Hum. Hered.* (in press).

Wright, S. (1921), Correlation and causation, *J. Agric. Res.* **20**:557–585.

Wright, S. (1931), Statistical methods in Biology, *J. Am. Stat. Assoc.* **26**:155–163.

Wright, S. (1968), *Evolution and the Genetics of Populations, Vol. 1, Genetic and Biometric Foundations*, The University of Chicago Press, Chicago.

Wright, S. (1978), *Evolution and the Genetics of Populations, Vol. 4, Variability within and among Natural Populations*, The University of Chicago Press, Chicago.

13

Half-Sib Analysis of Quantitative Data

CHING CHUN LI

1. Introduction

The nonexperimental study of population biology usually depends on the availability of data from the population under study. Thus, in a society where adoption of children is practiced, we may study foster parents and adopted children and compare them with true parents and children, in spite of the many pitfalls introduced by selective factors in the process of adoption. The study of adopted children would be impractical in a society where there are very few adoptions (except the cases where a childless uncle adopts his own nephew as a son).

There is a paucity of reported studies of half sibs in our scientific literature, because there have been comparatively few half sibs in our society and, perhaps also important, they are difficult to identify. Now the social behavior of our society has undergone considerable changes in the last generation. With early marriage, early divorce, and early remarriage, there are and will be a large number of half sibs in our society; they should be available for study just like twins and adopted children if they can be identified. It is gratifying to know that study of half sibs has already been underway on several campuses.

Half sibs differ from adopted children in many aspects, the most important of which is probably the fact that half sibs are genetically related while foster parents and adopted children are not. The genetic relationship between half sibs is as close as that between grandparents and grandchildren, and also as that between uncles and nephews, but with the distinctive advantage that they belong to the same generation.

CHING CHUN LI • Graduate School of Public Health, University of Pittsburgh, Pittsburgh, Pennsylvania 15261.

Half sibs may be classified in various ways. They may be "paternal" (with a common father) or "maternal" (with a common mother). And they may be reared together or reared apart, by the common parent or by one of the other two parents. So we see that the information on the various types of half sibs will enable us to study the father's and mother's effects on children as well as home and random environmental effects.

Furthermore, the information on the parents of half sibs would give us an opportunity to study the nature of assortative mating. Let P_0 be the common parent (say, the common mother) and P_1 and P_2 be the two successive fathers. If the measurements of a quantitative trait on all three parents are known, then we will have three observed correlations among the parents: $r(0, 1) = r(P_0, P_1)$, $r(0, 2) = r(P_0, P_2)$, and $r(1, 2) = r(P_1, P_2)$. If we distinguish the sex of the parents, there will be six observed correlations among the parents. Is $r(0,1)$ greater or smaller than $r(0.2)$? Is $r(1, 2)$ higher or lower than the product $r(0, 1) \cdot r(0, 2)$? Do $r(0, 1)$ and $r(0, 2)$ vary with the sex of the common parent? By comparing these correlations we will gain some understanding of the nature of assortative mating with respect to the quantitative trait under consideration.

One of the difficulties in studying the genetic and environmental effects on a quantitative trait is that there are usually more (unknown) parameters to be estimated that the equations furnished by the observed correlations between relatives, giving rise to indeterminacy — sometimes to a high degree of indeterminacy. The information on half sibs will contribute at least one additional equation to the system, thus alleviating the situation of indeterminacy. This, incidentally, also serves to remind us that in building models we are not free to include every factor that we wish to know, but have to limit ourselves within the range and availability of our observations. A proposal that involves many parameters and leads to indeterminacy does not help us to understand the presently available data, but may indicate what additional observations have to be made.

2. Variables and Notation

Due to the lack of generally agreed-upon notation, we shall say a few words about the symbolism employed in this chapter, although it is more or less the same as that adopted by the author previously. The reader will encounter some new letters. For instance, we use Z, instead of the usual P, to denote the observed phenotypic measurement of the quantitative trait of an individual. The reason is that we shall use P as a symbol for parent.

Similarly, we let Y denote the genotypic value (measurement) of an individual, instead of using G or H. In the genetic literature, some authors use G for genotypic value while others use G to denote the genic, or additive, or linear, or breeding value. In order to avoid confusion, again, we introduce a relatively new symbol, L, to denote the linear value (based on linearly fitted genic effects). Thus, we have a sequence of three variables: $L \rightarrow Y \rightarrow Z$, as indicated in Fig. 1.

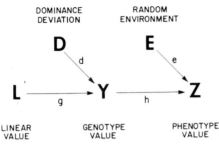

FIGURE 1. The genetic variables $(L + D = Y)$ and phenotype variables $(Y + E = Z)$ form the basic model in formulating kinship correlations.

Let D be the dominance deviation, so that $L + D = Y$. By the properties of linear regression, L and D of the same locus are always uncorrelated, so that $\sigma_L^2 + \sigma_D^2 = \sigma_Y^2$. They are also independent with those of other loci under panmixia. When there is no dominance, $D = 0$, and $L = Y$.

Environmental effects are difficult to describe, not mention to measure, because the "environment" consists of numerous types of elements. The elements which are beneficial to one trait may be harmful to another trait, so that a good environment in one aspect may be a poor environment in another. So, in studying quantitative traits, the environment must be defined relative to the particular trait under study. For instance, in studying tuberculosis, the temperature and humidity are relevant environmental factors; while in studying the color of the eye and hair, they are of little importance. It is one thing to enumerate environmental factors; it is quite another to prove its relevance.

Let E stand for the environmental elements that affect the development of the phenotype to a certain extent. In Fig. 1, E has been labeled "random environment"; by that we simply mean, as a first approximation, these environmental factors are uncorrelated with the genotype Y. Under these simple conditions, $Y + E = Z$, and $\sigma_Y^2 + \sigma_E^2 = \sigma_Z^2$.

Having explained the five variables in Fig. 1, we should also note the structure of the diagram as a whole. It is a conglomeration of two self-contained subdiagrams, each being complete by itself $(L + D = Y$, and $Y + E = Z)$. Let the lower case letters among the arrows of the diagram be path coefficients; then

(left portion)	(right portion)
$g^2 = \sigma_L^2/\sigma_Y^2$	$h^2 = \sigma_Y^2/\sigma_Z^2$
$d^2 = \sigma_D^2/\sigma_Y^2$	$e^2 = \sigma_E^2/\sigma_Z^2$
$g^2 + d^2 = 1$	$h^2 + e^2 = 1$

There is no necessary relationship between the fractions in the left portion and the fractions in the right portion of the diagram. In biological terms, the value of g^2 depends on the degree of dominance (the stronger the dominance, the smaller the g^2). Similarly, the value of h^2 depends on the extent of environmental influence (the stronger the environmental influence, the smaller the h^2). So, the magnitude of g^2 and h^2 are due to two entirely different reasons.

To stress the difference between these two causes, suppose a trait is determined almost entirely by the individual's genotype and is little influenced by external environmental factors ($E = 0$, and $Y = Z$, and $h^2 = 1$). The observed value of the parent–child correlation $r = 0.24 = \frac{1}{2}g^2$ in a random mating population would yield an estimate of "heritability" equal to $g^2 = 0.48$, indicating the presence of strong dominance ($d^2 = 0.52$). On the other hand, if there is no dominance $D = 0$, $L = Y$, and $g^2 = 1$) and the quantitative trait is influenced by environmental factors, the observed value of the parent–child correlation in a random mating population $r = 0.24 = \frac{1}{2}h^2$ would yield an estimate of "heritability" equal to $h^2 = 0.48$, indicating the presence of strong environmental influence ($e^2 = 0.52$). This illustrates the difference between interpretations of an observed correlation under different situations.

Probably in most cases both g^2 and h^2 are relevant and their product

$$g^2 h^2 \;=\; \frac{\sigma_L^2}{\sigma_Y^2}\,\frac{\sigma_Y^2}{\sigma_Z^2} \;=\; \frac{\sigma_L^2}{\sigma_Z^2}$$

frequently appears in the kinship correlation models. For instance, in a random mating population the observed parent–child correlation $r_{PO} = 0.24 = \frac{1}{2}g^2 h^2$ would yield an estimate of "heritability" of $g^2 h^2 = 0.48$, which includes both dominance and environmental effects. If we wish to obtain separate estimates of g^2 and h^2, then we need the additional information on sib–sib correlations; suppose it is $r_{OO} = (\frac{1}{4} + \frac{1}{4}g^2)h^2 = 0.27$. Solving these two equations simultaneously, we obtain $g^2 = 0.80$ and $h^2 = 0.60$, thus gaining a more detailed understanding of the kinship correlations.

From the above discussion we see there are really three types of "heritabilities" (g^2, h^2, and $g^2 h^2$), which are not always distinguished in the genetic literature. However, when we assume no dominance ($g^2 = 1$), then there is only one type of heritability, $g^2 h^2 = h^2$.

3. Correlation between Half-Sibs

It is comparatively easy to formulate a model for the correlation between half sibs in a random mating population. Assortative mating among the parents introduces considerable difficulty or uncertainty in model building for two reasons: one general and one specific. The general reason is the unknown cause or causes for the assortative mating. The specific reason is the lack of empirical knowledge about the correlations among the three parents of the half sibs. We shall discuss each briefly.

One suggestion is that the socioeconomic class is the overall cause for assortative mating, not the phenotype *per se*. The validity of this view depends largely on the particular quantitative trait under consideration. A necessary condition for its validity is that the trait must vary with the social classes. Another suggestion, the classic one, is that the assortative mating is primarily based on the measurement of the phenotype, the correlations between parental genotypes and environments being the consequences of the primary phenotypic correlation. Obviously there is merit to each suggestion and it is probable that both types of assortativeness exist in the loosely defined and highly mobile classes of our society. Wright (1978:367–369) discussed both models.

For the purpose of the present chapter, we assumed that assortative mating is primarily based on the phenotypic resemblance of the mates. For brevity we call this mating system *phenotypic assortative mating*. However, in the following discussion of the correlations among the three parents, we shall try to accommodate the social class theory also.

Consider the three parents with phenotype value Z, genotype value Y, and linear (additive) value L, as indicated in Fig. 2. Let $r_1 = r(Z_1, Z_0)$, $r_2 = r(Z_2, Z_0)$, and $r_{12} = r(Z_1, Z_2)$, where the subscript 0 indicates common parent — mother, say. These three phenotypic correlations among the three parents are assumed to be the primary causes of assorative mating (solid double headed arrows at the top of Fig. 2).

It is usually acceptable to take $r_1 = r_2 = r_{PP}$, where PP reads parent–parent (at the phenotype level). We wish to remind ourselves that even this is merely an assumption in the absence of hard empirical knowledge. The mating behavior of the common parent may change in successive marriages.

Let $m_1 = r(L_1, L_0)$, $m_2 = r(L_2, L_0)$, and $m_{12} = r(L_1, L_2)$ be the correlations between the linear values among the three parents. These correlations are

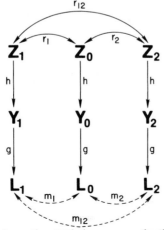

FIGURE 2. Phenotypic and genetic correlations among the three parents, where the subscript 0 indicates the common parent. Z = phenotype, Y = genotype, and L = linear or additive value as in Fig. 1.

consequences of the primary phenotypic correlations among the parents. They are indicated by dotted double-headed arrows at the bottom of Fig. 2 to indicate redundancy. Thus, $m_1 = g^2 h^2 r_1$ and $m_2 = g^2 h^2 r_2$. Our previous assumption of $r_1 = r_2 = r_{PP}$ leads to

$$m = m_1 = m_2 = g^2 h^2 r_{PP}$$

However, what the phenotypic correlation $r_{12} = r(Z_1, Z_2)$ between the two fathers should be is not immediately clear. There are a number of possibilities, depending on the mating behavior of the common parent (mother). On the one hand, r_{12} may be higher than r_{PP} if the common parent tends to choose the second mate very similar to the first one. On the other hand, r_{12} may be much lower than r_{PP}, being of the order of r_{PP}^2. (Note carefully this is *not* the same as saying $m_{12} = m^2$, which would make r_{12} still smaller, down to $g^2 h^2 r_{PP}^2$.)

Nagylaki (1978) assumes that the two fathers are correlated solely through the common mother. His argument that the partial correlation between the two fathers should be zero when the common parent is held constant ($r_{12.0} = 0$) leads to the result $r_{12} = r_1 r_2 = r_{PP}^2$. While this is certainly a possiblity, we recognize it is also an assumption because the vanishing of the partial correlation $r_{12.0}$ is an assumption.

Due to the lack of empirical evidence, we may entertain still other possibilities. The model we shall adopt in this chapter is based on the consideration of the assortative mating group, thus to a certain extent combining the social class concept with phenotypic assortative mating. Assuming no abrupt change in behavior of mate selection, we have not only $r_1 = r_2 = r_{PP}$ for the two marriages, but that the second father is chosen from the same assortative mating group as the first father. These two fathers, belonging to the same assortative group or social class, will be correlated to the same extent as the mates of the same group. Hence, our theory is simply that two individuals chosen from the same class are correlated to the same extent, marriage or no marriage. This leads to our model

$$r_{12} = r_1 = r_2 = r_{PP}$$

Consequently,

$$m_{12} = m_1 = m_2 = r_{PP} g^2 h^2 = m$$

The model shown above has been adopted by Li (1977, 1978) and Rao, Morton, and Yee (1974, 1976). Of course, the model is subject to change or modification in the face of empirical evidence (which has yet to come).

Now we are in a position to formulate a model for half-sib correlation (Fig. 3). We have used E to denote the environmental elements that influence the development of a phenotype, but uncorrelated with the genotype. We now use Γ to denote those environmental elements that exist in a family and thus are common to children reared together in the same family. This common family environment will contribute to the correlation between children reared together, whether they are full sibs, half sibs, nephews, cousins, or adopted (genetically unrelated) children. The path coefficient from this type of environment to phenotype is denoted by γ in Fig. 3. We recognize the existence of such Γ factors

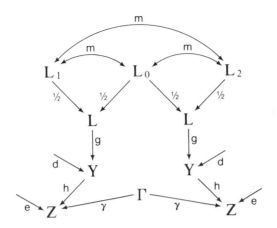

FIGURE 3. Correlation between half sibs, assuming all three parents are equally correlated. Both common familial environment and dominance are included. The phenotype (Z) and genotype (Y) values of the parents, already shown in Fig. 2, are omitted for brevity. The diagram begins with the L values of the parents (bottom of Fig. 2).

and their contribution to correlation between half sibs, without indicating their sources or causes. I wonder how important it is to say that these environmental factors are created by their parents.

Assortative mating also introduces complications to the inheritance properties of the dominance deviations. In Fig. 3 it is assumed that the dominance deviations of half sibs are uncorrelated; even if they were, the degree of correlation must be very low and its contribution to half-sib correlation is negligible. Then the phenotypic correlation between half sibs (O/O) will be

$$r_{O/O} = [r_{O/O} \text{ at } L \text{ level}] g^2 h^2 + \gamma^2$$
$$= \tfrac{1}{4}(1 + 3m)g^2 h^2 + \gamma^2 \tag{3.1}$$

where
$$m = r_{PP}g^2 h^2$$

While the formulation (3.1) is not comprehensive, it does contain four parameters: m is the genetic correlation between mates, g^2 the heritability affected by dominance, h^2 the heritability affected by environment, and γ^2 the common family influence.

4. Estimation of Parameters

Since there are four parameters, we need three other equations to obtain an estimate of the parameters. These are parent–parent, parent–child, and full-sib correlations. From Fig. 4 we have

$$\text{parent–parent:} \qquad r_{PP} = m/g^2h^2 \tag{4.1}$$

$$\text{parent–child:} \qquad r_{PO} = \tfrac{1}{2}(1 + r_{PP})g^2h^2 \tag{4.2}$$

$$\text{full-sibs:} \qquad r_{OO} = [\tfrac{1}{2}(1 + m)g^2 + \tfrac{1}{4}d^2]h^2 + \gamma^2 \tag{4.3}$$

$$\qquad\qquad = \tfrac{1}{4}(1 + g^2 + 2mg^2)h^2 + \gamma^2 \tag{4.3'}$$

where $d^2 = 1 - g^2$. In order to obtain the environmental component, we also need the equation for the complete determination of the phenotype:

$$h^2 + e^2 + \gamma^2 = 1 \tag{4.4}$$

instead of the usual $h^2 + e^2 = 1$.

Once given the observed values of the four kinship correlations, these equations may be readily solved. Equations (4.1) and (4.2) form a set by themselves for the two unknowns g^2h^2 and m. Solving,

$$g^2h^2 = \frac{2r_{PO}}{1 + r_{PP}}, \qquad m = \left(\frac{2r_{PO}}{1 + r_{PP}}\right)r_{PP}$$

Since g^2h^2 and m are known, so are the quantities

$$A = \tfrac{1}{4}(1 + 3m)g^2h^2, \qquad B = (1 + 2m)g^2h^2$$

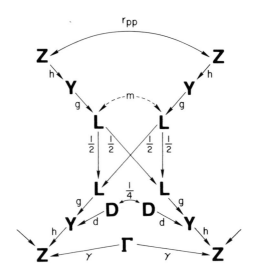

FIGURE 4. Parent–offspring and full sib correlations, assuming the dominance deviations of full sibs are correlated to the degree of 1/4.

Then, from (3.1),

$$\gamma^2 = r_{O/O} - A$$

and from (4.3'),

$$h^2 = 4r_{OO} - B - 4\gamma^2$$

Hence, $g^2 = (g^2 h^2)/(h^2)$ is also known. Finally, (4.4) gives $e^2 = 1 - h^2 - \gamma^2$. This completes the solution.

While the solving of the equations is an easy matter we should point out that it does not always give acceptable results for a given set of four values of kinship correlations. For instance, the solution may yield a g^2 greater than unity or a negative γ^2 for certain observed correlations. In such cases, we must re-examine both the model and the data. Either the model is inappropriate for the population under study, or there is some serious bias in the collection of data, or both.

5. Models and Populations

The correlation models (3.1) and (4.1)–(4.3'), are trying to cope with the general observation that full-sib correlations are usually *higher* than parent–child correlations. It is known that dominance and/or common family environment can make it so. Hence g^2 and γ^2 have been introduced into the models. This may not be appropriate in a different society, especially where the full-sib corre-lation is *lower* than the parent–child correlation. The recent study of two village populations in Gambia, West Africa, by Roberts, Billewicz, and McGregor (1978) illustrates the point clearly. In these Gambia villages a man is allowed to have four wives at any given time, and both divorce and wife inheritance are practiced. So there are both paternal and maternal half sibs available for study. Their main findings are summarized in Table 1.

It is seen from Table 1 that the parental correlation (0.096 ± 0.070) is not statistically significant, indicating that height is hardly a factor in mate selection in that part of Africa. This differs from that of the Western European popu-lations where the r_{PP} with respect to height is of the order of 0.28 to 0.30. Since all parents have been measured (over a period of time), the correlation r_{12} (Fig. 2) between successive fathers or successive mothers can be obtained, but it is not reported by the authors, thus depriving us of an opportunity of comparing r_{12} with r_1 and r_2. The half-sib correlation depends upon these three parental correlations. For instance, the term $3m$ in expression (3.1) would be $(r_1 + r_2 + r_{12})g^2 h^2$, if the r's were known. Only when they are not known we resort to assuming $r_{12} = r_1 = r_2 = r_{PP}$.

But the most striking feature of the results shown in Table 1 is that the full-sib correlations are lower than the parent–child correlations. A blind

Table 1. Correlations with Respect to Height in a West Africa
Population. Excerpted from Roberts, Billewicz, and McGregor (1978)

Parent–parent	Parent–child	
$r_{PP} = 0.096 \pm 0.070$	$r_{PO} = \begin{cases} \text{father–child,} & 0.463 \\ \text{mother–child,} & 0.487 \end{cases}$	

	Full sibs	Half sibs	Full sibs of the same families
$r_{OO} = \begin{cases} \text{males,} & 0.426 \\ \text{females,} & 0.331 \\ \text{both sexes,} & 0.406 \end{cases}$		$r_{O/O} = \begin{cases} \text{paternal,} & 0.140 \\ \text{maternal,} & 0.257 \end{cases}$	$r_{OO} = \begin{cases} 0.405 \\ 0.396 \end{cases}$

application of our models (3.1) and (4.1)–(4.4′) to these results would yield, not surprisingly, both $g^2 > 1$ and a negative γ^2, indicating the inapplicability of our models to a population where the culture pattern, mating system, conditions of nutrition, ways of nursing infants and rearing children, etc. are all different from the West European populations.

The phenomenon $r_{OO} < r_{PO}$ in a population with little phenotypic assortative mating is admittedly difficult to explain even assuming no dominance and no common home environmental effects. However, we may note that strong phenotypic assortative mating does make the full-sib correlation smaller than the parent–child correlation. Purely as a numerical example, let us take $r_{PO} = 0.475$, the average of the reported 0.463 and 0.487 in Table 1. When there is no dominance ($g^2 = 1$) and no common family environment ($\gamma^2 = 0$), we have $m = r_{PP}h^2$, and the expressions (4.2) and (4.3) would reduce to (Wright, 1921:153, 1978:386)

$$r_{PO} = \tfrac{1}{2}(1 + r_{PP})h^2 = 0.475$$

$$r_{OO} = \tfrac{1}{2}(1 + r_{PP}h^2)h^2 = 0.406$$

Solving,

$$r_{PP} = 0.5763 \quad \text{and} \quad h^2 = 0.6027$$

Thus, strong assortative mating and moderate heritability can account for the observed difference in parent–child and full-sib correlations; but this is not the case in Western Africa where the observed marital correlation is insignificantly low.

The phenomenon $r_{PO} > r_{OO}$, needless to say, requires further investigation. While there is no definitive explanation at the present moment, Roberts, Billewicz, and MacGregor (1978) suggested the variation of the within-sibship variance may be responsible for the lowering of the sib–sib correlations.

6. Half-Sib Analysis

The intra class correlation between half sibs are given in the lower right compartment of Table 1, together with that for full sibs of the same families from which the half sibs are obtained. The data on half sibs is a most distinctive

Table 2. The Pattern for Subdivision of Sum of Squares
in Analysis of Variance of Paternal Half Sibs when there
are 113 Fathers, 282 Mothers, and 583 Children. (Also
see Table 6 in Appendix.)

Variation	Degrees of freedom
Between fathers	$113 - 1 = 112$
Between mothers, within fathers	$282 - 113 = 169$
Between sibs, within mothers	$583 - 282 = 301$
Total	$583 - 1 = 582$

and welcome feature of the studies by Roberts, Billewicz, and McGregor (1978). The methodology adopted for the analysis of sib data by these authors is worth noting.

We shall use the paternal half sibs for concreteness in discussion. (For maternal half sibs we merely interchange father and mother.) There are 113 fathers, 282 mothers, and 583 offspring, consisting of both full and half sibs. The measurements of the children are subject to a natural hierarchical classification, for which an analysis of variance may be made. The preliminary subdivision of the sum of squares takes the form shown in Table 2 (see, e.g., Kempthorne, 1957:235–244, or Li, 1964, Chapter 9). The individuals in the second category (between mothers, within fathers) are half sibs, and those in the third category (between sibs, within mothers) are, of course, full sibs.

The authors did not describe the details; what I say here is the usual procedure in variance components analysis. For each category shown above, a mean square = (sum of squares)/(degrees of freedom) and its theoretically expected value are calculated. These expected values are in terms of σ_1^2 = variance between fathers, σ_2^2 = variance between mothers within fathers, and σ_3^2 = variance

Table 3. Variance Components and Intraclass Correlation of Full and
Half Sibs. Rearranged from Roberts, Billewicz, and MacGregor, 1978

Paternal half sibs			Maternal half sibs		
Source	Component		Source	Component	
Between fathers	0.1402		Between mothers	0.2568	
Between mothers, within fathers	0.2647	0.4049	Between fathers, within mothers	0.1389	0.3957
Between sibs, within mothers	0.5951		Between sibs, within fathers	0.6043	
Total	1.0000		Total	1.0000	

between sibs within mothers. Solve for these variances and then express them as fractions, $\sigma_i^2/(\sigma_1^2 + \sigma_2^2 + \sigma_3^2)$, $i = 1, 2, 3$, which add up to unity. These fractions are presumably the values given by the authors, reproduced here in Table 3. If so, the first fraction, 0.1402, is the intraclass correlation between paternal half sibs and the sum of the first two fractions, $0.1402 + 0.2647 = 0.4049$, is the intraclass correlation between full sibs (see Appendix). The same method holds for the maternal half sibs. It is these correlations that are given in the lower-right compartment of Table 1.

Roberts, Billewicz, and MacGregor (1978) do not obtain a single estimate of heritability from the body of data as a whole but calculated the heritabilities for each type of relatives separately, usually based on linear regression coefficients. For example:

Relative	Regression	Heritability
father–child	0.303	0.606
mother–child	0.424	0.848

where heritability is equal to twice the regression coefficient of child on parent. How are we to obtain an estimate of heritability from the variance components shown in Table 3? The authors think the variance components for paternal half sibs are more suitable for estimating heritability than the maternal ones. Their assumptions and calculations are shown in Table 4 (see Appendix also). According to the authors, the results based on paternal half sibs are the most reliable ones. Their general conclusion is that the heritability for height in the Gambia villages is about 56%.

7. Summary and Conclusion

Genetic and environmental variables have been defined and the meaning of three types of heritability clarified. The potential usefulness of studying half sibs has been discussed and one simple model for correlation between half sibs

Table 4. Results of analysis of half-sib data by Roberts,
Billewicz, and MacGregor (1978)

Component (Table 3)		Genetic		Family environment		Random environment
0.1402	=	0.1402				
0.2647	=	0.1402	+	0.1245		
0.5951	=	2(0.1402)			+	0.3147
1.0000	=	0.5608	+	0.1245	+	0.3147

presented. This, together with other kinship correlations, will enable us to estimate linear gene effect, dominance effect, common family environmental effects, and random environmental effects. One limitation is the assumption that environmental factors are uncorrelated with individual's genotype. It is emphasized that genetic and environmental parameters vary from population to population.

Reports on studies of half sibs are scarce. Hence, one recent study of a West Africa population which contains comprehensive data on half sibs has been reviewed with respect to both results and methodology. The purpose of the review is to stimulate interest in studying half sibs, not to be construed as an endorsement to the methodology or findings. On the contrary, I am sure that new models and new methodology will evolve as more empirical knowledge becomes available.

8. Appendix: Hierarchical Classification and Intraclass Correlation

8.1. The Linear Model

To facilitate description and to avoid abstractness, let us continue to use the paternal half sibs as an example. The structure of the hierarchical classification for such a case is shown in Table 5. For each sibship of father i and mother ij, the observed value $(y_{ij\alpha})$ of the quantitative trait of a child is assumed to be of the following linear model:

$$y_{ij\alpha} = u + f_i + m_{ij} + e_{ij\alpha} \qquad (A1)$$

where u is a constant, f_i is the effect of father i, m_{ij} is the effect of mother ij, and $e_{ij\alpha}$ is the variation for the individual α in sibship ij. Other assumptions concerning model (A1) will be given when we need them.

Before doing the analysis of variance it is desirable to obtain the various sums as shown in Table 5. Let n_{ij} be the number of children (and thus the number of observations) in the sibship of father i and mother ij. Then the total number of children of father i is $N_i = \Sigma_j n_{ij}$ and the grand total number of observations is

$$N. = \sum_i N_i = \sum_i \sum_j n_{ij}$$

Let us assume there are H fathers: $i = 1, 2, \ldots, H$. Let us also assume there are K mothers altogether in the data set of Table 5. Next, we obtain the various sums of the observed values of children. Thus,

$$Y_{ij} = \sum_\alpha y_{ij\alpha} = \text{total of a sibship } (ij)$$

Table 5. The Hierarchical Structure of Data

Father	Mother	Observed values of children			Number	Total	Number	Total
Father 1	$\begin{cases} \text{mother 11} \\ \text{mother 12} \end{cases}$	$\cdots$ $y_{11\alpha}$ $\cdots$ $\cdots$ $y_{12\alpha}$ $\cdots$			n_{11} n_{12}	$\left.\begin{array}{c} Y_{11} \\ Y_{12} \end{array}\right\}$	N_1	Y_1
Father i	$\begin{cases} \text{mother } i1 \\ \text{mother } i2 \\ \text{mother } i3 \end{cases}$	$\cdots$ $\cdots$ $\cdots$ $\cdots$ $y_{ij\alpha}$ $\cdots$ $\cdots$ $\cdots$ $\cdots$			n_{i1} n_{i2} n_{i3}	$\left.\begin{array}{c} Y_{i1} \\ Y_{i2} \\ Y_{i3} \end{array}\right\}$	N_i	Y_i
Father H	$\cdots$	$\cdots$ $\cdots$ $\cdots$			$\cdots$	$\cdots$	$\cdots$	$\cdots$
	Total	$\sum_i \sum_j \sum_\alpha y_{ij\alpha}$			$N.$	$Y.$	$N.$	$Y.$

$$Y_i = \sum_j Y_{ij} = \text{total of sibships of the same father}$$

$$Y. = \sum_i Y_i = \sum_i \sum_j Y_{ij} = \sum_i \sum_j \sum_\alpha y_{ij\alpha} = \text{grand total}$$

as shown in the bottom line of Table 5. Note that we simply write Y_i instead of $Y_{i.}$ for the total of sibships of the same father, as $Y_{.i}$ has no meaning for a hierarchical classification. The analysis of the data may then proceed according to the following steps.

8.2. Analysis of Variance

The analysis of variance requires the calculation of various "sums of squares" (*ssq*), each of which is associated with a number of degrees of freedom (*df*). To facilitate the calculation of such required sums of squares, it is best to first calculate the following quantities (A, B_1, B_2, C) based on the data exhibited in Table 5:

$$\begin{array}{cccc} A & B_1 & B_2 & C \\ = \sum_i \sum_j \sum_\alpha y_{ij\alpha}^2, & = \sum_i \sum_j \left(\dfrac{Y_{ij}^2}{n_{ij}} \right), & = \sum_i \left(\dfrac{Y_i^2}{N_i} \right), & = \dfrac{Y.^2}{N.} \quad \text{(A2)} \end{array}$$

These four quantities are arranged in descending order ($A > B_1 > B_2 > C$). These quantities have been called "areas" by Li (1964, Chapter 9), as they can be represented geometrically as areas in a natural way. Once these four basic quantities are calculated, the subsequent analysis follows easily, as the difference between two adjacent quantities is a required sum of squares in the analysis of variance (Table 6). The "mean square" (*msq*) is obtained as *ssq/df*.

The third source of variation in Table 6, viz., between individuals (within

Table 6. Preliminary Analysis of Variance of Data in Table 5. Quantities
A, B_1, B_2, C Are Those Given by Eq. (A2). H = Number of Fathers;
K = Number of Mothers. N = N. = Total Number of Children = Total
Number of Observations

Source of variation	Degrees of freedom df	Sum of squares ssq	Mean square msq
Between fathers (within population)	$H - 1$	$B_2 - C$	$(B_2 - C)/(H - 1)$
Between mothers (within fathers)	$K - H$	$B_1 - B_2$	$(B_1 - B_2)/(K - H)$
Between individuals (within mothers)	$N - K$	$A - B_1$	$(A - B_1)/(N - K)$
Total	$N - 1$	$A - C$	

mothers), is simply the variation among the children of the same father and the same mother; that is among the full sibs. It may also be designated succinctly as the "within-sibship" variation.

In the ordinary analysis of variance of experimental data, the variance ratio (F) would be used to test the significance of the major and minor classifications. In our present context, however, such a significance test would not have much meaning, as we know the fathers and mothers are all different genetically as well as environmentally. Furthermore, the "within-sibship" variation is also partially genetical and is not to be regarded as "experimental error." Our purpose here is to estimate the variances of the fathers, mothers, and the children. In other words, a variance component analysis, as described in the subsequent section, is called for.

8.3. Expected Values of Mean Squares

Since a mean square is expressed in terms of a sum of squares associated with degrees of freedom (Table 6), all we need to calculate are the expected values of the four quantities A, B_1, B_2, C. These are given in the upper portion of Table 7, from which the expected values of the mean squares may be obtained (lower portion of Table 7). The nonstatistical biologist may use the tabulated expected values directly without going through the derivations. However, the following details give us much understanding of the linear model and the technique of variance component analysis. First, we write out systematically the various totals in view of (A1):

individual: $\quad y_{ij\alpha} = u + f_i + m_{ij} + e_{ij\alpha}$

sibship (ij): $\quad Y_{ij} = n_{ij}u + n_{ij}f_i + n_{ij}m_{ij} + \sum_\alpha e_{ij\alpha}$

$$(A3)$$

sibships (i): $\quad Y_i = N_i u + N_i f_i + \sum_j n_{ij}m_{ij} + \sum_j \sum_\alpha e_{ij\alpha}$

grand total: $\quad Y. = N.u + \sum_i N_i f_i + \sum_i \sum_j n_{ij}m_{ij} + \sum_i \sum_j \sum_\alpha e_{ij\alpha}$

Table 7. Expected Values of Sum of Squares and Mean Squares

$$E(A) = E\left\{\sum_i \sum_j \sum_\alpha y_{ij\alpha}^2\right\} = N_. u^2 + N_. \sigma_f^2 + N_. \sigma_m^2 + N_. \sigma_e^2$$

$$E(B_1) = E\left\{\sum_i \sum_j \frac{Y_{ij}^2}{n_{ij}}\right\} = N_. u^2 + N_. \sigma_f^2 + N_. \sigma_m^2 + K\sigma_e^2$$

$$E(B_2) = E\left\{\sum_i \frac{Y_i^2}{N_i}\right\} = N_. u^2 + N_. \sigma_f^2 + \sum_i \left(\frac{\Sigma_j n_{ij}^2}{N_i}\right) \sigma_m^2 + H\sigma_e^2$$

$$E(C) = E\left\{\frac{Y_.^2}{N_.}\right\} = N_. u^2 + \frac{\Sigma_i N_i^2}{N_.} \sigma_f^2 + \frac{\Sigma_i \Sigma_j n_{ij}^2}{N_.} \sigma_m^2 + \sigma_e^2$$

Expected values of mean squares

Between fathers
(within population) $E(B_2 - C)/(H-1) = \sigma_e^2 + k_2\sigma_m^2 + k_3\sigma_f^2$

Between mothers
(within fathers) $E(B_1 - B_2)/(K-H) = \sigma_e^2 + k_1\sigma_m^2$

Between individuals
(within sibships) $E(A - B_1)/(N-K) = \sigma_e^2$

where

$$k_1 = \frac{1}{K-H}\left(N - \sum_i \frac{\Sigma_j n_{ij}^2}{N_i}\right)$$

$$k_2 = \frac{1}{H-1}\left(\sum_i \frac{\Sigma_j n_{ij}^2}{N_i} - \frac{\Sigma_i \Sigma_j n_{ij}^2}{N}\right)$$

$$k_3 = \frac{1}{H-1}\left(N - \frac{\Sigma_i N_i^2}{N}\right)$$

where u is a constant. In taking the expected values of the square of these totals, we assume that f_i, m_{ij}, and $e_{ij\alpha}$ are independent random variables with mean zero and variances σ_f^2, σ_m^2, and σ_e^2, respectively. Thus, $E(y_{ij\alpha}) = u = $ mean and

$$E(f_i^2) = \sigma_f^2, \qquad E(m_{ij}^2) = \sigma_m^2, \qquad E(e_{ij\alpha}^2) = \sigma_e^2,$$

The expected values of *all* product terms are zero on account of independence:

$$E(f_i m_{ij}) = 0, \qquad E(f_i e_{ij\alpha}) = 0, \qquad E(m_{ij} e_{ij\alpha}) = 0$$

and

$$E(f_i f_{i'}) = 0 \qquad E(m_{ij} m_{ij'}) = 0, \qquad E(e_{ij\alpha} e_{ij\alpha'}) = 0$$

where $i \neq i'$, $j \neq j'$, $\alpha \neq \alpha'$. With these assumptions, the expected values of the four quantities in (A2) may be readily obtained. For instance, the expectation of a single square is

$$E(y_{ij\alpha}^2) = E(u + f_i + m_{ij} + e_{ij\alpha})^2$$
$$= u^2 + \sigma_f^2 + \sigma_m^2 + \sigma_e^2$$

The sum of N. such expectations is

$$E(A) = E\left(\sum_i \sum_j \sum_\alpha y_{ij\alpha}^2\right) = N.u^2 + N.\sigma_f^2 + N.\sigma_m^2 + N.\sigma_e^2$$

which is the value given in Table 7.

Before proceeding to find the expectation of B_1 we note that

$$E\left(\sum_\alpha e_{ij\alpha}\right)\left(\sum_\alpha e_{ij\alpha}\right) = E(e + \cdots + e)(e + \cdots + e) = n_{ij}\sigma_e^2$$

because there are only n_{ij} square terms like $e_{ij\alpha}^2$ in the expansion, all other terms being of the type $e_{ij\alpha}e_{ij\alpha'}$ whose expectation is zero. Hence, the square of a sibship total (A3) has the expectation

$$E(Y_{ij}^2) = E\left(n_{ij}u + n_{ij}f_i + n_{ij}m_{ij} + \sum_\alpha e_{ij\alpha}\right)^2$$
$$= n_{ij}^2 u^2 + n_{ij}^2 \sigma_f^2 + n_{ij}^2 \sigma_m^2 + n_{ij}\sigma_e^2$$

Dividing the expectation above by n_{ij} throughout and then summing over all (ij) sibships, we obtain

$$E(B_1) = E\left\{\sum_i \sum_j \left(\frac{Y_{ij}^2}{n_{ij}}\right)\right\} = N.u^2 + N.\sigma_f^2 + N.\sigma_m^2 + K\sigma_e^2$$

where K = number of mothers = number of sibships. This is the second value given in Table 7.

The remaining expectations may be found in exactly the same manner. To clarify certain coefficients, an intermediate step is given below. From the total of the sibships of the same father given in (A3), we have

$$E(Y_i^2) = N.{}_i^2 u^2 + N.{}_i^2 \sigma_f^2 + \sum_j n_{ij}^2 \sigma_m^2 + N_i \sigma_e^2$$

Dividing the expectation above by N_i throughout and then summing over the fathers, we obtain $E(B_2)$ given in Table 7. Note the coefficient of σ_m^2 in $E(B_2)$ is, using the data of Table 5,

$$\sum_i \left(\frac{\Sigma_j n_{ij}^2}{N_i}\right) = \frac{n_{11}^2 + n_{12}^2}{N_1} + \cdots + \frac{n_{i1}^2 + n_{i2}^2 + n_{i3}^2}{N_i} + \cdots$$

which is clearer than the simpler expression $\Sigma_i \Sigma_j (n_{ij}^2/N_i)$, meaning the same thing, of course. Finally, from the grand total given in (A3), we have

$$E(Y^2) = N^2 u^2 + \sum_i N_i^2 \sigma_f^2 + \sum_i \sum_j n_{ij}^2 \sigma_m^2 + N. \sigma_e^2$$

Dividing the above by N. yields the expression for $E(C)$ in Table 7. This completes the derivation of the expectations of A, B_1, B_2, C.

To find the expected values of the mean squares, we note some regularities in the expressions in the upper portion of Table 7. First, every expected value has the term $N.u^2$, where u is the general mean of the population. Second, the coefficient of σ_e^2 in each expression is the number of degrees of freedom for the corresponding quantity; that is, the numbers $N., K, H, 1$, are the degrees of freedom for the quantities A, B_1, B_2, C, respectively. Since the sums of squares are the differences between two adjacent quantities (Table 6), the term $N.u^2$ cancels out in their expectations and the coefficients of σ_e^2 are exactly the degrees of freedom of the corresponding sums of squares. For example, the expected value of the within-sibship mean square (the third in Table 6) is

$$\frac{E(A - B_1)}{N. - K} = \frac{E(A) - E(B_1)}{N. - K} = \frac{(N. - K)\sigma_e^2}{N. - K} = \sigma_e^2$$

which is given in the bottom line of Table 7. For the same reason, the expected value of the other mean squares also contains the term σ_e^2.

In the difference $E(B_1 - B_2) = E(B_1) - E(B_2)$, the terms $N.u^2$ and $N.\sigma_f^2$ cancel out and only the terms involving σ_m^2 and σ_e^2 remain. Dividing this difference by $df = K - H$, we obtain the term σ_e^2 and the coefficient of σ_m^2 is

$$k_1 = \frac{N. - \Sigma_i \Sigma_j n_{ij}^2 / N_i}{K - H}$$

The coefficients k_2 and k_3 in the lower half of Table 7 are obtained the same way.

Since the numerical values of the mean square (Table 6) and the k coefficients (Table 7) are all known, the values of $\sigma_e^2, \sigma_m^2, \sigma_f^2$ may be readily solved from the equations in the lower half of Table 7. Now, suppose these variances have been found. Then the variance of the original observations may be estimated by

$$\sigma_y^2 = E(y_{ij\alpha}^2) - u^2 = \sigma_f^2 + \sigma_m^2 + \sigma_e^2 \qquad (A4)$$

where σ_f^2 is the variance of father's effect, σ_m^2 is the variance of mother's effect (within fathers), and σ_e^2 is the variance of individuals within sibships. At the risk of being repetitious, we remind the reader that the variance σ_e^2 is partially genetic and partially environmental in our present context (see A12), and it is not the "error" variance on replicated observations receiving the same "treatment" in experimental statistics.

8.4. Intraclass Correlation

Since the values of the variances σ_f^2, σ_m^2, and σ_e^2 have been found, we are now ready to calculate the intraclass correlation between half sibs and between full sibs. Children of the same father and different mothers are paternal half sibs. In our notation, they belong to sibships (ij) and (ij'), where $j \neq j'$. The covariance of half sibs is

$$\begin{aligned}
\text{cov (half sibs)} &= E(y_{ij\alpha} - u)(y_{ij'\alpha'} - u) \\
&= E(f_i + m_{ij} + e_{ij\alpha})(f_i + m_{ij'} + e_{ij'\alpha'}) \qquad \text{(A5)} \\
&= E(f_i^2) = \sigma_f^2
\end{aligned}$$

as all product terms have expectation zero. The variance of y has been given in (A4). Thus the correlation between half sibs is

$$r\text{(half sibs)} = \frac{\text{cov (half sibs)}}{\text{variance}} = \frac{\sigma_f^2}{\sigma_f^2 + \sigma_m^2 + \sigma_e^2} \qquad \text{(A6)}$$

This justifies the taking of the first fraction in Table 3 as the correlation between half sibs.

Full sibs are individuals who belong to the same sibship (ij) but $\alpha \neq \alpha'$. Their covariance is

$$\begin{aligned}
\text{cov (full sibs)} &= E(f_i + m_{ij} + e_{ij\alpha})(f_i + m_{ij} + e_{ij\alpha'}) \\
&= E(f_i^2) + E(m_{ij}^2) = \sigma_f^2 + \sigma_m^2
\end{aligned} \qquad \text{(A7)}$$

as all product terms have expectation zero. Hence the correlation between full sibs is

$$r\text{(full sibs)} = \frac{\text{cov (full sibs)}}{\text{variance}} = \frac{\sigma_f^2 + \sigma_m^2}{\sigma_f^2 + \sigma_m^2 + \sigma_e^2} \qquad \text{(A8)}$$

This justifies the taking of the sum of the first two fractions in Table 3 as the correlation between full sibs.

Needless to say, children of different fathers (and necessarily of different mothers) are unrelated and have zero correlation. This is formalized by saying $E(f_i f_{i'}) = 0$, where $i \neq i'$.

It may also be mentioned that for the subpopulation with a fixed father, we omit σ_f^2 from (A8) and obtain

$$r'\text{(full sibs)} = \frac{\sigma_m^2}{\sigma_m^2 + \sigma_e^2} \qquad \text{(A9)}$$

which is the usual formula for intraclass correlation for a simple one-way classification.

8.5. The Genetics Connection

The previous sections (analysis of variance, expected values of mean squares, and intraclass correlation) represent a purely statistical analysis of the data (Table 5) or any other set of data with a similar twofold hierarchical classification. There has been no genetical considerations, still less genetical interpretations. It is seemingly unconnected with our basic genetic model exhibited in Fig. 1 ($L + D = Y$ and $Y + E = Z$) in the text. The purpose of this section is to make the connection between the statistical results of the foregoing sections and the genetical model described in the text.

In making the genetics connection, we should be careful about the notation as we have used two separate systems of notation, each conventional in its own field. For instance, the letter e of $e_{ij\alpha}$ in the linear model (A1) is obviously not the e in the expression $h^2 + e^2 = 1$, where $e^2 = \sigma_E^2/\sigma_Z^2$ in the text. We use σ_e^2 to denote the variance of $e_{ij\alpha}$ within sibships (ij), and use σ_E^2 in the text to denote the variance of E, the environmental effect on the development of a phenotype Z. It is important to distinguish these two variances in the subsequent paragraphs.

Another common letter in the two systems of notation is m. In the text, m is the correlation between mates' genetic linear values L. In the Appendix, m_{ij} is the mother's effect (within fathers) on the quantitative trait of the children. From now on, however, we take $m = r(\text{mates'} L) = 0$, to be consistent with the previous assumption $E(f_i m_{ij}) = 0$. In other words, the assumption of the independence of f_i and m_{ij} implies random mating in the population. Hence the following results apply to random mating populations, as in the West African villages.

Finally, we recall that in the text the model is $L + D = Y$ and $Y + E = Z$ where Y is the genotype value and Z is the phenotype value. In the Appendix, we use $y = y_{ij\alpha}$ to denote the measurement of children (i.e., their phenotype value). Here we make the first genetics connection, viz.,

$$Z = y_{ij\alpha} \qquad \text{and} \qquad \sigma_Z^2 = \sigma_y^2 \qquad (A10)$$

where σ_y^2 is that given by (A4). Clearly, the sibship totals Y_{ij}, Y_i, and $Y.$ have nothing to do with the genotype value $Y = L + D$.

Now, from elementary population genetics (e.g., Li, 1976) we know that the covariance between full sibs is $\frac{1}{2}\sigma_L^2 + \frac{1}{4}\sigma_D^2$ and the covariance between half sibs is $\frac{1}{4}\sigma_L^2$, where L is the linear additive value and D the dominance deviation, assuming genotype and environment are uncorrelated. Equating these to (A7) and (A5), we have

$$\text{cov (full sibs)} = \sigma_f^2 + \sigma_m^2 = \frac{1}{2}\sigma_L^2 + \frac{1}{4}\sigma_D^2$$

$$\underline{\text{cov (half sibs)} = \sigma_f^2 \qquad\quad = \frac{1}{4}\sigma_L^2} \qquad (A11)$$

$$\text{subtracting} \qquad\quad \sigma_m^2 = \frac{1}{4}\sigma_L^2 + \frac{1}{4}\sigma_D^2$$

But the total phenotypic variance remains the same (A10), whatever the method of analysis. Hence the components of σ_e^2 may be obtained by subtraction.

The complete relationship is shown below:

$$
\begin{array}{lll}
\text{between fathers} & \sigma_f^2 = \tfrac{1}{4}\sigma_L^2 & \\[4pt]
\begin{array}{l}\text{between mothers}\\ \text{(within fathers)}\end{array} & \underline{\sigma_m^2 = \tfrac{1}{4}\sigma_L^2 + \tfrac{1}{4}\sigma_D^2} & \\[4pt]
\text{between sibships } \sigma_f^2 + \sigma_m^2 = \tfrac{1}{2}\sigma_L^2 + \tfrac{1}{4}\sigma_D^2 & & \text{(A12)}\\[4pt]
\text{within sibships} & \underline{\sigma_e^2 = \tfrac{1}{2}\sigma_L^2 + \tfrac{3}{4}\sigma_D^2 + \sigma_E^2} & \\[4pt]
\text{total} & \sigma_y^2 = \sigma_L^2 + \sigma_D^2 + \sigma_E^2 = \sigma_Z^2 &
\end{array}
$$

The sum of the first two components (between fathers and between mothers, within fathers) is the variance *between sibships*, which is also the covariance for full sibs. The within-sibship variance $\sigma_e^2 = \tfrac{1}{2}\sigma_L^2 + \tfrac{3}{4}\sigma_D^2 + \sigma_E^2$ justifies our previous statement that the variance within sibships is partially genetical and partially environmental. The total relationship (A12) shows the two different ways of subdividing the total variance.

Since the numerical values of σ_f^2, σ_m^2, and σ_e^2 are known from Table 7, the values of σ_L^2, σ_D^2, and σ_e^2 may be found from (A12). This will in turn enable us to calculate the various types of heritabilities. Thus,

$$
\begin{array}{lll}
g^2 = \sigma_L^2/\sigma_Y^2 & \quad & \text{dominance heritability}\\[4pt]
h^2 = \sigma_Y^2/\sigma_Z^2 & \quad & \text{environmental heritability}\\[4pt]
g^2 h^2 = \sigma_L^2/\sigma_Z^2 & \quad & \text{combined (net) heritability}
\end{array}
$$

In summary, the analysis of the type of data exhibited in Table 5 will not only give us the correlation between full sibs and half sibs from the same set of families, but also enable us to estimate the various types of heritabilities at the same time.

8.6. Genetic Variance between and within Sibships

The essential purpose of this section is to verify numerically some of the results obtained in the foregoing sections, especially those concerning the subdivision of the genetic variance ($\sigma_Y^2 = \sigma_L^2 + \sigma_D^2$) into between-sibships and within-sibships components. To work through a numerical example would be helpful to clarify the precise meaning and relationship of the various quantities such as σ_f^2, etc. To do this with minimum effort it is best to use an entire population rather than a set of sample observations, thus bypassing the problems of estimation. Since the environmental variance σ_E^2 appears only within sibships (A12), it may be ignored for our present purpose, so that we can concentrate on the allocation of the genetic variance.

Table 8. The Analysis of Genotype Variance $(\sigma_Y^2 = \sigma_L^2 + \sigma_D^2)$ of a Random Mating Population with Gene Frequencies $p = q = \frac{1}{2}$.

	Genotype AA	Aa	aa	Population	
	Frequency 1/4	1/2	1/4	mean	variance
Genotype value, Y	9	7	1	$\bar{Y} = 6.0,$	$\sigma_Y^2 = 9.00$
Linear value, L	10	6	2	$\bar{L} = 6.0,$	$\sigma_L^2 = 8.00$
Dominance deviation, D	-1	$+1$	-1	$\bar{D} = 0,$	$\sigma_D^2 = 1.00$

Table 9. The Allocation of Genetic Variance in a Random Mating Population, Table 8

Father	mother	frequency	Children's Y 9	7	1	Sibship mean	variance
AA	AA	1	1	0	0	9.0	0
	Aa	2	1	1	0	8.0	1.00
	aa	1	0	1	0	7.0	0
		4				mean 8.0 var 0.5	
Aa	AA	2	1	1	0	8.0	1.00
	Aa	4	1	2	1	6.0	9.00
	aa	2	0	1	1	4.0	9.00
		8				mean 6.0 var 2.0	
aa	AA	1	0	1	0	7.0	0
	Aa	2	0	1	1	4.0	9.00
	aa	1	0	0	1	1.0	0
		4				mean 4.0 var 4.5	

$$\text{Variance of group mean} = \sigma_f^2 = 2.00$$

$$\text{Mean of within-group variance} = \sigma_m^2 = 2.25 \quad \sigma_e^2 = 4.75$$

What we shall verify is true for any gene frequency, but we shall use $p = q = \frac{1}{2}$ to further reduce the arithmetic labor involved. The population under consideration is shown in Table 8. The structure of the families in the population is shown in Table 9. First, it is to be regarded as a hierarchical classification wherein each father has several mates. The mean and variance of each sibship is calculated. The sibships are grouped according to the father. Then the mean of the sibships of the same father is calculated for each father (8.0, 6.0, 4.0 with frequencies 4, 8, 4 respectively). The variance of such "father's mean" (= mean of sibships of the same father) is found to be

$$\text{(i)} \qquad \sigma_f^2 = 2.00 = \tfrac{1}{4}\sigma_L^2$$

Next, for each group of sibships of the same father, we calculate the variance (0.5, 2.0, 4.5, with frequencies 4, 8, 4, respectively) of the sibship means. The average of these variances is that "between mothers, within fathers," and it is readily found to be

$$\text{(ii)} \qquad \sigma_m^2 = 2.25 = \tfrac{1}{4}\sigma_L^2 + \tfrac{1}{4}\sigma_D^2$$

Now, let us regard Table 9 as an ordinary random mating table with nine types of sibships (no grouping by father). Then the variance of the sibship means (9, 8, 7, 8, 6, 4, 7, 4, 1) is that "between sibships." It will be found to be

$$\text{(iii) between sibships,} \qquad \sigma_f^2 + \sigma_m^2 = 4.25 = \tfrac{1}{2}\sigma_L^2 + \tfrac{1}{4}\sigma_D^2$$

Finally, the average value of the within-sibship variances (last column of Table 9) will be found to be

$$\text{(iv) within sibships,} \qquad \sigma_e^2 = 4.75 = \tfrac{1}{2}\sigma_L^2 + \tfrac{3}{4}\sigma_D^2$$

ignoring the environmental variance σ_E^2. When the genotype values 9, 7, 1 are subject to uncorrelated environmental fluctuations with variance σ_E^2, then the within sibship variance is $\sigma_e^2 = 4.75 + \sigma_E^2$.

This completes the clarification of the meaning of σ_f^2 and σ_m^2 and the verification of their relationship with σ_L^2 and σ_D^2. When there is no dominance, the genetic variance is equally allocated to between sibships and within sibships, a well-known result in population genetics. General accounts of analysis of variance and intraclass correlation may be found in Falconer (1960), Fieller and Smith (1951), and Smith (1957).

ACKNOWLEDGMENT

I express my grateful thanks to Professor Oscar Kempthorne, who has clarified several points for me during the preparation of the Appendix. The remaining errors are mine.

References

Falconer, D. S. (1960a), *Introduction to Quantitative Genetics*, Ronald Press, New York.

Falconer, D. S. (1960b), *Quantitative Genetics*, Ronald Press, New York.

Fieller, E. C., and Smith, C. A. B. (1951), Note on the analysis of variance and intraclass correlation, *Ann. Eugen.* 16:97–104.

Kempthorne, O. (1957), *An Introduction to Genetic Statistics*, John Wiley, New York. (Reprinted by Iowa State University Press, Ames, Iowa.)

Li, C. C. (1964), Chap. 9 of *Introduction to Experimental Statistics*, McGraw-Hill, New York.

Li, C. C. (1976), *First Course in Population Genetics*, Boxwood Press, Pacific Grove, California.

Li, C. C. (1977), Separation of common environment and dominance effects with classic kinship correlation models, *Soc. Biol.* **24**:259–266.

Li, C. C. (1978), Progress of the kinship correlation models, in *Genetic Epidemiology* (N. E. Morton and C. S. Chung, eds.), pp. 55–86, Academic Press, New York.

Nagylaki, T. (1978), The correlation between relatives with assortative mating, *Ann. Hum. Genet.* **42**:131–137.

Rao, D. C., Morton, N. E., and Yee, S. (1974), Analysis of family resemblance. II. A linear model for familial correlation, *Am. J. Hum. Genet.* **26**:331–359.

Rao, D. C., Morton, N. E., and Yee, S. (1976), Resolution of cultural and biological inheritance by path analysis, *Am. J. Hum. Genet.* **28**:228–242.

Roberts, D. F., Billewicz, W. Z., and McGregor, I. A. (1978), Heritability of stature in a West African population, *Ann. Hum. Genet.* **42**:15–24.

Smith, C. A. B. (1957), On the estimation of intraclass correlation, *Ann. Hum. Genet.* **21**:363–373.

Wright, S. (1921), Assortative mating based on somatic resemblance, *Genetics* **6**:144–161.

Wright, S. (1978), *Evolution and the Genetics of Populations*, Vol. 4, *Variability Within and Among Natural Populations*, University of Chicago Press, Chicago.

Mental Abilities

A Family Study

JOHN C. DeFRIES

1. Introduction

In the introductory chapter of *Hereditary Genius: An Inquiry Into Its Laws and Consequences*, Francis Galton (1869) began as follows: "I propose to show in this book that a man's natural abilities are derived by inheritance, under exactly the same limitations as are the form and physical features of the whole organic world " (p. 45). In this work, Galton demonstrated that relatives of eminent men (as subjectively evaluated by Galton) were more likely to be eminent than expected on the basis of chance alone; moreover, the closer the relationship to the most eminent man in the family, the higher the incidence of eminence.

Galton recognized that relatives of eminent men would share some social, educational, and financial advantages. He argued, however, that reputation is not due to environmental advantage, but to natural ability. One rather quaint argument against the hypothesis of environmental influence involved a comparison between the success of adopted kinsmen of Roman Catholic Popes and that of sons of eminent men. Although the former were given great social advantages, according to Galton, the latter were the more distinguished group.

In addition to the problem of cleanly separating genetic and environmental influences (a problem shared by current studies in human behavioral genetics),

---

JOHN C. DEFRIES ● Institute for Behavioral Genetics, University of Colorado, Boulder, Colorado 80309.   This report was supported in part by NICHD Grant No. HD-10333.

Galton's study lacked an objective index of mental ability. In order to rectify this shortcoming in subsequent research, Galton later developed a plethora of objective measures of human behavior, such as auditory thresholds, visual acuity, color vision, touch, smell, judgment of the vertical, judgment of length, weight discrimination, reaction time, and memory. [For a brief review of Galton's pioneering contributions to psychology and statistics, see McClearn and DeFries (1973).]

Of special significance to human behavioral genetics was Galton's (1875) introduction of the twin study method. In his book, *Inquiries Into Human Faculty and Its Development*, Galton (1883) summarized the evidence concerning the similarity of twins that were either "alike" or "unlike" at birth. Based upon evidence obtained from questionnaires and biographical material, Galton concluded that the similarity of members of 35 twin pairs who were similar at birth and who had been reared under similar conditions persisted after the twins had reached adulthood and gone their separate ways. In contrast, 20 sets of twins who were unlike at birth were not found to become more similar after being exposed to a similar environment.

Almost 100 years later, there is still disagreement concerning the effectiveness of the twin study method for separating genetic and environmental influences (cf. DeFries, Vandenberg, and McClearn, 1976; Lewontin, 1975). Nevertheless, twin studies have made many significant contributions to the field of human behavioral genetics and they continue to do so (see Loehlin and Nichols, 1976; Fuller and Thompson, 1978).

In recognition of his pioneering contributions, Galton has often been designated as the "father of mental testing" (Fuller and Thompson, 1978). A century of research in psychology, clearly foreshadowed by Galton, has demonstrated that cognition is multidimensional. The primary objective of this chapter is to communicate the principle that a multivariate approach is necessary in the study of mental abili*ties* (not mental abili*ty*). I shall begin by summarizing briefly the history of the development of cognitive test instruments and early family studies of specific cognitive abilities. This summary will be followed by a discussion of the genetics of spatial ability and an overview of the Hawaii Family Study of Cognition. [For a recent review of the genetics of specific cognitive abilities, see DeFries, Vandenberg, and McClearn (1976)].

2. Historical Developments

James McKeen Cattell, who coined the term "mental test" in 1890, worked with Galton in England and later brought his ideas to the United States. Cattell experimented with various ability measures, including keenness of eyesight and hearing, reaction time, afterimages, color vision, perception of pitch, and judgement of a 10-sec interval (Cattell and Farrand, 1896).

In 1904, an experimental psychologist at the Sorbonne, Alfred Binet, was appointed to a commission that had been assigned the task of formulating a national system of education for mentally retarded children. The commission concluded that no child should be sent to a special school unless an examination revealed that the child would be unable to profit from instruction in a regular school. Binet and Simon (1905, 1911) succeeded in developing a test that was effective for this purpose. The Binet–Simon test was later revised by Terman (1916) at Stanford University for administration in the United States.

Meanwhile, in England, Charles Spearman (1904) was attempting to provide a theoretical basis for the concept of intelligence. He developed a statistical procedure for measuring the extent to which correlated tests were measuring something in common and something that was test specific. In Spearman's "two-factor theory" of intelligence, the first factor was ascribed to general intelligence, whereas the second was a specific factor unique to each test.

Later investigators proposed the existence of other "group factors," the most prominent advocate being Thurstone (1938, 1947). In addition to developing a shortcut procedure for extracting factors from a correlation matrix, Thurston recommended rotating these factors to achieve "simple structure" (each test having loadings on only a few factors). Using these techniques, Thurstone identified seven uncorrelated factors (verbal meaning, verbal fluency, numerical ability, spatial ability, inductive reasoning, memory, and perceptual speed) in mental test data from several large studies. He later noted that a closer approach to simple structure could sometimes be achieved when factors were allowed to be correlated. Correlations among these "oblique" factors could then, in turn, be factor analyzed to produce higher-order-factor solutions. This hierarchical model of intelligence represented something of a compromise between Spearman's theory of one general plus many specific factors and Thurstone's original multiple-factor theory. Although more complex factorial structures, such as Guilford's 120 uncorrelated ability factors (Guilford and Hoepfner, 1971), have been postulated, what consensus there is seems to favor Thurstone's hierarchical model (Horn, 1976).

3. Previous Family Studies

The first family study of specific cognitive abilities was reported by Willoughby in 1927. A battery of six verbal and five nonverbal tests was administered to 141 children (12.5 to 13.5 years of age) and to members of their families. Average familial correlations for the verbal tests exceeded those for the nonverbal tests for all parent–offspring combinations and for two of three sibling comparisons. Five years later, Carter (1932) reported the results of another large family study of specific cognitive abilities. Two vocabulary and four arithmetic subtests were administered to members of 139 family groups which included one or more children over 12 years of age. Familial correlations again tended to be higher for the verbal tests.

For the next several decades, most family studies of cognition focused on measures of general intelligence. However, a resurgence of interest in the genetics of specific cognitive abilities has occurred, due at least in part to the success of twin studies (cf. Vandenberg, 1968). Williams (1975), for example, compared WISC data on 55 sons (10 years of age) to WAIS scores of their parents. In general, familial resemblance was greater for the verbal subtests than for the performance subtests, and this difference was especially marked between the verbal and performance IQ aggregates.

More recently, Loehlin, Sharan, and Jacoby (1978) adminstered a battery of cognitive tests (measuring verbal, numerical, perceptual speed, and spatial abilities) to 192 families in Tel Aviv, Israel. Complete data were obtained on both parents and two children (at least 13 years of age) in each family. In contrast to the results of previous studies, familial correlations for the verbal tests were not consistently higher than those for the nonverbal tests.

4. Genetics of Spatial Ability

The primary objective of the family study by Loehlin, Sharan, and Jacoby (1978) was to test the hypothesis that spatial ability is influenced by a sex-linked, recessive gene. In 1943, O'Connor observed that only about 25% of females scored above the median of males on a test of spatial ability, a result consistent with a hypothesis of sex-linked, recessive inheritance. Stafford (1961) later reported parent–child correlations for a spatial test which were also consistent with this hypothesis.

In contrast to the case of autosomal inheritance, the expected patterns of familial correlations for sex-linked characters depend upon the sex of the family members involved. The expected patterns of parent–offspring and sibling correlations for sex-linked, recessive characters are shown in Table 1. It may be seen in Table 2 that the order of parent–offspring correlations obtained by Stafford (1961) is in excellent agreement with this expectation. Parent–offspring correlations reported in four subsequent studies are also presented in Table 2. Only the small study by Hartlage (1970) yielded a pattern of correlations which closely approximates that observed by Stafford.

Yen (1975) utilized sibling correlations to test the hypothesis that spatial ability is influenced by a sex-linked, recessive gene. Four tests of spatial ability (spatial relations, paper form board, paper folding, and mental rotations) were administered to approximately 400 pairs of siblings who were high school students living in the San Francisco Bay area. The sex-linked, recessive pattern of correlations was obtained for all tests except spatial relations.

Table 1. Familial Correlations for Sex-Linked, Recessive Characters[a]

Parent–Offspring $r_{FS} < r_{MD} < r_{MS} = r_{FD}$ Sibling $r_{SD} < r_{SS} < r_{DD}$	$\begin{cases} F = \text{father's score} \\ S = \text{son's score} \\ M = \text{mother's score} \\ D = \text{daughter's score} \end{cases}$

Recent studies by Bouchard and McGee (1977) and by Loehlin, Sharan, and Jacoby (1978) have reported both parent–offspring and sibling correlations for tests of spatial ability. As may be seen in Table 3, their results provide little or no support for the sex-linkage hypothesis.

A rather sophisticated alternative test of sex-linkage was employed by Bock and Kolakowski (1973). They utilized maximum likelihood methods to resolve spatial score distributions for 380 boys and 347 girls into normalized components. Chi-square tests revealed significant departures when the data were fitted to a single normal distribution, but no significant departure from a two-component solution. From the fraction of individuals in the upper component of the boys' distribution, the frequency of the hypothesized recessive allele for high spatial ability (q) was estimated to be 0.5. Thus, the expected proportion of individuals in the upper component of the girls' distribution (q^2) was 0.25, a value close to the observed proportion of 0.20. Subsequent utilization of a similar approach by Yen (1975) and by Loehlin, Sharan, and Jacoby (1978) yielded rather mixed results. Thus, the latter investigators concluded that "the final word is not yet in on the 'spatial gene' " (p. 40).

One of the goals of the Hawaii Family Study of Cognition was to test the hypothesis that spatial ability is influenced by a sex-linked, recessive gene. The remainder of this chapter is devoted to a discussion of the Hawaii study.

Table 2. Parent–Offspring Correlations for Tests of Spatial Ability[a]

Author	Test	Father–son	Mother–daughter	Mother–daughter	Father–son
Stafford (1961)	Identical blocks	0.02(51)[b]	0.14(64)	0.31(50)	0.31(63)
Corah (1965)	Embedded figures	0.18(30)	0.02(30)	0.31(30)	0.28(30)
Hartlage (1970)	DAT space relations	0.18(25)	0.25(25)	0.39(25)	0.34(25)
Bock (1970)	Embedded figures	−0.05(25)	0.36(26)	0.18(26)	0.49(22)
Bock and Kolakowski (1973)	Guilford–Zimmerman Spatial visualization	0.15(99)	0.12(97)	0.20(115)	0.25(84)

[a] From DeFries et al. (1979a).
[b] Number of pairs is reported in parentheses.

Table 3. Familial Correlations for Spatial Tests[a]

Author/test	Father–son	Mother–daughter	Mother–son	Father–daughter	Spouse	Brother–sister	Brother–brother	Sister–sister
Bouchard and McGee (1977)								
Mental rotations	0.23	0.16	0.20	0.17	0.06	0.33	0.50	0.21
Number of pairs	185	196	204	172	144	249	132	112
Loehlin et al. (1978)								
Card rotations	0.27	0.40	0.27	0.32	0.28	0.24	0.44	0.52
Cube comparisons	0.16	0.19	0.04	0.17	0.01	0.32	0.43	0.14
Hidden patterns	0.40	0.22	0.44	0.38	0.21	0.39	0.76	0.55
Paper folding	0.27	0.21	0.24	0.30	0.09	0.17	0.44	0.44
Spatial composite	0.28	0.28	0.34	0.30	0.14	0.26	0.53	0.39
Number of pairs	183	201	183	201	192	99	42	51

[a] From DeFries et al. (1979a).

Table 4. Cognitive Tests, Test Times, and Reliabilities[a]

| Test | Test time | Reliability[b] | |
		Hawaiian battery	Korean battery
Vocabulary, primary mental abilities (PMA), or Korean version	3 min	0.96 (PUBL)	0.87 (KR-20)
Visual memory (immediate)	1-min exposure/ 1-min recall	0.58 (KR-20)	0.75 (KR-20)
Things (a fluency test)	2 parts/3 min each	0.74 (CRα)	0.71 (CRα)
Shepard–Metzler mental rotations (modified for group testing by Vandenberg)	10 min	0.88 (KR-20)	0.92 (KR-20)
Subtraction and multiplication	2 parts/2 min each	0.96 (CRα)	0.95 (CRα)
Elithorn mazes ("lines and dots"), shortened form	5 min	0.89 (PUBL)	–
Word beginnings and endings, Educational Testing Service (ETS), or Korean version	2 parts/3 min each	0.71 (CRα)	0.79 (CRα)
ETS card rotations	2 parts/3 min each	0.88 (CRα)	0.87 (CRα)
Visual memory (delayed)	1 min	0.62 (KR-20)	0.76 (KR-20)
PMA pedigrees (a reasoning test)	4 min	0.72 (PUBL)	–
ETS hidden patterns	2 parts/2 min	0.92 (CRα)	0.91 (CRα)
Paper form board	3 min	0.84 (KR-20)	0.85 (KR-20)
ETS number comparisons	2 parts/1½ min each	0.81 (CRα)	0.88 (CRα)
Whiteman test of social perception	10 min	0.69 (KR-20)	–
Raven's progressive matrices, modified form	20 min	0.86 (KR-20)	0.85 (KR-20)

[a] From Park *et al.* (1978).
[b] PUBL, from test manual; KR-20, Kuder–Richardson formula 20; CRα, composite reliability coefficient α (Guttman, 1945; Lord and Novick, 1968).

5. Hawaii Family Study of Cognition

In 1972, a large scale family study of specific cognitive abilities was initiated at the University of Hawaii. This study was a collaborative effort among eight coinvestigators, four from the University of Hawaii (G. C. Ashton, R. C. Johnson, M. P. Mi, and M. N. Rashad) and four from the University of Colorado (J. C. DeFries, G. E. McClearn, S. G. Vandenberg, and J. R. Wilson). During a four-year period, a battery of 15 tests of specific cognitive abilities (see Table 4) was administered to members of 1816 intact nuclear families (6581 individuals) living on the island of Oahu. Families consisted of both biological parents (60 years of age or younger) and one or more children (13 years of age or older). The two largest ethnic groups in our sample were Americans of Japanese ancestry and Americans of European ancestry (symbolized AJA and AEA, respectively.

The individual tests of specific cognitive abilities (printed on paper of different colors to facilitate monitoring of performance during administration) were bound into a booklet for use by each subject. Tests were group administered under highly standardized conditions (see Wilson, DeFries, McClearn, Vandenberg, Johnson, and Rashad, 1975). For example, a tape recording, synchronized with 35-mm slides, provided test instructions and controlled timing in all test sessions. The tests were administered in two, 1-h blocks, separated by a 10-min break during which refreshments were served.

In a cross-cultural study directed by a Korean national, Dr. Jong Park, a translation of this test battery was administered to 209 families in the Republic of Korea. Families were recruited from the city of Choon-Chun, capital of Kang-Wong-Do Province, which is located about 60 miles from Seoul and has a population of approximately 100,000. The Education Laboratory of the Department of Education (DOEL), Kang-Wong-Do Province, supervised family recruitment and test administration. In general, Korean families who participated in this study were highly comparable to the Hawaiian families with regard to such characteristics as age, education, and occupational level, although the range was somewhat less for the Korean subjects (see Park, Johnson, DeFries, McClearn, Mi, Rashad, Vandenberg, and Wilson, 1978).

The original plan was to test large groups of families in Korea under highly standardized conditions similar to those employed in Hawaii. However, this proved to be impossible due to the reluctance of the families to participate under these conditions. Except for one test session in which seven families participated, each family was tested separately in their home. Tests were administered by local elementary school teachers trained by the DOEL. Unfortunately, this difference in method of test administration may have vitiated the validity of any comparison of familial resemblance between the Korean and Hawaiian samples. When tests are administered to nuclear family groups, as was done in Korea, any factors which affect specific test sessions (e.g., any difference in the time of day, in the time limits for timed tests, in motivational level of family members engendered by different test administrators, etc.) will tend to increase between-family variance and therefore inflate measures of familial resemblance. Consequently, the method of test administration employed in Korea may have resulted in inflated measures of spouse similarity and parent—offspring resemblance.

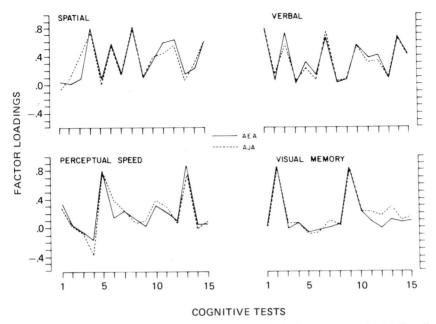

FIGURE 1. Loadings of 15 cognitive tests on four principal components in the Hawaii Family Study of Cognition (from DeFries *et al.*, 1974). AEA and AJA are Americans of European and Japanese ancestry, respectively.

5.1. Factor Structure

The first published report of the Hawaii study concerned AEA and AJA factor structures and was entitled, "Near Identity of Cognitive Structure in Two Ethnic Groups" (DeFries, Vandenberg, McClearn, Kuse, Wilson, Ashton, and Johnson, 1974). Phenotypic correlations among the 15 cognitive variables were obtained separately for the AEA and AJA samples and were then subjected to principal component analyses with varimax rotations. Communalities of one were used, and the number of axes retained for rotation was equal to the number of eigenvalues greater than one (Kaiser, 1960). Four readily interpretable components were obtained for each ethnic group: spatial, verbal, perceptual (numerical) speed, and visual memory. Principal component scores representing these four ability dimensions were subsequently computed for each individual.

Loadings of the 15 tests on the four principal components are shown graphically for AEA and AJA subjects in Fig. 1. It may be seen that the loading profiles for the two ethnic groups are highly similar. Coefficients of congruence for each dimension were 0.96 or higher. Subsequent analyses of larger AEA and AJA data sets (Wilson *et al.*, 1975) yielded even higher coefficients of congruence (0.99 or higher for each principal component). Thus, these results clearly indicate

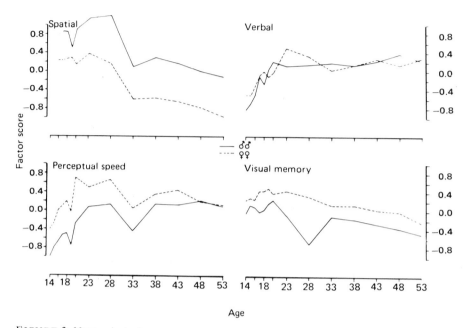

FIGURE 2. Mean principal components scores of males and females in the Hawaii Family Study of Cognition as a function of age (from Wilson *et al.*, 1975).

that the factor structures of the two ethnic groups tested in Hawaii are indeed nearly identical. When similar analyses were applied separately to data for males and females and for different age groups, the same factor structure emerged (Wilson *et al.*, 1975).

Corresponding analyses of the Korean data set revealed a similar, but not identical, factor structure (Park, 1975). Nevertheless, principal component scores corresponding to the spatial, verbal, perceptual speed, and visual memory abilities could also be obtained for the Korean sample.

5.2. Age and Sex Differences

Although the population mean IQ scores of males and females of different ages are defined as being identical (100), measures of specific cognitive abilities show pronounced age and sex differences. Such differences are clearly evident in Fig. 2, in which principal component scores of males and females tested in the Hawaii study are graphed separately as a function of age (yearly intervales from 14 through 20, and five-year blocks thereafter). Spatial ability manifests the well-known sex difference, with males achieving higher scores than females at all ages. A marked age effect may also be noted for spatial ability, with maximum scores being obtained by young adults. In contrast, verbal ability shows a rapid increase from 14 through about 20 years of age and then levels off during adulthood.

Table 5. Age-Adjusted Spouse Correlations for Principal Component Scores
in Three Ethnic Groups[a,b]

Principal components	Hawaiian AEA	Hawaiian AJA	Korean[c]
Spatial	0.13	0.03	0.43
Verbal	0.22	0.25	0.46
Perceptual speed[d]	0.11	−0.02	0.78
Visual memory	0.03	0.14	0.30
First principal component	0.23	0.15	0.72
Number of couples	870	311	209

[a] From Johnson et al. (1976b) and DeFries et al. (1979a).
[b] AEA and AJA are Americans of European and Japanese ancestry, respectively.
[c] Korean spouse correlations are significantly ($p \leqslant 0.05$) larger than corresponding Hawaiian correlations, except for AJA visual memory.
[d] AEA and AJA correlations are significantly ($p \leqslant 0.05$) different.

Somewhat surprisingly, no overall sex difference was observed for the verbal measure. With regard to perceptual speed and visual memory, however, both sex and age differences were found, with females and young adults generally obtaining higher scores than males and older adults.

Because the data summarized in Fig. 2 are cross sectional in nature (i.e., different individuals were measured at different ages), differences between age groups could be due in part to cohort differences. However, in a family study in which younger respondents are biological offspring of older respondents, the problem of cohort differences is lessened to some extent (see Wilson et al., 1975). Nevertheless, it remains to be seen whether or not longitudinal data would yield similar age curves.

The presence of these marked age effects suggested that the data should be age adjusted prior to other statistical analyses. For analyses of the final data set, which will be summarized in the following sections, a z-score banding technique was employed by which scores were standardized within age bands, thereby eliminating both linear and nonlinear differences among age groups. Width of each age interval was dictated by considerations of sample size (see DeFries, Johnson, Kuse, McClearn, Polovina, Vandenberg, and Wilson, 1979a; Park et al., 1978).

5.3. Assortative Marriage

Spouse correlations for the four varimax rotated principal component scores and for the first principal component (unrotated) are presented in Table 5. As stated previously, the individual tests included in the Hawaii battery are measures of specific cognitive abilities, not IQ or global intelligence. Nevertheless, the first principal component (unrotated) provides a measure which correlated 0.73 with WAIS full-scale IQ, a value about as high as the correlation of WAIS IQ with other measures of general intelligence (Kuse, 1977).

Spouse correlations for the Hawaiian couples in both ethnic groups are higher for verbal ability and for the first principal component than for the other specific cognitive abilities. Standard errors for the AEA and AJA spouse correlations are 0.03 and 0.06, respectively; thus, the majority of the coefficients are significantly greater than zero. Watkins (1978) recently obtained similar correlations (actually somewhat higher for verbal ability) when the same test battery was administered to a sample of newlyweds in California. These results suggest that the spouse similarities are due in fact to assortative mating and not to life experiences shared by married couples while they are living together.

Although the AEA and AJA spouse correlations are quite similar to each other and to those obtained by Watkins (1978), the values are somewhat lower than those reported by earlier investigators. In a recent review, Jensen (1978) reported that the unweighted mean of 43 spouse correlations for various tests of mental ability was 0.45. As previously discussed by De Fries *et al.* (1979a), several factors may account for the lower spouse correlations obtained in the Hawaii study. Since spouses are highly correlated for age, inadequate age adjustment may inflate spouse similarity when marked age effects are present. Recent studies by Johnson, DeFries, Wilson, McClearn, Vandenberg, Ashton, Mi, and Rashad (1976a) and Zonderman, Vandenberg, Spuhler, and Fain (1977) have demonstrated that age-adjusted data do yield lower spouse correlations. Moreover, the reduction was more marked in the latter study, in which the age range of the couples was greater. Thus, inadequate age adjustment may have inflated some of the spouse correlations summarized by Jensen.

A second factor which may account for the finding of lower spouse correlations in the Hawaii study is the nature of the tests. Individual tests in the Hawaii battery are measures of specific cognitive abilities, whereas most of the studies reviewed by Jensen (1978) measured global intelligence. However, it may be seen in Table 5 that the AEA and AJA spouse correlations for the first principal component (which correlates highly with WAIS full-scale IQ) are also relatively low. Thus, it appears that the difference in the nature of the tests does not account for the lower spouse correlations observed in the Hawaii study.

Finally, as stated previously, method of test administration may influence measures of familial resemblance. When tests are administered to individual family groups, measures of familial resemblance will be inflated if variance due to differences in ability level among families is confounded with that due to differences among test sessions. The extent to which tests were administered to individual family groups in the studies reviewed by Jensen (1978) is unknown. In any case, the results of administering the tests to large groups under highly standardized conditions in the Hawaii study suggest that assortative marriage for mental abilities may be less than previously believed.

Spouse correlations for the Korean couples are also presented in Table 5. It may be seen that Korean spouse correlations are significantly higher than those for all corresponding measures in Hawaii, except AJA visual memory. Recall that Korean subjects were tested primarily as nuclear family units in their own homes. Thus, the higher spouse correlations for Korean couples may be due to the difference in method of test administration. This hypothesis is supported by the fact that the highest Korean spouse correlation is for perceptual speed, a measure which should be most sensitive to differences among test sessions with regard to such factors as time limits and motivational levels of family members engendered by different test administrators. Differences in raw score variances between the Hawaiian and Korean samples, especially with regard to timed tests, are also consistent with this hypothesis.

It is conceivable, of course, that cultural differences could account for at least part of the difference between the Korean and Hawaiian spouse correlations. One cultural factor which could cause a greater spouse similarity in Korea is their custom of arranged marriages (see Johnson, Park, DeFries, McClearn, Mi, Rashad, Vandenberg, and Wilson, 1976b). Unfortunately, because of the difference in method of test administration, the relative importance of cultural factors cannot be assessed from these data.

5.4. Regression of Midchild on Midparent

"Familiality" has recently been defined by DeFries et al. (1979a) as familial resemblance due to genetic factors, environmental factors, or both. Obviously, familiality is necessary, but not sufficient, evidence for the presence of heritable variation.

In earlier family studies, parent–offspring resemblance was usually assessed by correlations. However, regressions are preferable to correlations for this purpose (DeFries, 1967). One advantage of the regression coefficient is that it is less affected by problems of restriction of range. Moreover, expectations for parent–child correlations are complex functions of the spouse correlation and the number of children per family, whereas the regression of offspring on midparent is not affected by these variables. In the absence of common (between-family) environmental influences and epistasis, single-parent/child (single child or midchild) covariance = midparent/child covariance = $\frac{1}{2} V_A(1 + t)$, where V_A is the additive genetic variance and t is the spouse correlation. Midparent variance $(V_{\bar{P}})$ is also a function of the spouse correlation, i.e., $V_{\bar{P}} = \frac{1}{2} V_P(1 + t)$. Thus, when between-family environmental influences are negligible, the regression of offspring on midparent $(b_{o\bar{P}})$ provides a direct estimate of heritability $(h^2 = V_A/V_P)$:

$$b_{o\bar{P}} = \frac{\frac{1}{2} V_A(1 + t)}{\frac{1}{2} V_P(1 + t)} = h^2$$

[For more detail, see McClearn and DeFries (1973) and DeFries et al. (1979a).]

It is important to note that between-family environmental influences are likely not to be negligible for mental abilities. Therefore, the regressions of

Table 6. Regressions of Midchild on Midparent for Principal Component Scores in Three Ethnic Groups[a]

Principal components	Hawaiian AEA[b]	Hawaiian AJA	Korean[c]
Spatial[d]	0.64	0.45	0.67
Verbal	0.61	0.55	0.73
Perceptual speed	0.46	0.38	0.74
Visual memory	0.43	0.25	0.55
First principal component[d]	0.62	0.43	0.64
Number of families	830	305	209

[a] From Park *et al.* (1978) and DeFries *et al.* (1979a).
[b] AEA and AJA are Americans of European and Japanese ancestry, respectively. Regressions are corrected for differences in test reliability.
[c] Korean coefficients are significantly ($p \leq 0.05$) larger than all corresponding AJA coefficients and that for AEA Perceptual Speed.
[d] AEA and AJA coefficients are significantly ($p \leq 0.05$) different.

midchild on midparent obtained in the Hawaii study should be regarded as measures of familiality and not as direct estimates of heritability.

The parent–offspring regressions presented in Table 6 have been adjusted for differences in test reliability. Such adjustment is essential if the coefficients are to be compared for evidence of differential familiality. The Spearman rank correlation between the adjusted AEA and AJA regression coefficients across the 15 individual tests is 0.76 (DeFries *et al.*, 1979a). It may be seen in Table 6 that parent–offspring regressions in both ethnic groups are moderately high for spatial ability and verbal ability, but somewhat lower for perceptual speed and visual memory. Thus, data obtained in the Hawaii study provide some evidence for differential familiality of different mental abilities. In a large twin study recently conducted by Loehlin and Nichols (1976), no evidence was found for differential heritability among various mental ability tests. Granting the validity of both results would imply that it is between-family environmental variance, not genetic variance, which differs in relative importance among various mental abilities.

It may also be seen in Table 6 that the regressions of midchild on midparent for the first principal component are 0.62 and 0.43 for AEA and AJA families, respectively. Since the regression of midchild on midparent provides an upper-bound estimate of heritability (assuming positive environmental covariance between parents and their children), these results suggest that the heritability of general intelligence in these populations is probably less than 0.6.

The Korean parent–offspring regressions (see Table 6) are significantly larger than those for all corresponding AJA measures and that for perceptual speed in the AEA group. As discussed previously with regard to the spouse correlations, this difference in familial resemblance is probably due at least in part to the difference in method of test administration. On the other hand, if differences in degree of assortative marriage actually do exist between the

Korean and Hawaiian samples, that could also account for a difference in parent—offspring resemblance. Assortative mating results in an increase in additive genetic variance in a population. Thus, if there is greater assortative marriage for mental abilities in Korea, the heritabilities could be higher for this reason. Of course, differences in between-family environmental influences could also be important.

Measures of AEA "cross familiality," which are a function of genetic correlations between the various ability dimensions, are discussed elsewhere (DeFries, Kuse, and Vandenberg, 1979b).

5.5. Spatial Ability

Single-parent/single-child correlations for the Hawaiian and Korean samples have recently been reported (DeFries et al., 1979a; Park et al., 1978). Of interest in the present context are the correlations for the relatively pure tests of spatial ability (mental rotations, paper form board, and card rotations) and for the spatial composite. These correlations, as well as those obtained in a study of a small mainland AEA sample (Spuhler, 1976), are presented in Table 7. None of the correlational patterns conforms to that expected for a sex-linked, recessive character (see Table 1).

Hawaiian AEA and AJA sibling correlations for the same measures are shown in Table 8. The AJA correlations are based upon relatively small sample sizes and are therefore rather unreliable. Nevertheless, the pattern of sibling correlations expected for a sex-linked, recessive character (see Table 1) was not obtained in either sample.

As discussed elsewhere (DeFries, Vandenberg, and McClearn, 1976), the ordering of familial correlations, by itself, does not provide a rigorous test of the sex-linkage hypothesis. With small samples, as in the study by Stafford (1961), the correlations may show the expected patterns, but differences among them may not be significant. On the other hand, due to vagaries of sampling, the expected correlational pattern may sometimes not be found even for a character which is sex-linked. It is clear that a more rigorous test of the hypothesis that a character is influenced by a sex-linked, major gene would be desirable. DeFries et al. (1979a) have recently suggested that such a test is provided by the application of hierarchical multiple regression analysis (see Cohen and Cohen, 1975) to family data.

Consider the model shown in Table 9, where child's score (C) is expressed as a function of three variables: child's sex $(S$, coded 1 or 2), mother's score (M), and father's score (F). It may be helpful to think of these three independent variables as being like main effects in an analysis of variance. Two-way interactions $(S \times M, S \times F, \text{ and } M \times F)$ are represented by products of variables from which the main effects have been linearly partialled. A three-way interaction $(S \times M \times F)$ is indicated by the product of the three independent

Table 7. Parent–Offspring Correlations for Spatial Tests and the
Spatial Composite[a]

Author/sample	Test	Father–son	Mother–daughter	Mother–son	Father–daughter
DeFries *et al.* (1979a)					
Hawaiian AEA	Mental rotations	0.20	0.30	0.13	0.20
	Paper form board	0.28	0.33	0.29	0.35
	Card rotations	0.26	0.34	0.21	0.23
	Spatial composite	0.33	0.38	0.29	0.31
	number of pairs	672	692	666	685
Hawaiian AJA	Mental rotations	0.20	0.11	0.17	0.24
	Paper form board	0.21	0.29	0.20	0.27
	Card rotations	0.24	0.17	0.10	0.11
	Spatial composite	0.26	0.22	0.20	0.32
	number of pairs	241	248	244	237
Park *et al.* (1978)					
Korean[b]	Mental rotations	0.22	0.46	0.26	0.41
	Paper form board	0.59	0.57	0.63	0.53
	Card rotations	0.12	0.61	0.36	0.54
	Spatial composite	0.33	0.53	0.37	0.45
	number of pairs	99–103	113–121	100–105	107–117
Spuhler (1976)					
Mainland AEA	Mental rotations	0.25	0.04	0.10	0.32
	Paper form board	0.37	0.24	0.12	0.35
	Card rotations	0.25	0.03	0.16	0.15
	Spatial composite	0.35	0.24	0.13	0.40
	number of pairs	81	81	81	81

[a] AEA and AJA are Americans of European and Japanese ancestry, respectively.
[b] Since pairwise deletion of data was employed, the number of pairs ranged as indicated for individual test and spatial composite scores.

variables, from which both the main effects and the two-way interactions have been partialled. B_1, the partial regression of child's score on child's sex, is a measure of the importance of sex differences. B_2 is the partial regression of child's score on mother's score, a measure of mother–child resemblance. Likewise, B_3, the partial regression of child's score on father's score is a measure of father–child resemblance.

As indicated in Table 9, the significance of the main effects, the two-way interactions, and the three-way interaction are tested sequentially. Thus, B_1, B_2, and B_3 are estimated from data for $C, S, M,$ and F during step 1. The products $SM, SF,$ and MF are then added to the equation during step 2. Finally, the product SMF is entered during step 3. The change in the multiple R^2 due to the products entered during this sequence is attributed to the respective interactions and may be tested for statistical significance.

Two-way interactions are indicative of a conditional relationship between

Table 8. Sibling Intraclass Correlations (± SE) for Spatial Tests and the Spatial Composite[a,b]

	Brother–sister	Brother–brother	Sister–sister
Hawaiian AEA			
Mental rotations	0.25 ± 0.07	0.35 ± 0.09	0.16 ± 0.09
Paper form board	0.35 ± 0.06	0.26 ± 0.10	0.20 ± 0.09
Card rotations	0.33 ± 0.06	0.17 ± 0.09	0.25 ± 0.09
Spatial composite	0.36 ± 0.06	0.29 ± 0.10	0.25 ± 0.09
Number of families	216	114	125
Hawaiian AJA			
Mental rotations	0.18 ± 0.12	0.16 ± 0.15	0.24 ± 0.17
Paper form board	0.28 ± 0.12	0.08 ± 0.14	0.19 ± 0.17
Card rotations	0.27 ± 0.12	0.33 ± 0.15	0.26 ± 0.17
Spatial composite	0.39 ± 0.12	0.17 ± 0.15	0.29 ± 0.17
Number of families	66	44	37

[a] From DeFries et al. (1979a).
[b] AEA and AJA are Americans of European and Japanese ancestry, respectively.

Table 9. Hierarchical Regression Model

$$\hat{C} = \underbrace{B_1 S + B_2 M + B_3 F}_{\text{(step 1)}} + \underbrace{B_4 SM + B_5 SF + B_6 MF}_{\text{(step 2)}} + \underbrace{B_7 SMF}_{\text{(step 3)}} + A$$

$\hat{C}$ = child's expected score
S = child's sex (coded 1 or 2)
M = mother's score
F = father's score
B_1 = partial regression of C on S (a measure of the importance of sex on child's score)
B_2 = partial regression of C on M (a measure of mother–child resemblance)
.
.
.
A = regression constant

the child's score and the two variables. For example, a significant B_4 would indicate that mother–child resemblance is a function of the child's sex. In like manner, a significant B_5 would indicate that father–child resemblance depends upon the child's sex. This, of course, is exactly what is expected for a character which is sex-linked. For such a character, B_7 should also be significant, since this would indicate that father–child and mother–child resemblances differ as a function of the child's sex.

Such a regression analysis was undertaken for the individual test and principal component scores obtained for the AEA and AJA samples in the Hawaii study (DeFries et al., 1979a). Considering the three relatively pure tests of spatial ability and the spatial composite, there are a total of 24 interactions which are informative with regard to sex linkage (4 variables × 3 interactions × 2 ethnic groups). Of these 24 interactions, only one was found to be significant: child's sex × mother's score (B_4), mental rotations, AEA ($p = 0.02$).

With 24 tests of significance, at least one would be expected to be significant at the 0.05 level purely by chance. Nevertheless, it is instructive to look at this significant result in greater detail. Once a significant interaction between child's sex and either father's score or mother's score is obtained, it is imperative to check the order of magnitude of the parent–child correlations. The reason for this is that these interactions may arise in different ways. Recall that a significant interaction between child's sex and mother's score indicates that mother–child resemblance differs as a function of the child's sex. Thus, a significant interaction between child's sex and mother's score could imply that mother–son resemblance exceeds mother–daughter resemblance (as expected for a sex-linked character) or *vice versa*. As may be seen in Table 7, AEA mother–child resemblance for performance on the mental rotations test does differ as a function of the child's sex. However, mother–daughter resemblance exceeds mother–son resemblance, and this is exactly opposite what is expected for a sex-linked character.

Ashton, Polovina, and Vandenberg (1979) have recently subjected data from the Hawaii study to complex segregation analyses, using the computer programs NUCLEAR and SKUMIX (MacLean, Morton, and Lew, 1975; MacLean, Morton, Elston, and Yee, 1976). Evidence was obtained that high spatial ability is influenced by a major gene. However, results of their analyses suggested autosomal dominance rather than sex linkage.

6. Summary and Conclusions

Results of the Hawaii Family Study of Cognition provide evidence concerning the familial nature of specific cognitive abilities. Spouse correlations for Hawaiian couples (both AEA and AJA) are somewhat lower than those reported in earlier studies. Factors which may account for this difference in spouse similarity include differences in adequacy of age adjustment, in the nature of the tests, and in method of test administration.

Large differences were found between spouse correlations obtained in Hawaii and those obtained for a cross-cultural sample tested in the Republic of Korea. Although some of the difference in spouse similarity may be due to cultural factors, such as the Korean practice of arranged marriages, it seems more likely that a difference in method of test administration is responsible for the higher Korean spouse correlations.

Regressions of midchild on midparent for both AEA and AJA families in Hawaii provide evidence of differential familiality for mental abilities. Spatial ability and verbal ability show greater familial resemblance than do perceptual speed and visual memory. Since parent—offspring resemblance is a function of common (between-family) environmental influences, as well as genetic factors, these results do not provide direct evidence for differential heritability. Other methodologies which more cleanly separate genetic and environmental influences, such as an adoption study currently being conducted by DeFries, Plomin, and Vandenberg, are required to provide such evidence.

Korean midparent—midchild regressions, like the spouse correlations, were found to exceed those obtained for the Hawaiian AEA and AJA families. This apparent difference in familiality may also be due to the difference in method of test administration. On the other hand, if there is more assortative marriage for mental abilities in Korea, that could also account for a difference in parent—offspring resemblance.

Considerable data were obtained in the Hawaii study to test the hypothesis that spatial ability is influenced by a sex-linked, major gene. Parent—offspring correlations, sibling correlations, and the results of a new hierarchical multiple regression technique for analyzing family data were unanimous in providing no support for the sex-linkage hypothesis. Results of complex segregation analyses (Ashton *et al.*, 1979) suggest a possible major-gene effect on spatial ability; however, the evidence is for an autosomal gene with dominance for high spatial ability rather than for a sex-linked recessive gene.

ACKNOWLEDGMENT

I thank Rebecca G. Miles for typing the manuscript and for her exceptional editorial assistance.

References

Ashton, G. C., Polovina, J. J., and Vandenberg, S. G. (1979), Segregation analysis of family data for 15 tests of cognitive ability, *Behav. Genet.*, 9:329–347.

Binet, A., and Simon, T (1905), Methodes nouvelles pour le diagnostic du niveau intellectual des anormaux, *Annee Psycholog.* 11:191–244, 245–366.

Binet, A., and Simon, T. (1911), La mesure de développement de l'intelligence chez les jeunes enfants, *Bull. Soc. Libre Étude Psychol. Enfant*, No. 70-71:187–248.

Bock, R. D. (1970), *A study of familial effects in certain cognitive and perceptual variables*, Final Report, Illinois Psychiatric Training Research Grant No. 17-317, University of Chicago, Chicago.

Bock, R. D., and Kolakowski, D. (1973), Further evidence of sex-linked major-gene influence on human spatial visualizing ability, *Am. J. Hum. Genet.* 25:1–14.

Bouchard, T. J., and McGee, M. G. (1977), Sex differences in human spatial ability: Not an X-linked recessive gene effect, *Soc. Biol.* 24:332–335.

Carter, H. D. (1932), Family resemblance in verbal and numerical abilities, *Genet. Psychol. Monog.* 12:3–10.

Cattell, J. M., and Farrand, L. (1896), Physical and mental measurements of the students of Columbia University, *Psychol. Rev.* 3:618–648.

Cohen, J., and Cohen, P. (1975), *Applied Multiple Regression/Correlation Analysis for the Behavioral Sciences*, Lawrence Erlbaum Associates, Hillsdale, New Jersey.

Corah, N. L. (1965), Differentiation in children and their parents, *J. Pers.* 33:300–308.

DeFries, J. C. (1967), Quantitative genetics and behavior: Overview and perspective, in *Behavior–Genetic Analysis* (J. Hirsch, ed.), pp. 322–339, McGraw-Hill, New York.

DeFries, J. C., and Plomin, R. (1978), Behavioral genetics, *Ann. Rev. Psychol.* 29:473–515.

DeFries, J. C., Vandenberg, S. G., McClearn, G. E., Kuse, A. G., Wilson, J. R., Ashton, G. C., and Johnson, R. C. (1974), Near identity of cognitive structure in two ethnic groups, *Science* 183:338–339.

DeFries, J. C., Vandenberg, S. G., and McClearn, G. E. (1976), Genetics of specific cognitive abilities, *Ann. Rev. Genet.* 10:179–207.

DeFries, J. C., Johnson, R. C., Kuse, A. R., McClearn, G. E., Polovina, J., Vandenberg, S. G., and Wilson, J. R. (1979a), Familial resemblance for specific cognitive abilities, *Behav. Genet.* 9:23–43.

DeFries, J. C., Kuse, A. R., and Vandenberg, S. G. (1979b), Genetic correlations, environmental correlations, and behavior, in *Theoretical Advances in Behavior Genetics: The Fifth Banff Conference on Theoretical Psychology* (J. R. Royce and L. P. Mos, eds.), Sijthoff & Noordhoff, Alphen aan den Rijn, The Netherlands.

Fuller, J. L., and Thompson, W. R. (1978), *Foundations of Behavior Genetics*, C. V. Mosby, St. Louis.

Galton, F. (1869), *Hereditary Genius: An Inquiry into its Laws and Consequences*, Macmillan, London. (Reprinted by Meridian Books, The World Publishing Company, Cleveland, 1962).

Galton, F. (1875), The history of twins as a criterion of the relative powers of nature and nurture, *J. R. Anthropol. Inst.* 5:391–406.

Galton, F. (1883), *Inquiries into Human Faculty and its Development*, Macmillan, London.

Guilford, J. P., and Hoepfner, R. (1971), *The Analysis of Intelligence*, McGraw-Hill, New York.

Guttman, L. (1945), A basis for analyzing test-retest reliability, *Psychometrika* 10:255–282.

Hartlage, L. C. (1970), Sex-linked inheritance of spatial ability, *Percept. Mot. Skills* 31:610.

Horn, J. L. (1976), Human abilities: A review of research and theory in the early 1970's, *Ann. Rev. Psychol.* 27:437–486.

Jensen, A. R. (1978), Genetic and behavioral effects of nonrandom mating, in *Human Variation: Biopsychology of Age, Race and Sex* (R. T. Osborne, C. E. Noble, and N. Weyl, eds.), pp. 51–105, Academic Press, New York.

Johnson, R. C., DeFries, J. C., Wilson, J. R., McClearn, G. E., Vandenberg, S. G., Ashton, G. C., Mi, M. P., and Rashad, M. N. (1976a), Assortative marriage for specific cognitive abilities in two ethnic groups, *Hum. Biol.* 48:343–352.

Johnson, R. C., Park, J., DeFries, J. C., McClearn, G. E., Mi, M. P., Rashad, M. N., Vandenberg, S. G., and Wilson, J. R. (1976b), Assortative marriage for specific cognitive abilities in Korea, *Soc. Biol.* 23:311–316.

Kaiser, H. F. (1960), The application of electronic computers to factor analysis, *Educ. Psychol. Meas.* 20:141–151.

Kuse, A. R. (1977), *Familial resemblances for cognitive abilities estimated from two test batteries in Hawaii*, unpublished doctoral dissertation, University of Colorado.

Lewontin, R. C. (1975), Genetic aspects of intelligence, *Ann. Rev. Genet.* 9:387–405.

Loehlin, J. C., and Nichols, R. C. (1976), *Heredity, Environment and Personality*, University of Texas Press, Austin.

Loehlin, J. C., Sharan, S., and Jacoby, R. (1978), In pursuit of the "spatial gene": A family study, *Behav. Genet.* 8:27–41.

Lord, F. M., and Novick, M. R. (1968), *Statistical Theories of Mental Test Scores*, Addison-Wesley, Reading, Massachusetts.

MacLean, C. J., Morton, N. E., and Lew, R. C. (1975), Analysis of family resemblance. IV. Operational characteristics of segregation analysis, *Am. J. Hum. Genet.* **27**:365–384.

MacLean, C. J., Morton, N. E., Elston, R. C., and Yee, S. (1976), Skewness in commingled distributions, *Biometrics* **32**:695–699.

McClearn, G. E., and DeFries, J. C. (1973), *Introduction to Behavioral Genetics*, Freeman, San Franciso.

O'Connor, J. (1943), *Structural Visualization*, Human Engineering Laboratory, Boston.

Park, J.-Y. (1975), *A study of multivariate cognition in Korea in relation to environmental and hereditary influences*, unpublished doctoral dissertation, University of Hawaii.

Park, J., Johnson, R. C., DeFries, J. C., McClearn, G. E., Mi, M. P., Rashad, M. N., Vandenberg, S. G., and Wilson, J. R. (1978), Parent–offspring resemblance for specific cognitive abilities in Korea, *Behav. Genet.* **8**:43–52.

Spearman, C. (1904), General intelligence, objectively determined and measured, *Am. J. Psychol.* **15**:201–293.

Spuhler, K. P. (1976), *Family resemblance for cognitive performance: An assessment of genetic and environmental contributions to variation*, unpublished doctoral dissertation, University of Colorado.

Stafford, R. E. (1961), Sex differences in spatial visualization as evidence of sex-linked inheritance, *Percept. Mot. Skills* **13**:428.

Terman, L. M. (1916), *The Measurement of Intelligence*, Houghton–Mifflin, Boston.

Thurstone, L. L. (1938), *Primary Mental Abilities*, University of Chicago Press, Chicago.

Thurstone, L. L. (1947), *Multiple-factor Analysis*, University of Chicago Press, Chicago.

Vandenberg, S. G. (1968), The nature and nurture of intelligence, in *Genetics* (D. C. Glass, ed.), pp. 3–53, Rockefeller University Press and Russell Sage Foundation, New York.

Watkins, M. (1978), Preliminary report on cognitive resemblance and education in newlyweds, *Behav. Genet.* **8**:573–574.

Williams, T. (1975), Family resemblance in abilities: The Wechsler scales, *Behav. Genet.* **5**:405–409.

Willoughby, R. R. (1972), Family similarities in mental-test abilities, *Genet. Psychol. Monog.* **2**:239–277.

Wilson, J. R., DeFries, J. C., McClearn, G. E., Vandenberg, S. G., Johnson, R. C., and Rashad, M. N. (1975), Cognitive abilities: Use of family data as a control to assess sex and age differences in two ethnic groups, *Int. J. Aging Hum. Devel.* **6**:261–276.

Yen, W. M. (1975), Sex-linked major-gene influences on selected types of spatial performance, *Behav. Genet.* **5**:281–298.

Zonderman, A. B., Vandenberg, S. G., Spuhler, K. P., and Fain, P. R. (1977), Assortative marriage for cognitive abilities, *Behav. Genet.* **7**:261–271.

Current Developments in Anthropological Genetics

Achievements and Gaps

DEREK F. ROBERTS

1. Introduction

The conference held in 1971 on "Methods and Theories of Anthropological Genetics" (Crawford and Workman, 1973) provides a useful datum against which the current developments can be appraised. By anthropological genetics is meant the study of the genetic variation that occurs within and between human populations, its origin, and the factors and processes that maintain it. Professor Spuhler (1973), in his summing-up, echoed the feelings of all when he said that the relatively new field of anthropological genetics — a blend of general genetics and the study of human populations — which took its effective beginnings in about 1950 had just reached its majority. He picked out a number of themes that could be traced in the contributions: the characterization of breeding populations and of their gene pools; variations of population structure; systems of mating; the processes of gene frequency change; the use of the increased knowledge of polymorphisms to examine genetic distances and genetic phylogeny; and computer simulation of genetic and demographic processes. In each of these there was vigorous growth. We all agreed that, in its 21 years, anthropological genetics had come of age.

DEREK F. ROBERTS • Department of Human Genetics, University of Newcastle upon Tyne, England

There are different conceptions of the age of majority, and different ages of biological maturity, while different parts of the organism mature at different times. With maturity comes a general slowing and cessation of growth; a period of achievement and increasing wisdom; it is preceded by the period of accelerated growth that goes by the name of adolescence. The different structures and tissues of the human body vary in their rates of growth, brain and head approaching adult development first, the protective tissues of the lymphoid system in early adolescence, while the muscles for performance and the reproductive tissues are the last. By analogy, perhaps in our subject the fundamental concepts and controlling mechanisms were laid down several decades ago; we have passed through the self-protective phase when it was necessary to argue the usefulness of our study, and perhaps in 1971 we were still in the exuberant adolescent phase of our development. We are now concentrating on achievements, applying vigorously our limbs (our methods) to the tasks of anthropological genetics (solution of problems) in the light of our concepts (our theory). We are already thinking of reproduction, training of future generations, to whom we now have something worthwhile to offer.

With maturity, after the differentials of earlier growth comes the balance of the parts. Success and achievement in adulthood depends largely upon the health of this balance. We need to enquire whether we have attained this or whether our growth has been dysplastic. This as I see it is the function of the present volume.

2. Historical Material

The first two chapters on the use of historical material in genetic studies illustrate achievement despite a major limitation; as Swedlund says, "in studying the genetics of historical populations . . . there are no genes — a fact that must be disconcerting to the most optimistic." The sophisticated analyses of historical material for genetic purposes and the questions that are asked are therefore different from those in other types of population genetic study. For skeletal material, the primary genetic interest is indirect — through demographic and morphometric analyses — though there is a minor direct relevance in the presence and differing incidences of genetic disease detectable in bone. The illustrations given are quite removed from Howell's (1973) pioneer use of cranial measurements for establishing phylogenetic trees based on discriminant functions, though the problems these pose with their general continental orientation, correlating with geography better than did the genetic arborization of Cavalli-Sforza and Edwards (1963), still remain to be resolved.

Weiss provides us with a clear and critical warning not to read too much into paleodemographic material, and this all of us who have worked with skeletal remains will echo. Difficulties not only relate to the antiquity of the material. I recollect examining the material from the grave of the crew of a bomber which had been shot down in 1943 in a raid over Germany. We knew the names and features of the members of the crew, and there was no difficulty in identifying their remains. But with them there was in addition the skeleton of a young woman, for whom there was no evidence at all from the official or local records — perhaps she was a member of the Resistance who had been despatched without trace. The quirk of the stranger in the burial, albeit then only five years old, reminds us that there may have been similar quirks in other earlier burials.

Weiss, besides drawing attention to the advances in method over the last decade, points out a major finding of genetic importance in paleodemographic analysis, namely, that early selection was primarily through differential mortality, and that it was about the time of the rise of agricultural states that this became a less, and fertility a more, effective force in determining the variance in reproduction. Both factors, however, remained important until very recently, with the rise of modern medical science, so that today natural selection must now act mainly through fertility. A second main finding is that the general biological pattern of aging and death has remained quite constant for a very long time. Hence the age patterns of contemporary degenerative diseases represent the inherent aging biology of man.

Swedlund's excellent review of genetic uses of historical population documentation reminds us that they range far more widely than studies of population structure and the mating patterns that they produce, and suggests greater attention to questions of selection through the analysis of differential fertility and mortality. His Deerfield cohort study is particularly useful with its suggestion of the protective effect of exposure to epidemics. His suggestion of the potential usefulness of historical demography in the study of the distribution of disease along family and community lines is timely. Here there are already notable examples, for instance the distribution of porphyria in South Africa (Dean, 1971), where the several thousand patients with the disease all descend from either Gerrit Jansz van Rooyen who came to the Cape in 1685, or his wife Ariaantje van den Berg. But it is not only as an example of the founder effect that this disease, rare in Europe, so frequent in South Africa, is of interest. It is the finding by Dean that the gene for porphyria was not apparently deleterious. The gene today is deleterious in that those who have it are particularly susceptible to some drugs of modern medicine, notably barbiturates and sulphonamides, and in the absence of these it is likely to have done little harm during the reproductive years. Certainly the porphyrics historically in South Africa appear to have had the same large number of children as the nonporphyric families, or indeed, slightly larger numbers than usual.

3. Evolution

The rise of sociobiology in the 1970's has provided a major evolutionary topic for discussion (Sahlins, 1977), and it would have been quite wrong for a series of this nature to have ignored it. It is particularly pleasing to see Harpending drawing attention to the "certain amount of sloppy logic in the exuberance of sociobiology." He points out a major difficulty in such studies, the lack of any solid generalization, like Fisher's fundamental theorem of natural selection, to be of help in dealing with social variables. Nonetheless, to take a much discussed problem, the evolution of selfishness or altruism, he successfully shows that which of these is selected for is dependent on an equilibrium point defined in terms of fitness, benefit, cost, the amount of migration and population size, and, what is most important, that the emergence of altruism and selection for it are dependent upon a structured population and the effects of chance, for without chance in a totally deterministic system there will be fixation for selfishness. Here he has applied the methods of argument, standard in anthropological genetics, and extended them to cultural transmission and the interaction between it and genetic transmission, to produce a characteristically thought-provoking contribution.

Livingstone's review is quite different. He examines broadly the data relating to the selectionist vs. the neutralist controversy over the explanation of gene frequency differences. He reminds us that perhaps frequencies at most loci are not in equilibrium, and that differences in genotypic fitness between populations have been demonstrated with respect to some loci and are much more widespread than is generally considered in evolutionary models. Only with such differences can the well-established differences in frequency of genes such as that for cystic fibrosis be explained, at very low frequency in Orientals, but very high frequency in Britain (approximately 1 in 1600 live births affected, and 1 in 20 of the population being carriers). It is this high frequency, which cannot be attributed to mutation pressure, that provides the strongest indication that in Britain there may be a polymorphic balance at the cystic fibrosis locus. His simulation runs as always are very illuminating, this time not only in showing the importance of family size for the fate of particular alleles, but also arriving at the quite consistent if limited probability of retention of lethals. Again, though he does not make the point explicitly, this will account well for the fact that different isolates are characterized by high frequencies of different lethals, and of course supports Penrose's (1959) early statement that much of modern man's burden of deleterious recessives is attributable to the great increase in population size over the last few centuries.

Narrowing the discussion further is Schanfield's chapter on the HLA and Gm systems in relation to major anthropotaxonomy. It is depressing to learn from him of the imminent reduction of facilities for intensive Gm testing on account of retrenchment in two out of the four existing laboratories. It is particularly important therefore to enquire before this occurs whether the right questions have been asked. One can only be impressed by the contrast in the clinical interest between the HLA and Gm systems, and indeed the growth in knowledge of the HLA system has been largely stimulated by its obvious associations with disease. One would have thought that with the present increase in interest in immunogenetics, and the Gm antigen locations, that their role, say, in the development of immune complexes and the immunological response to diseases would also have been a major growing point. How far do the Gm and HLA differences in frequency account for morbidity differences between populations and differential survival of individuals? What are the mechanisms of the established associations – is it that some HLAs protect against a particular disorder or that others increase susceptibility? Surely they cannot all be attributed to linkage with other more directly relevant genes. Part of the limited anthropological attention to the HLA system was undoubtedly, as Schanfield points out, attributable to the difficulty of testing remote populations, but today with modern methods it is quite possible to take portable equipment into the field, obtain the specimens, separate out the white cells, freeze them down, and then transport them to the laboratory as we have done in our studies in Orkney. The major problem is population specificity, the absence in non-European populations of so many of the antigens common in Western Europeans, so the converse is also probable; hence one is unlikely to find in the major sources of supply of HLA antisera, the serum of pregnant women in Western Europe and North America, antisera to the antigens most characteristic of, say, Australian aborigines or Semang.

MacCluer's chapter takes one of the major components of evolution, differential fertility, and applies to it the method of analysis, simulation, in which she has perhaps done more than anybody in anthropological genetics. She sets out the topics where this approach may be used to advantage, and gives clear warning of what it cannot be expected to do. Her examination, for example, by the program KINSIM of the effect of migration on population structure, and by POPSIM of the effects of age structure and mating patterns on evolution and growth of small populations, are of direct relevance to the historical studies that Swedlund reviewed. The special purpose model designed for Huntington's chorea is particularly interesting, and I should greatly like to see applied to it the data from East Anglia, where Dr. Caro has compiled remarkably complete historical material which reduces the total population distribution to the descendants of a few families enmeshed in an intricate web of relationships, though it would probably be necessary to adjust the gene frequency upwards to a more realistic level and also take account of marrying in by remote if unknown consanguinity. Whether or not one agrees with Harpending's criticism, there is no doubt that simulation is a useful generator of questions in the unexpected findings that it produces, and which then demand a return to the biological data to enquire if they are true or are artifacts of the assumptions in the procedure.

4. Analytical Theory

There is a group of chapters which concern pure theory. A general review is that of Reich and his colleagues on genetic epidemiology, which explores the population distribution not only of simple genetic traits but also non-Mendelian phenotypes, taking into account their familial occurrence and relevant environmental variables. The object of genetic epidemiology is to discover the combinations of variables and their respective loadings that will allow the best prediction that an individual will develop a given disorder; having identified the key variables, they can be modified in the expectation that this will prevent the disorder. Reich first reviews methods of analysis (segregation and linkage) that will allow the detection of major loci. Then he turns to complex traits and the applications of path analysis in their resolution, and shows how the effect of transmissible cultural factors can be taken into account by the TAU and BETA models. One can only look forward eagerly to the results of applications of such analyses to specific problems.

Lalouel's useful review of measures of distance between populations reminds us of the increasing rate of advance in this field of knowledge; very slow at first so that Pearson's coefficient of racial likeness stood alone, despite all its shortcomings, for years and indeed decades, but gathering momentum during the 1950's to give the enormous progress of the 1960's and 1970's. Recent progress seems to have been greatly accelerated with the development of the bioassay of kinship of Morton and his several associates, and the introduction of multidimensional scaling, whose fundamentals Lalouel's chapter so clearly sets out.

At the opposite end of the spectrum is the discussion by Cannings, Thompson, and Skolnik of pedigree analysis. Although the fundamental tool in all genetic analysis, for decades this was considered at only the most elementary level, and its development for application to more complex systems (e.g., population genealogies, variations in penetrance) was strangely neglected. How wide a variety of situations can be encompassed in pedigree analysis is well shown by this chapter, which demonstrates that the computation of likelihoods is feasible for models involving the complexities of such factors as assortative mating, common environments, and a variety of modes of transmission. This chapter is essentially forward looking, and the results of its application are eagerly awaited.

Other chapters include illustrations of application, as well as the theory of the methods themselves. Rao and Morton survey an area of major development in this decade, path analysis. It is clearly going to be of primary importance, for example, in understanding the theory of assortative mating, and in particular distinguishing between social and phenotypic homogamy. Of the examples given, particularly interesting is the application to periodontal health, both for its findings of zero genetic heritability, and the demonstration that nuclear families are sufficient for the differentiation of biological and cultural inheritance. However, the fact (b-c ridge count) that two heritabilities each defined as a proportion sum to more than unity suggests that there is a little smoothing to be done.

In this section comes Elston's chapter on segregation analysis. Having formulated his genetic models in terms of the joint genotypic distribution of mating individuals, relations between phenotype and genotype, the mode of inheritance and the sampling method employed, he sets out the likelihoods and discusses testing of hypotheses. His concluding two examples of applications of segregation analysis in man, the inheritance of serum cholesterol levels and the ability to taste phenylthiocarbamide, show how powerful this method is going to be in elucidating the problems of inheritance of many a trait which has so far proved to be recalcitrant. I particularly look forward to the extension of the analysis to threshold characters, the category into which so many familial clinical disorders appear to fall.

A special case is that discussed by C. C. Li, half-sib analysis of quantitative data. He rightly points out the paucity of reported studies of half sibs in the scientific literature, largely because of the rarity of half sibs in our society, and suggests that with the change in social behavior we can expect an increased number. This paucity also reflects, of course, the ethnocentricity of so much genetic investigation. In many human societies half sibs are indeed common, not only because of the polygamous breeding structure, but also because of the intensity of mortality in primitives, so that it is a fortunate child who retains both his biological parents until he himself is adult. My colleagues and I were particularly appreciative of Professor Li's kind words on our West African height study (Roberts, Billewicz, and McGregor, 1978), and in return perhaps I may supply the details he notes. As is implicit in our text, it was unfortunately not possible to measure all parents; many of them were already dead at the beginning of the study. However, there were 43 families where Li's requirement of correlations in height between successive fathers or successive mothers can be obtained. The correlations for these are as follows:

father with first wife:	$r = +0.134$
father with second wife:	$r = +0.129$
first wife with second wife:	$r = +0.119$

These are clearly not different from the overall interspouse correlation of $r = 0.096 \pm 0.070$ that we employed, and certainly suggests no change in the assortative mating between father with first wife and father with second wife. They do give, however, a slightly different value for Li's $3m \, (= 0.382)$, slightly higher than ours of 0.288. We think it would not be correct to employ these values, however, in our estimates, since they relate to such a small part of our data, and we felt it more proper to use the total amount instead of this small sample.

Finally there is a small group of chapters where methods are reviewed by application instead of derivation or description. This includes DeFries' study, which, after tracing the historical development of methods of examination of mental abilities from Galton's earlier advocacy of twin analysis, shows how intrafamilial correlations have been used, with particular reference to the Hawaii family study of cognition. The difficulties of administering tests in comparable ways to different ethnic units, and of interpreting intrafamilial correlations in terms of heritability as classically defined, are clearly indicated. There now emerges little support for any major X-linked gene effect on spatial ability.

The chapter by Jorde is much broader, a remarkably comprehensive and well-documented review of studies of population structure. Again, one is impressed at the amount of advance, refinement, and application in the last decade. Such advance, moreover, is observed across the whole field — genetic effects of population subdivision, hierarchical and temporal subdivision, measures of population differentiation, and determinants of population structure. Jorde reminds us quite properly of a conspicuous gap; despite all the theoretical and applied analyses, there appears to be a lack of any serious attempt to study the biosocial processes which underlie population structure. Again, it is particularly gratifying to see his final point, the importance of random, statistically indeterminate events, not because it is illustrated specifically from our own work but because of its importance. For so many hundreds of centuries of human history man and his ancestors must have subsisted in small groups particularly subject to such events, and they must have played an extremely important part in the evolutionary shuffling and rearrangement of gene pools. Who knows, it may indeed have been such an event that gave man his 23 pairs of chromosomes by establishing the fusion of the two acrocentrics of his immediate ancestors!

5. Overview

One cannot help but be impressed at this collection of works, and at the amount of activity that they show in many areas of anthropological genetics. It is of course quite impossible to be comprehensive in such a selection, and before answering the question as to the balance of our subject posed at the outset, we need to look at other topics where there is intensive work so far not mentioned.

5.1. New Polymorphisms

The enormous progress in knowledge of genetic polymorphisms in man that brought a new dimension to evolutionary thought, though it apparently reached its climax in the 1960's, has by no means ceased. The traditional pattern is being followed, namely, the identification of variants of a substance, establishment of their inherited basis, establishment of gene frequencies in the population in which they were discovered, and then much more slowly identification of gene frequencies in other populations to sketch out the world map of frequency distribution. For the older, established polymorphisms the map is reasonably complete, but for many the frequencies are still in the process of documentation, and indeed for some there is virtually no information yet, for example, soluble aconitase, alpha-L-fucosidase, galactose-1-phosphate uridyl transferase, and uridine monophosphate kinase. But there is more yet to be discovered, as the result of modern technical advances. For example, development of isoelectric focusing has shown that the apparently simple Mendelian phosphoglucomutase polymorphism at locus 1 is in fact more complex and that what was taken to be a single allele (PGM_1^1) is heterogeneous; use of radioactive ligands in electrophoresis has brought to light the transcobalamine-2 variation (Daiger, Labowe, Parsons, Wang, and Cavalli-Sforza, 1978). Then in addition to polymorphisms detectable in the adult, others occur during fetal growth and development; polymorphic isoenzyme variants are relevant at a particular stage of development only, and then disappear (Roberts, 1978). The biological advantages and disadvantages attaching to almost all of these remain to be discovered.

A particularly interesting major discovery is the genetic variation in human complement, the series of proteins normally present in serum, which are activated by antibody–antigen interaction, and which "complement" the action of antibodies in defence against invasive proteins. Genetic heterogeneity has been shown for the C1-esterase inhibitor, C2, C3 proactivator, C3, C4, C6, and C7 components. Of these, the only one whose world distribution of variants has been at all investigated is C3. This shows little variation in frequency between populations within any continental group, but almost all the variation occurs between continental groups. Where the data are sufficient, the gradient of frequencies does not appear to be a regular cline but appears to be stepped, with zones of negligible variation separated by quite steep transitional zones. This must indicate irregularities in gene flow or variations in selective efficacy, so that the pattern of distribution poses very real evolutionary problems as to its explanation.

5.2. Ecogenetic Studies

One area in anthropological genetics that is developing very successfully is semi-ecological, and here there appear to be three common strategies. One is to single out some trait of complex determination, and use contrasting ecological conditions to identify the relative importance of genetic and environmental determinants. A second strategy is to examine migrants, comparing a particular trait amongst those who migrate with their relatives who have remained in the home environment. An extension of this which has been remarkably successful is the study of sibs who have been brought up in different environments, examining the correlations of a particular trait on the one hand with their biological parents and on the other with their adoptive relatives. A successful example of the first of these strategies is the Harvard Solomon Islands project, particularly in respect to blood pressure and its interaction with genetics and culture (Page, Damon, and Moellering, 1974). For the second there is the Tokelau Island migrant study, showing lack of significant change in serum cholesterol despite other evidence of environmental changes in habitat (Prior, Stanhope, Evans, and Salmond, 1974), and the recent work on multiple sclerosis, or rather its lack, in immigrants to Britain from other continents (Dean, personal communication). The third is well illustrated by the studies of genetic influences in alcoholism (Goodwin, Schulsinger, Hermansen, Guze, and Winokur, 1973).

5.3. Some Gaps

There are, however, several areas in which it seems to me more attention to population analysis appears promising. One such area is chromosome variation. At the beginning of the present decade there was a major advance, the discovery that human chromosomes stain differentially and show characteristic banding patterns. These developments have been particularly relevant in clinical genetics, but they have also helped to elucidate the chromosome changes that have occurred in the course of human and primate evolution, and one can insert on the hominoid phylogeny diagram the segments at which each major chromosomal change occurred. It is perhaps unlikely that major variations in chromosome structure will be found between human populations. However, another area of advance in karyotyping has been the demonstration of chromosome polymorphisms. Normal members in Western European populations show variation in the intensity of fluorescence and in morphology, for example, in size of the short arms, stalk and satellites of chromosome 21; here I think it would be interesting to seek differences in frequency of these variants from one population to another. The biological significance of such variants of course remains to be determined.

Yet another area is linkage mapping of man. This has come about as the result of the increased number of polymorphic markers available for testing, so that direct pedigree studies have allowed ever more informative linkage analyses. It is also traceable to the remarkable advances in somatic cell genetics, particularly cell hybridization techniques, and to deletion mapping, in which those patients with deletion of a particular chromosomal segment are examined for a variety of marker systems and any locus where heterozygosity is identified is not situated in the deleted segment. The present map of the human chromosomes would have been inconceivable a decade ago. In a further decade how much further may our knowledge have advanced? Will it allow us to detect minor chromosome rearrangements, particularly inversions, differing in frequency from one population to another?

A third area where there is great scope is in the removal of our ethnocentric emphasis in genetic analysis. The population and breeding structures of mankind and their ecologies still retain appreciable variation, which provides opportunity for the solution of genetic problems not possible in our hungry and expanding western ways. Doubtless all who read this series will be stimulated to think of a number of other areas in anthropological genetics that are not yet fully exploited.

6. Conclusion

To return to our opening analogy, it is quite obvious that we are still experiencing all phases of development. The chapters illustrate clearly in different fields the simultaneous consolidation and achievement of adulthood, the vigor of youth, the infant emergence of new concepts, possibly the approach of death. It is obvious from these chapters that there has been no slowing and cessation of activity in anthropological genetics. Rather, it appears that this activity is likely to continue, and with it in many areas the increased wisdom of maturity, seeking refinement, with more self-criticism instead of exuberance. Whether this activity is balanced is a different matter. Certainly the contributions show that it is more balanced now than formerly — witness first the number of instances where the new procedures have been applied to practical problems and have not been established in isolation, and secondly, the interrelations that emerge repeatedly and unexpectedly among the several presentations.

There is one particular source of imbalance that I sense. As one who has been fortunate enough to enjoy the stimulation and discomforts of field studies, and has learned to appreciate the extent of his own ignorance and blessings from the personal contact with others of different culture, I should be very reluctant to see anthropological genetics become an armchair discipline. From the contributions presented here there is indeed a suggestion that this is happening. This is not entirely our fault, for despite the rapidity of modern travel there are a host of difficulties, financial and political, that make getting to the field today a very different procedure from what it was thirty years ago. A second, related, possible imbalance that I sense from some of the presentations is that theory is way ahead of application. It may well be that this impression is due to the structure of the offerings, for I understand that there will follow a sequence of case reports and studies of application of method, and to this I look forward with eager anticipation. I am less concerned at this, since for decades there was collection of data without adequate theory, and I am sure that the direction of the tilt of the present incomplete balance, if it exists, is preferable. But perhaps this itself will encourage the next generation of investigators into the field.

References

Cavalli-Sforza, L. L. and Edwards, A. W. F. (1963), Analysis of human evolution, in *Genetics Today*, (S. J. Geerts, ed.) *Proceedings of the 11th International Congress on Genetics (The Hague)*, Vol. 3. pp. 923–933.

Crawford, M. H., and Workman, P. L. (eds.) (1973), *Methods and Theories of Anthropological Genetics*, University of New Mexico Press, Albuquerque.

Daiger, S. P., Labowe, M. L., Parsons, M., Wang, L., and Cavalli-Sforza, L. (1978), Detection of genetic variation with radioactive ligands, *Am. J. Hum. Genet.* **30**:202–214.

Dean, G. (1971), *The Porphyrias*, Pitman, London.

Goodwin, D. W., Schulsinger, F., Hermansen, L., Guze, S. B., and Winokur, G. (1973), Alcohol problems in adoptees raised apart from alcoholic biological parents, *Arch. Gen. Psychof.* **28**:238–243.

Howells, W. W. (1973), Cranial variation in man. A study by multivariate analysis of patterns of difference among recent human populations, *Pap. Peabody Mus. Archaeol. Ethnol. Harv.* 67.

Page, L. B., Damon, A., and Moellering, R. C., Jr. (1974), Antecedents of cardiovascular disease in six Solomon Islands societies, *Circulation* **49**:1132–1146.

Penrose, L. S. (1959), Natural selection in man: some basic problems, in *Natural Selection in Human Populations*, (D. F. Roberts and G. A. Harrison, eds.) pp. 1–10, Pergamon, London.

Prior, I. A. M., Stanhope, J. M., Evans, J. G., and Salmond, C. E. (1974), The Tokelau Island migrant study, *Int. J. Epidem.* **3**:225–232.

Roberts, D. F. (1978), The genetics of human fetal growth, *Postgrad. Med. J.* **54**:107–113.

Roberts, D. F., Billewicz, W. Z., and McGregor, I. A. (1978), Heritability of stature in a West African population, *Ann. Hum. Genet.* **42**:15–24.

Sahlins, M. (1977), *The Use and Abuse of Biology: An Anthropological Critique of Sociobiology*, Tavistock, London.

Spuhler, J. N. (1973), Anthropological Genetics: an overview, in *Methods and Theories of Anthropological Genetics* (M. H. Crawford and P. L. Workman, eds.), pp. 423–451, University New Mexico Press, Albuquerque.

Index